BARBARA O'NEILL
LOST BIBLE OF HERBAL REMEDIES

The Supreme Compendium of Herbal Healing, Ancient Secrets and Recipes Perfected for Today's Health Needs

Leila Dania

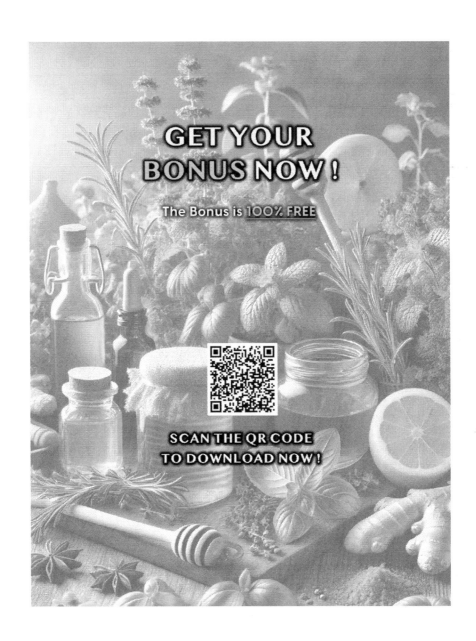

Table of Contents

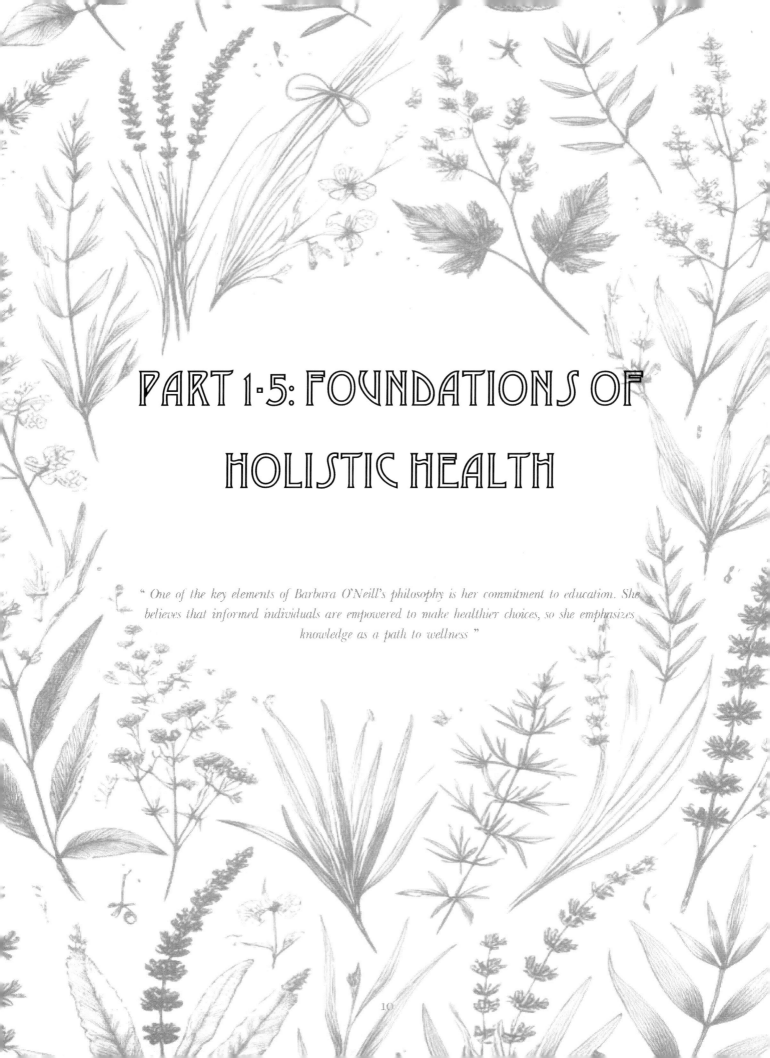

PART 1-5: FOUNDATIONS OF HOLISTIC HEALTH

" One of the key elements of Barbara O'Neill's philosophy is her commitment to education. She believes that informed individuals are empowered to make healthier choices, so she emphasizes knowledge as a path to wellness "

Chapter 1: Embracing a Holistic Health Philosophy

Barbara O'Neill has become a beacon for those interested in natural health, advocating for a wellness philosophy that integrates the body's innate healing power with holistic remedies. Her approach combines scientific understanding with centuries-old wisdom, providing a comprehensive perspective on health that is accessible and highly applicable. In this chapter, we delve into her principles, methods, and practical applications, examining how her philosophy of wellness goes beyond symptomatic relief to address root causes, empower individuals, and foster lasting health improvements.

Barbara O'Neill's Approach to Wellness

Barbara's journey into natural health is fueled by her commitment to helping people find true, sustainable wellness. Her method encourages individuals to see the body as an interconnected system, where every function, nutrient, and habit plays a role in overall health. This concept lays the foundation for a lifestyle that respects natural rhythms and healing processes, offering a holistic alternative to modern medicine's frequent focus on isolated treatments. Let's explore the core tenets of her approach and understand how it can be implemented in our daily lives to foster optimal well-being.

A Foundation of Knowledge and Empowerment

One of the key elements of Barbara O'Neill's philosophy is her commitment to education. She believes that informed individuals are empowered to make healthier choices, so she emphasizes knowledge as a path to wellness. Her teachings cover everything from basic human anatomy and physiology to the role of specific nutrients in health, the impact of toxins, and how lifestyle factors like sleep, stress, and physical activity contribute to wellness. By understanding how the body functions and what it needs, individuals can make conscious, informed choices that enhance their well-being rather than detract from it.

For instance, Barbara teaches the importance of liver health and detoxification as a foundation for overall wellness. The liver plays a critical role in processing and eliminating toxins, and Barbara's approach includes dietary adjustments, herbal supplements, and lifestyle practices that support liver function. For example, incorporating herbs like milk thistle, dandelion root, and turmeric into the diet can assist in liver detoxification, while reducing the intake of processed foods and alcohol helps lessen the liver's burden.

In addition to the liver, Barbara focuses on digestive health as a cornerstone of wellness. She explains that proper digestion and nutrient absorption are essential for energy, immunity, and mental clarity. Through her teachings, she guides people to identify and avoid foods that may be causing inflammation or digestive distress. For many, this means reducing or eliminating processed foods, sugar, and gluten, which can be hard for some to digest and may contribute to health issues like fatigue, headaches, and skin problems. Instead, Barbara encourages whole foods, rich in fiber and nutrients, that support digestion and gut health.

The Power of Natural Remedies and Preventive Care

Barbara's approach also emphasizes the power of natural remedies—especially herbal medicine—in promoting health and preventing disease. She champions herbs not as a replacement for medical intervention when needed, but as a complement to lifestyle and dietary changes that support the body's resilience and self-healing abilities.

A typical example Barbara advocates is using echinacea to boost the immune system during cold and flu season, or applying aloe vera topically for skin healing. Her methodology is grounded in a philosophy of prevention, where people are encouraged to use natural remedies not only in response to ailments but as part of a proactive wellness routine. For example, rather than waiting until a sore throat or sinus infection develops, she suggests daily habits like drinking herbal teas, using immune-supportive herbs, and ensuring adequate hydration as preventive measures that contribute to the body's defense mechanisms.

For those struggling with stress—a common modern ailment with vast implications for physical health—Barbara often recommends adaptogenic herbs such as ashwagandha and rhodiola. Adaptogens are unique in their ability to help the body adapt to stress, reducing its negative impacts on immunity, digestion, and mental clarity. By integrating these herbs into daily routines, individuals can enhance their ability to manage stress naturally, without relying solely on pharmaceuticals or external solutions.

Holistic Health in Everyday Life

A standout feature of Barbara's philosophy is its emphasis on practical application. Rather than treating health as an abstract concept, she breaks it down into actionable steps, helping people transform their daily routines in a way that supports lasting wellness. She often advocates for incremental changes, such as replacing processed snacks with raw nuts and fruits or incorporating a daily herbal tea ritual, which are easier to maintain and build up over time.

Barbara's approach is particularly resonant for those who feel overwhelmed by the demands of modern life. She understands that wellness isn't achieved through grand gestures but through consistent, small steps that align with a holistic philosophy. For example, she encourages morning routines that might include a few minutes of meditation, stretching, and a nutritious breakfast rich in protein and whole foods. Each element of the routine is designed to nurture the body and mind, fostering a sense of balance and resilience that permeates the rest of the day.

A Lifestyle of Connection and Awareness

At the heart of Barbara O'Neill's wellness philosophy is the concept of awareness—both of one's own body and of the interconnectedness between human health and the natural environment. She emphasizes that good health doesn't exist in isolation from nature, which provides resources for nourishment and healing. Her teachings often include recommendations for seasonal eating, grounding exercises, and spending time outdoors, all of which help individuals connect with nature in meaningful ways.

For example, Barbara advises incorporating seasonal, locally-sourced fruits and vegetables into the diet whenever possible. Eating in harmony with the seasons not only supports local ecosystems but also provides the body with the nutrients it most needs at different times of the year. In winter, this might mean focusing on warming foods like root vegetables, while in summer, lighter, hydrating fruits and leafy greens are beneficial.

Barbara also teaches awareness of the self through practices like mindfulness and stress reduction techniques. She explains that by tuning into one's physical sensations, emotional responses, and mental states, individuals can better understand their unique health needs. For instance, many people report that certain foods or lifestyle habits exacerbate symptoms like fatigue or irritability. By developing self-awareness, they can identify these triggers and adjust their routines accordingly, leading to a more balanced and healthy life.

In a world where the pace of life often leaves us feeling disconnected, the concept of a holistic, interconnected approach to health—the Mind-Body-Spirit connection—holds a profound place in natural wellness. This idea stems from the understanding that our minds, bodies, and spirits are not separate entities working in isolation but are intimately linked and impact one another in powerful ways. When we address and nurture all three aspects, we unlock the potential for healing that goes beyond treating symptoms to foster a state of balance and harmony.

The Mind-Body-Spirit connection is rooted in ancient healing traditions that emphasize the role of balance in well-being. Traditional Chinese Medicine (TCM), Ayurveda, and Indigenous medicine all recognize that health cannot be isolated to the body alone; the mind and spirit play equal roles. By connecting these elements through natural remedies, lifestyle adjustments, and mindfulness practices, we empower ourselves to achieve health that is both sustainable and truly transformative.

Understanding the Connection: The Interplay of Mind, Body, and Spirit

The mind, body, and spirit each have unique functions, yet they communicate and respond to each other constantly. When we experience stress, for example, our mental state can trigger physical symptoms, like headaches, tense muscles, or even digestive issues. On the other hand, physical pain can affect our mood, while spiritual emptiness or a lack of purpose can influence both our mental and physical states, manifesting as fatigue, anxiety, or restlessness.

- **Mind:** The mind processes thoughts, emotions, and memories. It serves as the control center, guiding how we interpret and respond to the world. Mental health, including resilience, focus, and emotional stability, significantly influences our physical health.
- **Body:** The body houses all physiological processes, from digestion to immunity. It responds to mental states, holding onto stress in physical forms such as tension, fatigue, or illness. Likewise, the body's well-being affects mental clarity and spiritual openness.

- **Spirit:** Often considered the most abstract aspect, spirit relates to our sense of purpose, connectedness, and inner peace. While it may be intangible, it significantly impacts both mental and physical health. Those who feel a deep sense of purpose and spiritual connection often experience improved well-being and longevity.

The interaction between these three parts is what forms the essence of holistic health. Neglecting one area often leads to imbalances that can manifest in any part of the system. For instance, unaddressed mental stress can weaken the immune system, leading to chronic illness, while a sedentary lifestyle may contribute to depressive symptoms. The goal of natural healing is to bring these aspects into harmony, creating a foundation of wellness that is resilient and adaptable to life's challenges.

The Role of Natural Herbal Remedies in the Mind-Body-Spirit Connection

Natural herbal remedies offer powerful support in enhancing the Mind-Body-Spirit connection, especially when combined with mindful practices. Many herbs contain active compounds that support physical health while promoting mental clarity and spiritual calm. Unlike synthetic medicines, which often target only one symptom or area, herbal remedies are versatile and work on multiple levels, supporting the whole person rather than merely suppressing symptoms.

- **For the Mind:** Adaptogens like Ashwagandha and Rhodiola can help reduce stress by balancing cortisol levels, fostering mental clarity, and enhancing resilience. Herbs such as Valerian root, Lavender, and Lemon Balm promote relaxation, aiding those who struggle with anxiety and sleep issues. For those seeking sharper mental focus, Ginkgo Biloba has long been used to improve cognitive function and memory.
- **For the Body:** Herbs like Turmeric and Ginger are known for their anti-inflammatory properties, supporting overall physical health and reducing symptoms that may arise from mental and spiritual imbalances. Echinacea and Elderberry strengthen the immune system, protecting the body against illness. These herbs work with the body's natural systems to promote health, providing gentle support that aligns with the body's own healing abilities.
- **For the Spirit:** Sacred herbs, such as Holy Basil (Tulsi) and Sage, have been used for centuries in spiritual practices to promote inner peace and grounding. These herbs support spiritual practices by calming the mind and body, making it easier to connect with one's inner self. For those who engage in meditation or other spiritual practices,

herbs like Mugwort and Damiana can deepen the experience, fostering a sense of openness and connection to the world around us.

By integrating these natural remedies into daily routines, individuals can support each aspect of their being, working towards a state of balance. Herbal remedies can be consumed as teas, used in aromatherapy, or applied topically, providing versatile options for different lifestyles and preferences.

Practical Steps to Strengthen the Mind-Body-Spirit Connection

Achieving harmony between the mind, body, and spirit is a personal journey, yet there are practical steps that can guide individuals on this path. While natural remedies provide a strong foundation, incorporating additional holistic practices enhances their effects.

1. **Mindfulness and Meditation:** These practices calm the mind, reduce stress, and foster self-awareness. Meditation has been shown to lower blood pressure, reduce anxiety, and improve mental clarity. By practicing mindfulness, individuals can learn to respond to life's challenges with resilience and equanimity, which benefits both mental and physical health.

2. **Breathing Exercises:** Deep breathing techniques, such as diaphragmatic breathing, can have a profound effect on mental and physical health. These exercises stimulate the vagus nerve, which helps to regulate the nervous system, reduce stress hormones, and improve heart rate variability. Regular breathing exercises create a state of calm, aiding in better decision-making and enhancing one's spiritual awareness.

3. **Physical Activity:** Exercise is crucial not just for physical health but also for mental clarity and spiritual growth. Activities like yoga and Tai Chi emphasize the Mind-Body-Spirit connection by combining movement with mindful breathing. Even simple practices like daily walking can clear the mind, relieve stress, and foster a sense of gratitude and connectedness.

4. **Journaling and Reflection:** Writing down thoughts, emotions, and experiences can help in understanding mental patterns, identifying sources of stress, and clarifying one's purpose. Reflection allows for spiritual growth by deepening one's awareness of personal values and goals.

5. **Nature Immersion:** Spending time in nature can have a transformative effect on mental, physical, and spiritual health. Studies show that nature reduces stress and promotes a sense of well-being. Whether it's a walk in the park, gardening, or simply

sitting under a tree, connecting with nature helps individuals feel part of something larger than themselves.

Building a Sustainable Mind-Body-Spirit Routine

Creating a routine that incorporates the Mind-Body-Spirit connection is essential for long-term well-being. However, sustainability is key—practices should feel natural, enjoyable, and enriching rather than forced or overwhelming. Begin by choosing one or two practices that resonate most, whether it's incorporating an herbal tea ritual, practicing meditation, or spending time outdoors.

Over time, as these practices become second nature, individuals can gradually add other elements. The goal is not perfection but consistent, compassionate care for oneself. Life's stresses and challenges are inevitable, but with a strong foundation in the Mind-Body-Spirit connection, individuals can navigate these with greater resilience and inner peace.

Balance in Daily Life

Living a balanced life is the foundation of wellness. The concept of balance goes beyond managing time or meeting basic needs; it involves nurturing every aspect of oneself, including physical health, emotional well-being, and mental clarity. Achieving balance requires deliberate choices, lifestyle adjustments, and a proactive approach to wellness. It's about understanding that every decision we make—from the food we eat to the way we spend our time—affects our overall quality of life. Here, we explore practical strategies, rooted in natural remedies and lifestyle habits, to cultivate a balanced life.

Balance doesn't mean perfection; it means finding equilibrium. For many, life's demands often tip the scales, leading to stress, fatigue, and disconnection from personal needs. A balanced life invites us to regularly pause, assess, and make changes that prioritize our health and happiness. Each person's path to balance is unique, but certain principles can guide anyone toward a more harmonious life.

Recognizing the Role of Physical Health

Physical health forms the cornerstone of a balanced life. When the body is strong and energized, it supports mental clarity and emotional resilience. Prioritizing physical health begins with basic wellness practices: a balanced diet, regular exercise, and adequate rest.

However, these practices are not one-size-fits-all. Each individual has unique needs based on lifestyle, body type, and health goals.

One of the easiest and most impactful ways to support physical health is through diet. Embracing whole foods, rich in nutrients, can stabilize energy levels, boost immunity, and support mental clarity. Natural remedies also play a significant role. For instance, including herbs like ginger and turmeric in meals can reduce inflammation and improve digestion. These herbs offer a gentle yet effective approach to wellness, integrating natural health into daily routines without the need for drastic changes.

Alongside diet, physical activity is essential for balance. Regular exercise, whether through gentle yoga or brisk walking, stimulates the release of endorphins—hormones that promote happiness and reduce stress. Physical activity doesn't require an intense gym routine; simple, consistent movement can improve mood and strengthen the body. For example, a daily 20-minute walk in nature can rejuvenate the body, support cardiovascular health, and reduce stress.

Rest is equally critical. In our fast-paced culture, sleep is often sacrificed, leading to physical and mental exhaustion. Quality sleep allows the body to repair and the mind to process emotions and experiences. When sleep is prioritized, people feel more energetic, focused, and capable of handling daily stressors. For those struggling with sleep, natural remedies like chamomile tea or lavender oil can encourage relaxation without the side effects of synthetic sleep aids.

Emotional Well-being: The Heart of Balance

While physical health is foundational, emotional well-being is equally vital. Emotions are powerful drivers of behavior and decision-making. Balancing emotions requires awareness, acceptance, and healthy coping strategies. A balanced emotional state allows individuals to respond to life's challenges calmly and constructively.

Practices like mindfulness and meditation help cultivate emotional balance. Mindfulness encourages individuals to stay present, reducing anxiety about the future or regrets about the past. Meditation, even for a few minutes a day, can soothe the mind and help people reconnect with their inner selves. These practices don't require special equipment or training—just a willingness to pause and focus on the present moment. For example, taking five deep breaths before reacting to a stressful situation can help shift the emotional response from reactive to reflective.

In addition, natural remedies can support emotional well-being. Certain herbs, like valerian root and passionflower, are known for their calming effects, making them beneficial for those who struggle with stress or anxiety. Incorporating these herbs into a nightly routine, perhaps through a warm tea, can provide gentle support for the nervous system and encourage emotional balance.

Building strong relationships also contributes to emotional wellness. Connecting with loved ones provides a sense of belonging and reduces feelings of isolation. Spending time with friends or family can foster positive emotions, creating a network of support during challenging times. It's important to remember that balance includes setting boundaries; it's perfectly acceptable to decline social obligations to preserve energy and mental space.

Mental Clarity: A Balanced Mind for a Balanced Life

Mental clarity is crucial in maintaining life balance. A balanced mind makes it easier to prioritize tasks, set realistic goals, and stay focused. In today's world, distractions are constant, from social media notifications to work demands. Cultivating mental clarity involves both reducing external distractions and nurturing internal focus.

Establishing a daily routine supports mental clarity. A structured day with set times for activities helps the mind stay organized. For example, creating a morning routine that includes hydration, light stretching, and a moment of intention-setting can set a positive tone for the rest of the day. Morning routines don't need to be complex; even a simple ritual can provide a sense of grounding.

Mental clarity can also be supported by natural supplements. Herbs like ginkgo biloba and rosemary are traditionally used to improve focus and memory. Ginkgo, for instance, enhances circulation to the brain, which can support cognitive functions. Adding these herbs to meals or taking them in supplement form can provide gentle mental support without relying on stimulants.

Reducing digital distractions is another step toward mental clarity. Excessive screen time, especially before bed, can lead to mental fatigue. Setting aside specific times to check emails or social media can help reduce constant interruptions. Likewise, engaging in offline activities like reading or journaling can rest the mind and promote a sense of calm.

Creating Daily Rituals for Balance

Rituals bring intention and mindfulness to daily life. Unlike routines, which are often automatic, rituals involve a conscious focus on each activity, transforming mundane tasks into moments of self-care and reflection. Daily rituals don't have to be elaborate; they can be as simple as savoring a cup of herbal tea in the morning or journaling before bed.

For example, practicing gratitude each evening can shift the focus from stress to appreciation. Writing down three things to be grateful for can elevate mood and foster a positive outlook. Gratitude rituals cultivate a mindset of abundance, encouraging people to focus on what's going well rather than on challenges.

Rituals can also involve nature. Spending time outdoors, whether through gardening, hiking, or simply sitting in the sun, nurtures the body and soul. Nature has a grounding effect that reconnects individuals to the earth, creating a sense of peace. Even a few minutes spent observing a sunrise or breathing in fresh air can bring balance to the day.

The Importance of Self-Compassion

Self-compassion is essential for a balanced life. It involves treating oneself with the same kindness and understanding one would offer a friend. Too often, people hold themselves to unrealistic standards, leading to feelings of inadequacy. Self-compassion encourages a gentler, more forgiving approach, especially during times of struggle.

Practicing self-compassion means allowing space for rest without guilt, recognizing personal achievements, and forgiving oneself for mistakes. When people approach themselves with kindness, they are less likely to experience burnout or stress. Simple acts of self-care, like taking breaks, enjoying a hobby, or setting boundaries, contribute to this sense of compassion.

For instance, someone who feels overwhelmed by a busy schedule might allow themselves a few minutes each day for a quiet activity they enjoy, like drawing or listening to music. These small moments of self-care are acts of self-compassion that support balance and well-being.

Integrating Balance into Relationships and Work

Balance isn't only a personal journey; it extends to relationships and work. Healthy relationships provide mutual support, respect, and growth. However, relationships can also be a source of stress when boundaries aren't clear. Maintaining balance in relationships means knowing when to give and when to take time for oneself.

In work life, balance involves setting realistic goals, managing time effectively, and knowing when to step back. Overcommitting can lead to burnout, making it harder to enjoy personal life. Creating a work-life balance is essential for overall well-being. This might involve setting limits on work hours, taking lunch breaks away from the desk, or setting boundaries with colleagues.

For instance, dedicating weekends to personal interests, rather than work, reinforces the boundary between professional and personal life. Engaging in hobbies or spending time with loved ones during weekends helps recharge the mind and body for the week ahead.

Psychological Benefits of Holistic Health

Holistic health is not only about treating the body but also about nurturing the mind and spirit. This approach recognizes that mental well-being is intricately connected to physical and emotional health. By focusing on holistic health, individuals can improve psychological resilience, reduce stress, and enhance overall life satisfaction. Understanding the psychological benefits of holistic health is key to adopting practices that promote mental clarity, emotional stability, and a sense of fulfillment. For many, this journey leads to a healthier mindset and a stronger foundation for facing life's challenges.

Holistic health approaches have long been used to alleviate mental health struggles and promote emotional well-being. Practices such as herbal remedies, mindfulness, and balanced nutrition offer powerful tools for supporting psychological health. Unlike conventional treatments that often target symptoms in isolation, holistic health encourages individuals to address root causes, which often stem from lifestyle, stress, or imbalances in diet and environment. By addressing these underlying factors, holistic health empowers individuals to make lasting changes that not only alleviate symptoms but also improve mental and emotional health.

Reducing Stress Through Holistic Health Practices

Stress is one of the most common mental health challenges in today's fast-paced world, impacting millions of people in the United States alone. Chronic stress can lead to a host of psychological issues, including anxiety, depression, and insomnia. By adopting holistic health practices, individuals can reduce stress and cultivate a greater sense of calm. Herbal remedies, such as adaptogens, have been used for centuries to help the body cope with stress by balancing cortisol levels and supporting the adrenal system.

For example, **Ashwagandha** is a well-known adaptogen that has shown promising results in reducing cortisol, the body's primary stress hormone. By lowering cortisol, Ashwagandha helps to reduce the physical symptoms of stress, such as fatigue, while also promoting mental clarity and focus. Similarly, herbs like **Lemon Balm** and **Valerian Root** have calming properties, making them valuable allies for those struggling with anxiety or sleep disturbances. Regular use of these herbs, often in the form of teas or tinctures, can support the nervous system and foster a state of relaxation.

Mindfulness and meditation practices also play a significant role in reducing stress. Studies have shown that even a few minutes of daily meditation can help reduce symptoms of anxiety and improve emotional resilience. Meditation allows individuals to observe their thoughts without attachment, fostering a sense of mental clarity and peace. Combined with natural remedies, mindfulness can help individuals shift their perspective, learning to manage stressors with greater ease and adaptability.

Enhancing Emotional Stability with Balanced Nutrition

Emotional stability is essential for mental health, and holistic health emphasizes the importance of nutrition in maintaining this balance. The brain requires specific nutrients to function optimally, including vitamins, minerals, and fatty acids. Deficiencies in these nutrients can lead to mood swings, irritability, and even depression. Holistic health promotes a balanced diet that includes whole foods, such as fruits, vegetables, nuts, and seeds, to support emotional well-being.

For instance, foods rich in **Omega-3 fatty acids**—found in flaxseeds, walnuts, and fish oil—are known to support brain health and reduce symptoms of depression. Omega-3s play a vital role in brain structure and function, and studies suggest they can improve mood by reducing inflammation in the brain. Similarly, **Magnesium** is another critical nutrient that supports emotional stability. Known as the "relaxation mineral," magnesium helps calm the nervous system, reduce anxiety, and improve sleep quality. Many individuals find relief from anxiety and irritability simply by incorporating magnesium-rich foods, such as leafy greens, nuts, and whole grains, into their diets.

In addition to these essential nutrients, certain herbs can also support emotional stability. **St. John's Wort**, for example, has been traditionally used to treat mild to moderate depression. By balancing serotonin levels in the brain, this herb can improve mood and reduce symptoms of depression without the side effects often associated with prescription medications. However, it's essential for individuals to consult healthcare providers before using St. John's Wort, as it can interact with other medications. Other mood-supporting herbs, like **Passionflower** and **Chamomile**, can be used as teas to promote relaxation and reduce irritability.

Promoting Self-Awareness and Personal Growth

One of the most significant psychological benefits of holistic health is the promotion of self-awareness and personal growth. Many holistic practices, such as journaling, meditation, and self-reflection, encourage individuals to look inward and explore their thoughts, emotions, and motivations. This process fosters a greater sense of self-awareness, which is essential for personal growth and emotional resilience.

Journaling is a powerful tool for self-awareness, allowing individuals to express their thoughts and feelings openly. By regularly journaling, people can identify patterns in their behavior and emotional responses, gaining insights into what triggers stress or negative emotions. Over time, this self-awareness helps individuals make intentional changes that support their mental well-being. For example, someone who notices a pattern of feeling anxious after consuming caffeine may decide to reduce their intake to improve their emotional balance.

Mindfulness practices also support self-awareness by helping individuals stay present and observe their thoughts without judgment. When practiced regularly, mindfulness can reduce anxiety, improve focus, and foster a sense of calm. Many find that mindfulness leads to personal growth by helping them let go of past regrets and worries about the future, focusing instead on the present moment. This shift in perspective encourages a healthier mental state and reduces the likelihood of being overwhelmed by stress or negative emotions.

Building Resilience and Coping Skills

Resilience is the ability to bounce back from challenges and adapt to change. Holistic health promotes resilience by providing individuals with tools to manage stress, process emotions, and maintain a positive outlook. Herbal remedies, such as adaptogens, support the body's natural stress response, while mindfulness practices and emotional awareness foster mental resilience. This combination creates a foundation for strong coping skills, enabling individuals to navigate life's ups and downs with greater ease.

Adaptogens like **Rhodiola** and **Holy Basil** (Tulsi) are particularly helpful in building resilience. These herbs support the adrenal glands, which play a crucial role in the body's response to stress. By strengthening the adrenal system, adaptogens help individuals respond to stress in a balanced manner, reducing the risk of burnout and fatigue. Regular use of adaptogens can improve mental clarity and focus, enabling individuals to tackle challenges with a calm and resilient mindset.

In addition to herbal support, techniques like deep breathing and visualization can enhance resilience by reducing stress levels and promoting relaxation. Deep breathing exercises, such as diaphragmatic breathing, activate the parasympathetic nervous system, helping the body enter a state of relaxation. This practice is particularly helpful for those who struggle with anxiety or feel overwhelmed by stress. Visualization, where individuals imagine themselves successfully navigating a challenging situation, can also build confidence and mental resilience, making it easier to cope with adversity.

Fostering a Sense of Purpose and Spiritual Fulfillment

A sense of purpose and spiritual fulfillment is essential for mental well-being. Holistic health acknowledges that humans are more than their physical bodies and minds; spiritual health plays a significant role in overall happiness and life satisfaction. By exploring spiritual practices, individuals can connect with a sense of purpose that provides meaning and motivation in life. This connection is often associated with improved mental health, as individuals who feel a sense of purpose are better able to manage stress and maintain a positive outlook.

Spiritual practices can take many forms, from meditation and prayer to spending time in nature or engaging in creative activities. For some, a simple practice of gratitude can foster a deep sense of purpose by helping them appreciate the positive aspects of their lives. By focusing on gratitude, individuals shift their mindset from lack to abundance, fostering a more positive outlook. This shift is particularly helpful for those struggling with depression or feelings of emptiness.

Herbs such as **Holy Basil** and **Mugwort** are often used in spiritual practices to promote mental clarity and inner peace. Holy Basil, known as the "Queen of Herbs," is revered in Ayurvedic medicine for its ability to balance mind, body, and spirit. It is believed to enhance spiritual connection, reduce stress, and improve mood, making it a valuable tool for those seeking a greater sense of purpose. Mugwort, on the other hand, is often used in rituals and meditation to promote vivid dreams and spiritual insights.

Encouraging Social Connections and Community Support

Holistic health also emphasizes the importance of social connections and community. Humans are inherently social beings, and meaningful relationships play a vital role in mental and emotional health. Holistic practices often encourage individuals to build strong social networks, as these connections can provide support during challenging times and contribute to a sense of belonging. By fostering social connections, individuals can improve their psychological resilience and reduce feelings of isolation or loneliness.

Community support can take many forms, from joining a local wellness group to participating in online communities focused on holistic health. These connections provide a space for individuals to share experiences, seek advice, and offer support to one another. Many holistic health practices, such as group meditation or yoga classes, create opportunities for people to connect on a deeper level, building friendships that contribute to emotional well-being. For those new to holistic health, joining a community can be an excellent way to stay motivated and explore new practices with others who share similar goals.

Through these various approaches, holistic health supports psychological well-being in a way that is comprehensive and sustainable. By addressing the mind, body, and spirit, individuals can create a foundation of mental resilience, emotional stability, and a deeper sense of fulfillment. Holistic health offers a pathway to mental well-being that respects the individual's unique needs and goals, empowering each person to take an active role in their mental health journey.

Chapter 2: Core Principles of Natural Healing

The human body is an extraordinary organism equipped with built-in mechanisms for healing and regeneration. From the repair of broken bones to the fighting off of infections, our bodies are constantly working to maintain health and restore balance. These self-healing mechanisms operate on multiple levels, involving complex processes that range from cellular repair to immune responses. Understanding these natural abilities can empower individuals to support their body's healing efforts through lifestyle choices, diet, and natural remedies.

Self-Healing Mechanisms of the Body

The ability to self-heal is intrinsic to all human beings and is an integral part of our survival. When supported through holistic practices, natural remedies, and a balanced lifestyle, these mechanisms can function at their best, offering resilience against disease and promoting longevity. Here, we'll explore the body's primary self-healing mechanisms and how we can nurture them for optimal health.

The Immune System: The Body's First Line of Defense

The immune system plays a crucial role in the body's ability to heal itself. This complex network of cells, tissues, and organs works together to detect and neutralize harmful pathogens such as bacteria, viruses, and fungi. When the immune system is functioning optimally, it protects the body against infections, accelerates wound healing, and minimizes inflammation. However, a weakened immune system can lead to frequent illnesses and slower recovery times.

Supporting immune health starts with a diet rich in vitamins, minerals, and antioxidants. Nutrients such as vitamin C, zinc, and selenium are vital for immune function. For example, vitamin C found in citrus fruits and green leafy vegetables enhances the production of white blood cells, which are crucial in fighting infections. Zinc, present in foods like pumpkin seeds and chickpeas, aids in immune cell development and communication, while selenium, found in nuts and fish, supports antioxidant activity.

Herbal remedies can also bolster immune health. Echinacea, elderberry, and astragalus are known for their immune-boosting properties. Echinacea, for example, has been shown to reduce the severity and duration of colds. By incorporating these herbs into daily routines—perhaps as teas, tinctures, or supplements—individuals can provide gentle, ongoing support to their immune system. Maintaining a strong immune system means the body is better equipped to handle infections and heal more effectively.

The Process of Inflammation: A Healing Response

Inflammation is one of the body's primary healing responses. When an injury occurs, or an infection is detected, the immune system triggers an inflammatory response to contain and eliminate harmful agents. This process involves an increase in blood flow to the affected area, which delivers essential nutrients and white blood cells to aid in repair. While acute inflammation is beneficial and essential for healing, chronic inflammation can have detrimental effects on health.

A common example of the healing power of inflammation is the swelling and redness that occurs around a cut or scrape. The warmth and redness signal that the body is sending resources to fight infection and repair tissue. However, when inflammation becomes chronic, often due to factors such as stress, poor diet, or exposure to toxins, it can lead to conditions like arthritis, cardiovascular disease, and even cancer.

To support healthy inflammation levels, anti-inflammatory foods and herbs can be incorporated into the diet. Turmeric, ginger, and green tea are potent anti-inflammatory agents. Curcumin, the active compound in turmeric, is known for its ability to reduce inflammation and has been used traditionally to treat conditions such as arthritis and digestive disorders. By adding turmeric to meals or taking it as a supplement, individuals can harness its benefits to manage inflammation and support the body's natural healing process.

Cellular Regeneration: The Body's Renewal Process

Every day, the body is engaged in the process of cellular regeneration. Cells are constantly being replaced, repaired, or regenerated to maintain optimal function. Skin cells, for example, renew approximately every 28 days, while liver cells regenerate every six months.

This process of renewal is critical for healing as it ensures that damaged cells are replaced, allowing tissues and organs to recover and function effectively.

The regenerative process is particularly evident in the skin's healing of cuts and scrapes. When the skin is wounded, blood clotting begins to prevent further bleeding, and new cells are produced to close the wound. This cycle of regeneration is crucial not only for wound healing but also for the long-term maintenance of organs and tissues.

Supporting cellular regeneration requires adequate nutrition, hydration, and rest. Antioxidant-rich foods, such as berries, leafy greens, and nuts, protect cells from oxidative damage and promote healthy cell function. Additionally, hydration is essential, as water is involved in cellular transport and waste removal, which are vital for regeneration. Getting sufficient sleep is another critical component; during sleep, the body focuses on repair and regeneration, making rest indispensable for self-healing.

Detoxification: The Body's Natural Cleansing System

Detoxification is the body's way of removing toxins and waste products. The liver, kidneys, lungs, skin, and lymphatic system all play roles in filtering out harmful substances that enter the body from the environment, food, and even metabolic processes. A well-functioning detoxification system is essential for maintaining health and preventing disease.

The liver is perhaps the most well-known detox organ, as it processes and neutralizes toxins. The kidneys filter waste from the blood, while the skin eliminates toxins through sweat. The lymphatic system, a network of vessels and nodes, also helps by transporting waste away from tissues. Ensuring these systems function effectively is essential for self-healing.

Herbs like dandelion root, milk thistle, and burdock are renowned for their detoxifying properties. Dandelion root aids in liver health by promoting bile production, which is necessary for digestion and toxin breakdown. Milk thistle is often used to protect liver cells from damage, while burdock supports kidney function. By incorporating these herbs into the diet or as supplements, individuals can support their body's natural detox processes and foster self-healing.

The Role of the Nervous System in Healing

The nervous system, particularly the parasympathetic branch, is deeply involved in the healing process. Often called the "rest and digest" system, the parasympathetic nervous system conserves energy and promotes relaxation, which is essential for recovery and regeneration. When the body is in a state of chronic stress, it operates in the "fight or flight" mode, which inhibits the healing response and can lead to a range of health issues.

Practices like meditation, deep breathing, and yoga activate the parasympathetic nervous system, encouraging a state of relaxation where healing can occur. Meditation, for instance, has been shown to reduce cortisol levels, which is beneficial for reducing inflammation and supporting immune function. Yoga not only strengthens the body but also promotes mental and emotional balance, enhancing overall well-being.

To nurture the nervous system, certain adaptogenic herbs like ashwagandha and rhodiola can be helpful. These herbs help the body adapt to stress by regulating the adrenal glands, which produce stress hormones. When used consistently, adaptogens can foster resilience against stress, allowing the nervous system to maintain a healing state more effectively.

Microbiome Balance: Supporting Gut Health

The microbiome—the community of bacteria and other microorganisms living in the gut—plays a significant role in the body's ability to heal. A balanced microbiome supports digestion, immune function, and even mental health. The beneficial bacteria in the gut help break down food, absorb nutrients, and prevent the growth of harmful pathogens.

An imbalanced microbiome, often caused by poor diet, antibiotics, or stress, can lead to digestive issues, weakened immunity, and inflammation. Probiotics and prebiotics are essential for maintaining a healthy microbiome. Probiotics, found in fermented foods like yogurt, sauerkraut, and kimchi, introduce beneficial bacteria into the gut. Prebiotics, such as fiber-rich foods like bananas, garlic, and oats, provide nourishment for these bacteria, encouraging a balanced and thriving microbiome.

The gut's connection to the immune system is particularly profound, as approximately 70% of the immune cells reside in the gut. By supporting gut health, individuals also support immune function, enhancing the body's ability to ward off infections and heal itself more efficiently.

The Endocrine System and Hormonal Balance

Hormones regulate a vast array of functions in the body, including metabolism, mood, and immune response. The endocrine system, responsible for hormone production and regulation, plays a critical role in self-healing. When hormone levels are balanced, the body operates smoothly, but imbalances can disrupt immune function, energy levels, and mental health.

For instance, cortisol, the stress hormone, has a significant impact on inflammation and immune response. Chronic stress can lead to elevated cortisol levels, which suppress immune function and slow down healing. To support hormonal balance, practices like reducing stress, getting adequate sleep, and consuming a nutrient-rich diet are essential.

Certain herbs, like holy basil and maca root, support the endocrine system by balancing hormone production. Holy basil, an adaptogen, helps regulate cortisol levels, making it beneficial for managing stress. Maca root is often used to support energy and mood, as it may help balance hormones like estrogen and testosterone. Integrating these herbs into a daily routine can provide gentle support for the endocrine system, promoting hormonal harmony and enhancing self-healing.

The Power of Positive Mindset and Emotional Healing

Mental and emotional health significantly influence the body's healing processes. Positive emotions such as gratitude, optimism, and love have been shown to boost immune function, reduce inflammation, and enhance overall health. Conversely, chronic stress, anxiety, and unresolved trauma can suppress immune function and hinder the body's ability to heal.

Practices like journaling, gratitude exercises, and visualization can foster a positive mindset and emotional well-being. For example, journaling about things one is grateful for can shift focus from stressors to blessings, promoting mental clarity and emotional balance. Visualization, where one imagines themselves in a state of health and vitality, can also be powerful in activating the body's natural healing abilities.

Flower essences, like those from the Bach Flower Remedies, are another tool for emotional healing. These gentle remedies, made from flowers, are believed to work on an energetic level to support emotional balance. For instance, rescue remedy, a popular Bach Flower blend, is often used during times of emotional distress to promote calmness and resilience. These natural remedies offer subtle support for emotional healing, contributing to the body's overall ability to self-heal.

Role of Mindfulness in Healing

Mindfulness has emerged as a powerful tool for healing in recent decades, offering individuals a way to connect with their present moment, reduce stress, and improve physical and mental well-being. At its core, mindfulness is about cultivating awareness of one's thoughts, emotions, and physical sensations without judgment. This practice provides a pathway to healing by allowing individuals to understand and manage their internal experiences, fostering a greater sense of balance and resilience. Within the framework of holistic health, mindfulness serves as a bridge that links mental clarity with physical wellness, offering a way to address root causes of discomfort and pain rather than merely treating symptoms.

Mindfulness has roots in ancient traditions, particularly within Buddhist and yogic practices. Today, it has been adapted to suit a variety of wellness settings, from clinical therapy to self-care routines. Numerous studies demonstrate the effectiveness of mindfulness in reducing anxiety, alleviating depression, and managing pain. By focusing on the present moment, mindfulness empowers individuals to become active participants in their healing journey. It enhances the body's natural capacity to heal by reducing stress hormones, improving immune function, and fostering a positive mindset. For those incorporating herbal remedies into their wellness routines, mindfulness serves as a complementary practice that can amplify the benefits of natural healing.

Understanding the Connection Between Mindfulness and Healing

To appreciate the role of mindfulness in healing, it's essential to understand how the mind and body interact. The human body has a built-in capacity to heal, regulated by complex systems such as the immune, endocrine, and nervous systems. However, chronic stress, negative emotions, and unprocessed trauma can disrupt these systems, leading to an array of physical and psychological ailments. Mindfulness helps individuals reconnect with their bodies and minds, creating an environment conducive to healing by reducing the impact of stress and promoting relaxation.

One of the primary ways mindfulness aids healing is by regulating the **stress response**. When a person experiences stress, the body releases cortisol and adrenaline, hormones that prepare it for fight or flight. While this response is essential in dangerous situations, chronic stress keeps the body in a state of heightened alert, which can lead to inflammation, digestive issues, and a weakened immune system. Mindfulness practices such as meditation and deep breathing activate the **parasympathetic nervous system**, shifting the body into a relaxed state where healing and repair can occur. By reducing stress levels, mindfulness helps to lower inflammation and supports immune function, enabling the body to heal more effectively.

Mindfulness also encourages a **positive mindset**, which is crucial for healing. A significant aspect of mindfulness is non-judgmental awareness, where individuals observe their thoughts and emotions without labeling them as "good" or "bad." This perspective allows individuals to approach their thoughts with curiosity and acceptance rather than fear or resistance. Research shows that a positive mindset can speed up recovery times, reduce pain perception, and even improve the outcomes of medical treatments. By fostering self-compassion and acceptance, mindfulness enables individuals to approach their health challenges with a resilient and open mind, enhancing the overall healing process.

Practical Techniques for Incorporating Mindfulness into Daily Life

Mindfulness can be incorporated into daily life in numerous ways, from formal meditation practices to simple moments of awareness throughout the day. These practices offer individuals a means of reducing stress, managing emotions, and fostering a sense of calm, all of which support healing. Here are some effective ways to incorporate mindfulness into a daily routine:

1. **Mindful Breathing**: Breathing exercises are among the most accessible forms of mindfulness and can be practiced anywhere. Diaphragmatic breathing, also known as belly breathing, is a technique where individuals breathe deeply from the diaphragm, expanding the belly on each inhale and contracting it on the exhale. This type of breathing activates the parasympathetic nervous system, promoting relaxation. By focusing solely on the breath, individuals can bring their attention to the present moment, which helps to reduce anxiety and create a sense of calm.

2. **Body Scan Meditation**: This meditation guides individuals through a process of focusing on each part of the body, from head to toe, noticing any sensations, tension, or discomfort without judgment. The body scan encourages relaxation and helps individuals develop a deeper connection with their physical state. By tuning into the body, individuals can become more aware of where they hold tension and begin to release it, supporting physical healing.

3. **Mindful Eating**: Eating mindfully involves paying attention to the flavors, textures, and smells of food, as well as the experience of chewing and swallowing. This practice

encourages individuals to slow down and appreciate their meals, which can improve digestion and reduce stress. Mindful eating also helps individuals recognize hunger and fullness cues, promoting a healthier relationship with food. By fostering a sense of gratitude for nourishment, mindful eating supports physical and emotional health.

4. **Walking Meditation**: Walking meditation is a form of mindfulness where individuals focus on the sensations of walking, such as the feel of the ground under their feet, the rhythm of their steps, and the movement of their muscles. This practice encourages a state of presence and awareness, reducing stress and promoting mental clarity. Walking meditation can be practiced anywhere, making it an ideal mindfulness exercise for those who prefer movement over sitting still.

5. **Journaling for Self-Reflection**: While not traditionally considered a mindfulness practice, journaling allows individuals to process their thoughts and emotions in a mindful way. By writing down their experiences and reflecting on them, individuals can gain insights into their mental state and identify patterns that may be contributing to stress or anxiety. Journaling also fosters self-awareness and helps individuals approach their thoughts with curiosity and compassion.

Enhancing the Effects of Herbal Remedies with Mindfulness

Mindfulness can significantly enhance the effects of herbal remedies, creating a holistic approach to healing that addresses both the mind and body. When individuals practice mindfulness while using herbal remedies, they become more attuned to their body's responses, which can deepen the healing experience. For example, taking a calming herbal tea, such as chamomile or lavender, with mindfulness can help individuals fully experience the effects of the herbs, noticing the relaxation that follows and appreciating the subtle flavors and aromas.

Combining mindfulness with herbal remedies can also improve adherence to wellness routines. By approaching their health practices with intention and awareness, individuals are more likely to stay consistent, which is essential for achieving long-term benefits. Mindfulness encourages individuals to check in with themselves, helping them notice if they need a specific herb or practice to support their current state. For instance, someone who feels anxious may choose an herbal tea with adaptogens like ashwagandha, while someone struggling with sleep may opt for valerian root.

Mindfulness as a Tool for Emotional Healing

Beyond physical health, mindfulness is a powerful tool for emotional healing. Many individuals carry unprocessed emotions or past traumas that contribute to mental and physical health issues. Mindfulness offers a way to process these emotions by creating a safe space for them to surface without judgment. Through mindfulness practices, individuals can observe their emotions, acknowledge them, and let them go, which can alleviate the mental burden associated with unresolved emotions.

Loving-kindness meditation is a form of mindfulness that specifically focuses on emotional healing. This meditation involves sending feelings of love, compassion, and forgiveness to oneself and others. By practicing loving-kindness, individuals can release feelings of resentment, anger, or sadness that may be affecting their mental and physical well-being. This practice fosters emotional resilience and helps individuals develop a healthier relationship with their emotions.

Mindfulness also encourages **emotional regulation**, which is the ability to manage and respond to emotions in a healthy way. Through mindfulness, individuals learn to pause before reacting, giving themselves time to process their emotions and choose a constructive response. This skill is particularly valuable for those dealing with chronic stress, anxiety, or anger. By improving emotional regulation, mindfulness supports mental clarity and reduces the likelihood of stress-related health issues.

Cultivating a Mindful Lifestyle for Long-Term Healing

Adopting a mindful lifestyle can lead to lasting changes in overall health and well-being. While formal mindfulness practices, such as meditation, are highly beneficial, mindfulness can be integrated into virtually any activity, from brushing one's teeth to talking with a friend. By bringing awareness and presence into everyday actions, individuals can reduce stress and improve their quality of life.

Creating a mindful lifestyle may begin with small, intentional changes. For example, individuals can start by setting aside five minutes each day to practice mindful breathing or meditation. As they become more comfortable with these practices, they can gradually incorporate mindfulness into other areas of their life, such as work, exercise, and personal relationships. The goal is to make mindfulness a natural part of daily life, rather than something that requires effort or discipline.

A mindful lifestyle also encourages individuals to make choices that align with their values and goals. When people are mindful of their thoughts and actions, they are more likely to engage in behaviors that support their well-being. This includes choosing nutritious foods, setting healthy boundaries, and engaging in activities that bring joy and fulfillment. By living mindfully, individuals create an environment that supports healing on a physical, mental, and emotional level.

Mindfulness is a journey, not a destination. It requires patience, consistency, and self-compassion. However, the benefits of mindfulness for healing are profound and far-reaching. By embracing mindfulness, individuals can experience a greater sense of peace, resilience, and overall well-being, empowering them to take control of their health and live a life that is balanced, fulfilled, and in harmony with their true selves.

Chapter 3: Nutrition as Medicine

Whole foods are the foundation of a healthy, balanced diet and have been celebrated for their nutritional density, natural flavors, and the powerful support they offer to the body's self-healing mechanisms. In an era of highly processed foods, preservatives, and artificial additives, whole foods stand out as the simplest and most effective way to nourish the body, support wellness, and prevent disease. They provide essential vitamins, minerals, fiber, and other nutrients in their natural, unprocessed forms, offering a stark contrast to refined and artificial foods that often lack these vital elements.

Importance of Whole Foods

Whole foods include fresh fruits and vegetables, whole grains, nuts, seeds, legumes, and unprocessed meats and fish. These foods are minimally altered from their natural state, preserving their original nutritional content and avoiding the chemical additives that are often found in processed foods. The impact of whole foods on health is profound; they support everything from immune health to digestive function, cardiovascular wellness, and mental clarity.

Nutrient Density and Bioavailability

One of the primary benefits of whole foods is their nutrient density. Nutrient-dense foods are packed with essential vitamins and minerals that the body needs to function optimally. Unlike processed foods, which are often filled with empty calories from sugars and unhealthy fats, whole foods offer a wealth of nutrients per calorie. This means that individuals can obtain the nutrients they need without consuming excessive amounts of food, which is especially beneficial for maintaining a healthy weight and avoiding nutrient deficiencies.

In addition to being nutrient-dense, whole foods often have a high level of bioavailability. Bioavailability refers to how easily nutrients are absorbed and utilized by the body. Many whole foods contain vitamins and minerals in forms that the body can efficiently process, allowing them to be absorbed more readily. For instance, the iron found in leafy green vegetables is more easily absorbed by the body when consumed with foods rich in vitamin C, such as bell peppers or oranges. This natural synergy in whole foods enhances nutrient absorption, providing more effective nourishment than many fortified or artificially enriched processed foods.

An example of the nutrient density of whole foods can be seen in a handful of almonds. Almonds contain healthy fats, protein, fiber, and important vitamins like vitamin E, which is a powerful antioxidant. This nutrient profile makes almonds a much better choice than a processed snack like a bag of chips, which may be high in calories but low in actual nutritional value. By choosing whole foods like almonds over processed options, individuals can fuel their bodies with nutrients that support sustained energy, mental clarity, and overall wellness.

Fiber: A Critical Component of Whole Foods

Fiber is an essential nutrient found exclusively in plant-based whole foods. It plays a crucial role in digestive health, helps regulate blood sugar levels, and supports heart health. There are two types of fiber: soluble and insoluble. Soluble fiber dissolves in water to form a gel-like substance, which helps lower cholesterol and blood sugar levels. Insoluble fiber, on the other hand, adds bulk to the stool, promoting healthy digestion and regular bowel movements.

A diet rich in fiber from whole foods, such as fruits, vegetables, whole grains, and legumes, provides benefits that processed foods lack. Processed foods are often stripped of their natural fiber during manufacturing, making them less beneficial for digestive health and potentially leading to issues such as constipation, irregular blood sugar levels, and increased risk of cardiovascular disease.

For example, choosing a whole grain like quinoa over refined grains like white rice offers more fiber, which can help with satiety, stabilize blood sugar levels, and lower cholesterol. Fiber-rich whole foods also feed the beneficial bacteria in the gut, which play a significant role in immune function, mental health, and overall wellness. Unlike fiber supplements, which provide isolated fiber without the accompanying nutrients, whole foods offer a complete nutritional package that works synergistically within the body.

Antioxidants: Protecting the Body from Oxidative Stress

Whole foods are also rich in antioxidants, compounds that protect the body from oxidative stress and inflammation. Oxidative stress occurs when there is an imbalance between free radicals—unstable molecules that can damage cells—and antioxidants, which neutralize these harmful molecules. Chronic oxidative stress has been linked to numerous health conditions, including heart disease, cancer, and neurodegenerative disorders.

Fruits and vegetables, especially those with vibrant colors like berries, spinach, and sweet potatoes, are particularly high in antioxidants. Each color in fruits and vegetables indicates the presence of specific antioxidants, such as beta-carotene in orange foods like carrots, which supports eye health, and anthocyanins in purple foods like blueberries, which promote brain health.

Incorporating a variety of colorful whole foods into one's diet ensures a broad range of antioxidants, each offering unique health benefits. For instance, including leafy greens like kale and spinach provides antioxidants like lutein and zeaxanthin, which are essential for eye health. Regularly consuming these foods can help protect against conditions like macular degeneration and cataracts, which are more common as individuals age.

Whole Foods and Blood Sugar Regulation

Whole foods play a critical role in stabilizing blood sugar levels, an important factor in preventing and managing diabetes. Processed foods, particularly those high in refined sugars and carbohydrates, cause rapid spikes in blood sugar levels, which can lead to insulin resistance over time. Insulin resistance is a precursor to type 2 diabetes and is associated with various metabolic disorders.

Whole foods, especially those high in fiber, help slow down the digestion and absorption of sugars, resulting in more stable blood sugar levels. For instance, an apple, which contains natural sugars along with fiber, vitamins, and minerals, has a different impact on blood sugar than apple juice. The fiber in the apple slows down sugar absorption, preventing the rapid spike in blood sugar that occurs with juice. This slower absorption rate helps the body maintain steady energy levels, reducing the risk of energy crashes and cravings.

Legumes, such as lentils and chickpeas, are excellent whole food choices for blood sugar regulation. They have a low glycemic index, meaning they are digested slowly and have minimal impact on blood sugar. Incorporating legumes into meals can help individuals feel full for longer periods, stabilize blood sugar, and provide essential nutrients like protein, iron, and B vitamins, making them a powerful addition to a balanced diet.

Supporting Heart Health with Whole Foods

Whole foods, particularly fruits, vegetables, whole grains, and nuts, have been shown to reduce the risk of heart disease. The fiber, antioxidants, and healthy fats found in whole foods contribute to improved cholesterol levels, lower blood pressure, and reduced inflammation, all of which are factors that protect heart health.

Nuts and seeds, such as walnuts and flaxseeds, are high in omega-3 fatty acids, which have anti-inflammatory properties and support cardiovascular health. Omega-3s help reduce triglycerides, lower blood pressure, and prevent the formation of blood clots. Including a handful of walnuts in the diet, for example, can provide these heart-protective benefits while also delivering protein and fiber.

In addition to nuts and seeds, whole grains like oats are known for their heart health benefits. Oats contain a type of soluble fiber called beta-glucan, which has been shown to lower cholesterol levels. Starting the day with a bowl of oatmeal topped with fruits and nuts offers a heart-healthy, nutrient-dense breakfast that supports energy, satiety, and cardiovascular wellness.

Whole Foods and Mental Health

The connection between diet and mental health is gaining recognition, with whole foods emerging as a key factor in supporting emotional well-being and cognitive function. Diets rich in processed foods and refined sugars have been associated with a higher risk of depression and anxiety, while whole foods provide the nutrients necessary for brain health.

Foods rich in omega-3 fatty acids, such as salmon and chia seeds, have been shown to support brain function and improve mood. Omega-3s are essential fats that play a role in cell membrane integrity, particularly in brain cells, and have anti-inflammatory effects that can reduce symptoms of depression.

Leafy greens, berries, and nuts are also beneficial for mental health. Berries, high in antioxidants, protect the brain from oxidative stress, which can lead to cognitive decline. Leafy greens provide folate, a B vitamin essential for neurotransmitter function and mental clarity. Including these foods in one's diet can enhance mood, support memory, and promote long-term brain health.

Practical Strategies for Incorporating Whole Foods

Transitioning to a diet rich in whole foods may seem challenging at first, but with gradual changes, it can become a sustainable lifestyle. One effective strategy is to start with simple swaps, replacing processed items with whole foods. For instance, replacing white bread with whole grain bread or using brown rice instead of white rice adds fiber and nutrients to meals without drastically changing the flavor.

Meal preparation can also support a whole foods diet. Preparing meals in advance with ingredients like fresh vegetables, lean proteins, and whole grains allows for convenient, nutritious meals throughout the week. For snacks, keeping options like fresh fruit, nuts, and seeds readily available can make it easier to avoid processed options.

Shopping the perimeter of the grocery store is another tip for choosing whole foods, as fresh produce, meats, and dairy products are often located along the outer edges, while processed foods are found in the inner aisles. By focusing on the perimeter, shoppers can prioritize whole food options and make healthier choices.

Incorporating whole foods into daily life promotes not only physical health but also mental and emotional wellness. Whole foods provide the body with essential nutrients in their most natural forms, supporting a balanced, sustainable approach to health. The simple act of choosing whole foods over processed options can lead to profound benefits, enhancing energy, preventing disease, and fostering overall wellness.

Nutrient-Rich Foods

The foundation of good health is built upon nutrient-rich foods that fuel the body, support mental clarity, and foster emotional balance. Eating nutrient-dense foods provides the body with the essential vitamins, minerals, and compounds it needs to function optimally, boost immunity, and support natural healing processes. Nutrient-rich foods form the backbone of holistic health, as they are free from the processed ingredients and additives that can lead to inflammation and chronic illness. By focusing on whole, natural foods, individuals can harness the power of nutrition to heal and maintain a balanced mind, body, and spirit.

Nutrient-rich foods are those that deliver a high level of vitamins, minerals, and other vital nutrients relative to their calorie content. These include fruits, vegetables, whole grains, nuts, seeds, and lean proteins, all of which are packed with nutrients that support different aspects of health. For individuals seeking natural healing and wellness, prioritizing these foods helps ensure that the body has the resources it needs to repair itself, ward off disease, and maintain high energy levels.

The Importance of Micronutrients in Health and Healing

Micronutrients, which include vitamins and minerals, are essential for the body's biochemical processes. Although they are needed in smaller amounts than macronutrients like carbohydrates, proteins, and fats, they play an outsized role in maintaining health and facilitating healing. Without adequate levels of these nutrients, the body cannot perform functions such as hormone production, immune response, and cellular repair.

Vitamins are organic compounds that play vital roles in growth, immunity, and metabolic function. For example, Vitamin C is a powerful antioxidant that helps the body fend off infections and supports collagen production, essential for skin health and wound healing. Vitamin D, often referred to as the "sunshine vitamin," supports bone health by aiding calcium absorption and is critical for immune function. Vitamin B12, found primarily in animal products, is essential for neurological health and red blood cell formation.

Minerals are inorganic elements such as calcium, magnesium, and iron that are essential for numerous bodily functions. Calcium supports strong bones and teeth, while magnesium plays a critical role in muscle function, mood regulation, and sleep quality. Iron is necessary for red blood cell production and oxygen transport, making it crucial for energy levels and cognitive function. A deficiency in any of these minerals can lead to health issues such as fatigue, poor immunity, and weakened bones.

When individuals consume nutrient-rich foods, they obtain these vital vitamins and minerals, helping the body function at its best. For those focused on natural healing, maintaining optimal levels of micronutrients is essential for supporting the body's natural resilience and recovery processes.

Superfoods: Nutrient-Dense Options for Enhanced Health

"Superfoods" is a term often used to describe foods that are exceptionally rich in nutrients and provide unique health benefits. While there is no official scientific definition for superfoods, they are generally recognized for their high levels of antioxidants, healthy fats, fiber, and phytochemicals. Incorporating superfoods into a diet can amplify the healing effects of nutrition, providing the body with concentrated sources of beneficial compounds that support both physical and mental health.

Some popular superfoods include:

- **Blueberries**: Known for their high antioxidant content, blueberries protect cells from oxidative damage, which is linked to aging and various diseases. They are also a good source of vitamin C and fiber, supporting immune health and digestion.

- **Spinach**: Spinach is rich in iron, calcium, and magnesium, making it a powerful ally for bone health, muscle function, and energy production. It also contains folate, a B vitamin that supports brain health and mood regulation.

- **Salmon**: High in omega-3 fatty acids, salmon is an excellent choice for heart and brain health. Omega-3s reduce inflammation and support cognitive function, making salmon a valuable food for those looking to support long-term health.

- **Chia Seeds**: These tiny seeds are packed with fiber, omega-3 fatty acids, and protein, making them a nutrient-dense addition to meals. They help maintain stable blood sugar levels and provide lasting energy.

- **Sweet Potatoes**: Rich in beta-carotene, a precursor to vitamin A, sweet potatoes support eye health and immune function. Their high fiber content also promotes digestive health, making them a nutritious and filling option.

By incorporating superfoods like these into daily meals, individuals can enhance the nutrient density of their diet, supporting healing and overall well-being. However, it's important to remember that no single food can provide all the nutrients the body needs, which is why a varied and balanced diet is essential.

Nutrient-Rich Foods for Specific Health Needs

For individuals seeking natural remedies for specific health concerns, certain nutrient-rich foods can target and support different bodily functions. By choosing foods tailored to their unique needs, individuals can maximize the healing potential of their diet. Below are some examples of nutrient-rich foods that support common health goals:

1. **Immune Support**: To support the immune system, focus on foods rich in vitamins C and E, zinc, and antioxidants. Oranges, strawberries, bell peppers, and broccoli are excellent sources of vitamin C, while almonds and sunflower seeds provide vitamin E. Zinc, found in pumpkin seeds and legumes, plays a vital role in immune function and wound healing.

2. **Digestive Health**: Foods high in fiber, such as leafy greens, apples, and whole grains, support a healthy digestive system by promoting regular bowel movements

and nurturing gut bacteria. Fermented foods, like yogurt, kefir, and sauerkraut, contain probiotics that help maintain a balanced gut microbiome, essential for overall health.

3. **Heart Health**: Foods rich in omega-3 fatty acids, such as walnuts, flaxseeds, and fatty fish, support cardiovascular health by reducing inflammation and lowering cholesterol levels. Whole grains, like oats and brown rice, also support heart health by providing fiber that can help regulate blood pressure and cholesterol.

4. **Bone Health**: Calcium, magnesium, and vitamin D are critical for strong bones. Leafy greens like kale and spinach, dairy products, and fortified plant-based milks provide these nutrients. Including these foods regularly in a diet helps maintain bone density and reduce the risk of osteoporosis.

5. **Skin Health**: Foods high in antioxidants and healthy fats promote healthy skin by reducing inflammation and protecting against UV damage. Avocados, rich in vitamin E and healthy fats, nourish the skin, while tomatoes, which contain lycopene, offer natural sun protection.

Practical Ways to Incorporate Nutrient-Rich Foods into Daily Life

For those transitioning to a more nutrient-dense diet, practical strategies can help make the process enjoyable and sustainable. Integrating nutrient-rich foods into meals doesn't have to be complicated; even small adjustments can make a significant impact on health.

One effective approach is to **start the day with a nutrient-rich breakfast**. Smoothies made with leafy greens, berries, chia seeds, and a source of protein like Greek yogurt or nut butter provide a well-rounded meal packed with vitamins, minerals, and fiber. Adding superfoods like spirulina or wheatgrass powder can enhance the nutrient content further, offering a concentrated dose of vitamins and antioxidants.

For lunch and dinner, **build meals around vegetables** and lean proteins. A balanced plate might include a large portion of leafy greens or other colorful vegetables, a source of protein such as grilled salmon or beans, and a serving of whole grains like quinoa or brown rice. This combination provides a range of nutrients that support energy levels, immune health, and mental clarity.

Another strategy is to **use herbs and spices** to add flavor and nutrition to meals. Turmeric, for example, is known for its anti-inflammatory properties and can be added to soups, stir-fries, and teas. Ginger, another anti-inflammatory spice, is excellent for digestion and can be used fresh in smoothies or grated over salads.

For snacks, choosing **nutrient-dense options** like nuts, seeds, and fresh fruit can provide lasting energy and prevent blood sugar spikes. Almonds, for instance, are high in healthy fats and protein, making them a filling snack that also supports heart health. Fresh fruit like apples or berries satisfies sweet cravings while delivering fiber and antioxidants.

The Role of Hydration in Nutrient Absorption and Overall Health

While nutrient-rich foods are essential, hydration also plays a critical role in health and healing. Water is necessary for almost every bodily function, including digestion, nutrient absorption, and temperature regulation. Without adequate hydration, the body cannot transport nutrients effectively or remove waste products, which can hinder overall health.

For optimal hydration, aim to drink at least eight glasses of water per day, adjusting for activity levels and climate. Herbal teas, such as chamomile, peppermint, and ginger, offer a hydrating alternative to water and provide additional health benefits. Chamomile, for instance, supports relaxation, while peppermint aids digestion. These teas are caffeine-free, making them ideal for hydration without the dehydrating effects of caffeine.

Incorporating foods with high water content can also support hydration. Fruits like watermelon, cucumber, and oranges have high water content and provide electrolytes, helping to maintain fluid balance in the body. These hydrating foods are especially beneficial during warmer months or after physical activity.

Mindful Eating and the Benefits of Savoring Nutrient-Rich Foods

Mindful eating is an approach that encourages individuals to savor their meals, paying attention to flavors, textures, and the body's hunger and fullness cues. This practice supports a healthier relationship with food and enhances the enjoyment of nutrient-rich meals. When individuals eat mindfully, they are more likely to feel satisfied with their food choices and less likely to overeat.

Mindful eating also allows individuals to recognize the benefits of nutrient-rich foods in real time, noticing how these foods affect their energy levels, mood, and overall well-being. For example, someone who incorporates a nutrient-dense lunch may find that they have more sustained energy throughout the afternoon, compared to a meal high in refined sugars and empty calories. This awareness reinforces healthy eating habits and encourages individuals to prioritize nutrient-rich options.

Incorporating nutrient-rich foods into daily life is a powerful step toward holistic health and natural healing. By choosing foods that nourish both the body and mind, individuals can support their well-being, resilience, and vitality in a way that is sustainable and deeply rewarding.

Greens and Antioxidants

The power of greens and antioxidants in promoting health and vitality is well-documented. Leafy greens, vibrant vegetables, and antioxidant-rich herbs play a crucial role in supporting the body's immune function, reducing inflammation, and protecting cells from damage caused by free radicals. These foods are rich in vitamins, minerals, and phytonutrients that not only support essential bodily functions but also prevent chronic diseases, improve energy levels, and enhance overall wellness. Greens and antioxidants are foundational to any natural healing regimen and should be prioritized in daily dietary habits.

Greens like spinach, kale, and arugula, along with brightly colored vegetables such as bell peppers and carrots, provide the body with essential antioxidants. These antioxidants include vitamins like vitamin C and E, and other powerful compounds such as beta-carotene and flavonoids. The unique properties of each green and antioxidant contribute to a symbiotic effect, where nutrients work together to boost the body's self-healing capabilities and fortify the immune system against common and complex health challenges.

Understanding Free Radicals and Antioxidants

Before delving into specific greens and their benefits, it's essential to understand the role of antioxidants in combating free radicals. Free radicals are unstable molecules that result from various sources, including pollution, UV exposure, and metabolic processes. While free radicals are a natural byproduct of bodily functions, an excess can lead to oxidative stress, damaging cells, proteins, and DNA. This stress is associated with aging, inflammation, and various chronic diseases like cancer, heart disease, and neurodegenerative disorders.

Antioxidants, present abundantly in greens, neutralize free radicals, preventing or minimizing cellular damage. They donate electrons to free radicals, stabilizing these molecules and inhibiting the harmful chain reactions they cause. By incorporating greens rich in antioxidants into the diet, one can provide the body with a natural defense against oxidative stress, promoting long-term health and resilience.

Leafy Greens: Nutritional Powerhouses

Leafy greens are among the most nutrient-dense foods available, packed with essential vitamins and minerals that support overall health. Spinach, kale, and Swiss chard are excellent examples of greens that contain high levels of antioxidants. These greens offer a range of nutrients, from vitamin A and C to folate and iron, each contributing uniquely to bodily functions.

For example, spinach is loaded with beta-carotene, a precursor to vitamin A that supports vision health and immune function. It also contains lutein and zeaxanthin, antioxidants known to protect against eye-related disorders such as macular degeneration. Kale, another nutrient powerhouse, offers high levels of vitamin C and K, along with various phytonutrients that support heart health and reduce inflammation.

In addition to vitamins, leafy greens are rich in chlorophyll, a pigment with numerous health benefits. Chlorophyll helps detoxify the body, supports liver health, and has potential anti-cancer properties. Its molecular structure closely resembles hemoglobin, the oxygen-carrying molecule in red blood cells, which may explain why chlorophyll is believed to improve oxygen transport in the body.

Including a variety of leafy greens in the diet ensures a broad spectrum of antioxidants and phytonutrients. For example, a salad with spinach, arugula, and Swiss chard provides diverse nutrients, supporting immune function, energy production, and cellular health. For those new to greens, blending spinach or kale into smoothies is a simple and delicious way to increase intake without altering meal routines dramatically.

Cruciferous Vegetables: Detoxification and Antioxidant Support

Cruciferous vegetables, such as broccoli, Brussels sprouts, and cauliflower, are not only packed with antioxidants but also contain compounds that support the body's natural detoxification processes. These vegetables are rich in sulforaphane, a compound known for its anti-inflammatory and cancer-fighting properties. Sulforaphane activates enzymes in the liver that help neutralize harmful toxins, assisting the body in managing the daily influx of environmental and dietary pollutants.

Broccoli, for instance, is an excellent source of both vitamin C and sulforaphane. Vitamin C, a powerful antioxidant, supports immune function and helps the body repair tissue, while sulforaphane provides protection against inflammation and certain cancers. Studies suggest that regular consumption of cruciferous vegetables can reduce the risk of various cancers, particularly those affecting the digestive tract.

Incorporating these vegetables into daily meals can be as simple as roasting or steaming them as a side dish. For those looking to enhance the flavor, a drizzle of olive oil, a dash of herbs, or a squeeze of lemon can complement the natural taste while adding additional antioxidants, such as oleic acid from olive oil and vitamin C from lemon.

Herbs and Microgreens: Concentrated Sources of Antioxidants

Herbs and microgreens are often overlooked as sources of antioxidants, but they pack a powerful nutritional punch in small quantities. Microgreens like sunflower sprouts, pea shoots, and radish greens are young versions of vegetables and herbs, harvested shortly after sprouting. These tiny greens are nutrient-dense, offering higher concentrations of vitamins, minerals, and antioxidants compared to their mature counterparts.

Herbs such as parsley, cilantro, and basil are also rich in antioxidants. Parsley, for example, contains myricetin, a flavonoid with anti-inflammatory and cancer-fighting properties. Cilantro has detoxifying effects, particularly for heavy metals, while basil provides essential oils with antibacterial and antioxidant benefits. Adding fresh herbs to dishes not only enhances flavor but also boosts the antioxidant content, contributing to overall health.

Microgreens can be easily incorporated into salads, sandwiches, and smoothies, while fresh herbs can be used as garnishes or blended into sauces. Growing microgreens at home is a simple way to ensure a constant supply of these nutrient-dense greens. A small indoor tray can yield a fresh batch of microgreens in about a week, providing an affordable and sustainable source of antioxidants.

Antioxidants in Colored Vegetables: The Power of Diversity

While greens are incredibly beneficial, it's essential to incorporate a rainbow of vegetables into the diet to maximize antioxidant intake. Each color in fruits and vegetables represents different antioxidants, contributing to various health benefits. For instance, orange and red vegetables like carrots, bell peppers, and tomatoes are high in beta-carotene and lycopene, antioxidants known for supporting skin health and reducing cancer risk.

Yellow and orange vegetables, such as sweet potatoes and pumpkin, are rich in carotenoids, which support immune health and vision. Red and purple vegetables, like beets and eggplant, contain anthocyanins, which have anti-inflammatory properties and support heart health. By combining greens with a range of colored vegetables, individuals can achieve a broader spectrum of antioxidants, enhancing the overall protective effects of their diet.

For example, a stir-fry with spinach, bell peppers, and carrots provides a blend of antioxidants that support eye health, immune function, and cellular repair. This colorful approach not only makes meals visually appealing but also ensures a diverse intake of phytonutrients, each offering unique benefits to the body's systems.

Practical Tips for Incorporating Greens and Antioxidants into Daily Life

Incorporating greens and antioxidant-rich foods into daily life doesn't have to be complicated. Small changes in meal preparation can significantly boost antioxidant intake, providing more protection against oxidative stress and supporting overall wellness. For example, starting the day with a green smoothie that includes spinach, kale, and berries is an easy way to consume several servings of greens and antioxidants at once. Adding a banana or an apple can enhance flavor while providing natural sweetness.

Salads offer a versatile way to increase greens intake. A salad can include various leafy greens, microgreens, and colorful vegetables like carrots, bell peppers, and radishes. Adding nuts and seeds, such as almonds or sunflower seeds, contributes healthy fats and additional antioxidants, creating a balanced, nutrient-dense meal. A simple homemade dressing with olive oil, lemon juice, and fresh herbs like basil or parsley can further enhance the antioxidant content.

For those with limited time, green powders made from dehydrated greens can be a convenient alternative. While fresh greens are ideal, green powders provide concentrated nutrients that can be added to smoothies, soups, or even water. It's essential to choose high-quality powders that retain the integrity of the nutrients, ensuring maximum health benefits.

Benefits of Antioxidants Beyond Physical Health

While antioxidants are primarily known for their role in preventing physical diseases, they also contribute to mental and emotional well-being. Oxidative stress doesn't only affect the body; it impacts the brain, potentially leading to cognitive decline and mood disorders. By protecting brain cells from oxidative damage, antioxidants can support mental clarity, memory, and emotional resilience.

For instance, flavonoids found in blueberries and leafy greens have been shown to improve cognitive function and reduce the risk of age-related cognitive decline. Regular consumption of these foods can enhance focus, support learning, and even improve mood. For individuals dealing with stress or anxiety, antioxidant-rich foods can provide neuroprotective effects that help the brain manage stress more effectively.

Antioxidants also support skin health by combating the free radicals that lead to premature aging and skin damage. Greens like kale and arugula, rich in vitamins A and C, promote collagen production, enhancing skin elasticity and reducing wrinkles. Including a variety of antioxidant-rich foods in the diet can help achieve a natural, healthy glow, further supporting the body's appearance as it ages.

Cultivating a Habit of Green and Antioxidant Consumption

Making greens and antioxidants a staple in daily life requires consistency and creativity. Rather than viewing greens as an occasional side dish, incorporating them into every meal can become a natural habit. For example, greens can be added to breakfast through an omelet with spinach and tomatoes, lunch through a colorful salad, and dinner by adding broccoli or green beans to a main dish.

Snacking on vegetables and antioxidant-rich fruits, such as carrot sticks, cherry tomatoes, or blueberries, can replace processed snacks with nutrient-dense options. Prepping vegetables in advance and keeping them accessible in the fridge makes it easy to reach for a healthy snack, supporting a balanced and antioxidant-rich diet throughout the day.

For families with children, making greens and antioxidants a regular part of meals can set the foundation for lifelong healthy eating habits. Engaging children in the process, such as by letting them choose a vegetable or helping prepare a smoothie, can increase their interest in and acceptance of these foods.

Essential Fats for Healing

Essential fats, often referred to as essential fatty acids, are crucial for maintaining health, supporting mental clarity, and promoting healing throughout the body. Unlike some nutrients, essential fats cannot be synthesized by the body and must be obtained through diet. These healthy fats are found in foods such as fish, nuts, seeds, and oils, and they play a central role in reducing inflammation, supporting brain function, and improving cardiovascular health. For anyone on a journey toward natural healing, understanding the benefits of essential fats and incorporating them into the diet is key.

There are two main types of essential fatty acids: **omega-3** and **omega-6** fats. Both are vital for health, but they must be consumed in a balanced ratio to support optimal function. Unfortunately, the modern Western diet often contains an excess of omega-6 fats relative to omega-3s, which can lead to inflammation and various health issues. By focusing on omega-3-rich foods and ensuring a healthy balance of these fats, individuals can harness the power of essential fats to support healing and prevent chronic disease.

Omega-3 Fatty Acids: The Foundation of Anti-Inflammatory Healing

Omega-3 fatty acids are a type of polyunsaturated fat that has been widely studied for its health benefits. Known for their anti-inflammatory properties, omega-3s are crucial for heart health, brain function, and reducing symptoms associated with inflammatory conditions such as arthritis. Omega-3s are primarily found in fatty fish like salmon, mackerel, and sardines, as well as in plant-based sources such as flaxseeds, chia seeds, and walnuts.

There are three main types of omega-3 fatty acids: **ALA (alpha-linolenic acid)**, **EPA (eicosapentaenoic acid)**, and **DHA (docosahexaenoic acid)**. Each type plays a distinct role in health and healing:

- **ALA** is primarily found in plant sources and must be converted by the body into EPA and DHA to be used effectively. However, this conversion process is limited, making it important to consume EPA and DHA directly when possible.

- **EPA** is known for its strong anti-inflammatory effects and is especially beneficial for heart health. It helps to reduce inflammation in blood vessels and can lower the risk of heart disease.

- **DHA** is a major structural component of the brain and retina, making it essential for cognitive function, eye health, and mental clarity.

For those looking to increase their intake of omega-3s, fatty fish are the most bioavailable source of EPA and DHA. Including fish in the diet two to three times per week can provide a steady supply of these essential fats. For those following a plant-based diet, chia seeds, flaxseeds, and hemp seeds are excellent sources of ALA, although it may be beneficial to consider an algae-based omega-3 supplement to ensure adequate levels of EPA and DHA.

Omega-6 Fatty Acids: Balancing Essential Fats for Optimal Health

While omega-3 fatty acids receive a lot of attention for their health benefits, omega-6 fatty acids are also essential for health. Omega-6s play a role in brain function, skin health, and bone density. However, they are more common in the diet than omega-3s and are often found in processed foods and cooking oils such as corn oil, soybean oil, and sunflower oil. This overabundance of omega-6 fatty acids in the typical Western diet can create an imbalance that promotes inflammation, which is why it's important to moderate intake and prioritize high-quality sources.

Linoleic acid is the primary omega-6 fatty acid found in the diet. When consumed in moderation and from healthy sources, linoleic acid can support health. Sources of omega-6 fatty acids that are beneficial include nuts, seeds, and plant oils in their whole form, such as evening primrose oil, borage oil, and blackcurrant seed oil. These oils contain gamma-linolenic acid (GLA), a type of omega-6 fatty acid that has anti-inflammatory properties and may be helpful for conditions like arthritis and eczema.

The key to harnessing the benefits of omega-6 fatty acids lies in balancing them with omega-3s. Health experts recommend a **ratio of about 4:1 of omega-6 to omega-3**, although many people consume a ratio closer to 20:1. To restore balance, individuals can reduce their intake of processed foods and oils high in omega-6s and focus on incorporating more omega-3-rich foods.

Essential Fats and Cardiovascular Health

One of the most well-documented benefits of essential fats, particularly omega-3s, is their impact on cardiovascular health. Omega-3 fatty acids have been shown to reduce the risk of heart disease by lowering triglycerides, reducing blood pressure, and preventing the formation of blood clots. EPA and DHA help to improve endothelial function, which keeps blood vessels flexible and responsive, allowing for efficient blood flow and reducing the risk of artery hardening.

For individuals with a family history of heart disease or high cholesterol, incorporating omega-3-rich foods like salmon, walnuts, and flaxseeds can be especially beneficial. Studies have found that a diet high in omega-3s can lower the risk of heart disease by reducing levels of LDL (bad) cholesterol while increasing HDL (good) cholesterol. Additionally, the anti-inflammatory effects of omega-3s help to protect the cardiovascular system by reducing the buildup of plaque in the arteries.

Omega-6 fatty acids also play a role in cardiovascular health but should be consumed mindfully to avoid inflammation. When balanced properly with omega-3s, omega-6 fats can support heart health by maintaining cholesterol levels and providing energy. However, consuming too many omega-6 fats from processed oils and fried foods can counteract these benefits and contribute to cardiovascular issues.

Essential Fats for Brain Health and Cognitive Function

Essential fats are critical for brain health and cognitive function. DHA, in particular, is a major structural component of the brain and is crucial for the development and maintenance of cognitive function. It supports the growth of neurons and plays a role in neurotransmission, which is essential for memory, learning, and mood regulation. Low levels of DHA have been linked to cognitive decline and an increased risk of neurodegenerative diseases such as Alzheimer's.

For individuals looking to support mental clarity and prevent cognitive decline, incorporating omega-3-rich foods is essential. Consuming fatty fish like salmon or sardines at least twice a week can provide the necessary levels of DHA to support brain health. For those who do not consume fish, an algae-based supplement can be an effective alternative, as it provides a plant-based source of DHA.

EPA also plays a role in mental health by reducing inflammation and supporting mood stability. Studies have shown that EPA can be effective in reducing symptoms of depression, making omega-3 fatty acids a natural option for those looking to support their mental health. By reducing inflammation in the brain and promoting healthy neurotransmitter function, omega-3s help to foster a stable mood and prevent the cognitive symptoms associated with mental health disorders.

Essential Fats and Skin Health

The skin is the body's largest organ, and essential fats play a key role in maintaining its health and resilience. Omega-3 and omega-6 fatty acids help to keep the skin hydrated, improve elasticity, and reduce inflammation, which can alleviate conditions like acne, eczema, and psoriasis. Essential fats contribute to the skin's lipid barrier, which prevents moisture loss and protects against environmental irritants.

DHA and EPA from omega-3s are particularly beneficial for reducing skin inflammation and improving hydration. Individuals with dry or inflamed skin may notice improvements by incorporating more omega-3-rich foods or supplements into their diet. Omega-6 fatty acids, such as gamma-linolenic acid (GLA) found in evening primrose oil and borage oil, also support skin health by providing anti-inflammatory benefits and promoting smooth, supple skin.

For practical application, individuals can incorporate essential fats into their diet by consuming sources like salmon, chia seeds, flaxseeds, and walnuts. For those with specific skin concerns, adding a GLA supplement may provide additional support, helping to reduce symptoms of conditions like eczema or dry skin.

Essential Fats and Joint Health

Inflammation is a major factor in joint pain and stiffness, especially for those with arthritis or other inflammatory conditions. Essential fats, particularly EPA and DHA, have been shown to reduce inflammation in joints, improving mobility and reducing discomfort. Omega-3 fatty acids work by inhibiting the production of inflammatory molecules called cytokines, which can lead to chronic inflammation and pain when left unchecked.

Incorporating essential fats into the diet can be beneficial for individuals experiencing joint pain or those looking to prevent joint degeneration. Studies have found that omega-3 supplementation can reduce morning stiffness, swelling, and pain associated with rheumatoid arthritis, allowing individuals to maintain mobility and quality of life. A diet that includes fatty fish, chia seeds, and flaxseeds provides a natural source of these anti-inflammatory fats, helping to keep joints flexible and pain-free.

For individuals with arthritis or inflammatory joint conditions, focusing on a balanced intake of omega-3s and reducing omega-6 intake can further support joint health. Many people find that a diet rich in omega-3s allows them to reduce their dependence on anti-inflammatory medications, making essential fats a valuable component of natural pain management.

Practical Tips for Including Essential Fats in Your Diet

Incorporating essential fats into a daily diet doesn't have to be complicated. Here are some practical strategies to help individuals increase their intake of omega-3 and healthy omega-6 fats:

1. **Add fatty fish to your weekly meals**: Aim to include fatty fish, such as salmon, mackerel, or sardines, in your diet two to three times per week. These fish are rich in EPA and DHA, providing a bioavailable source of omega-3s.

2. **Incorporate plant-based omega-3 sources**: For those who do not consume fish, chia seeds, flaxseeds, and walnuts offer plant-based sources of ALA. These foods can be added to smoothies, salads, and oatmeal for a nutritious boost.

3. **Use healthy oils**: Swap out processed cooking oils like soybean or corn oil for healthier options like olive oil, avocado oil, or coconut oil. These oils contain beneficial fats and can help maintain a balanced intake of essential fatty acids.

4. **Consider supplements if needed**: For individuals who struggle to get enough omega-3s through diet alone, fish oil or algae-based supplements provide a convenient option to ensure adequate intake of EPA and DHA.

5. **Reduce intake of processed foods**: Processed foods and fast foods are often high in omega-6 fatty acids from refined oils. By reducing consumption of these foods, individuals can create a better balance between omega-3 and omega-6 fats, supporting overall health.

By understanding the benefits of essential fats and making mindful choices, individuals can harness the healing power of these nutrients.

Chapter 4: Basic Herbal Recipes

Elderberry, also known by its scientific name *Sambucus nigra*, has a long-standing reputation as a powerful natural remedy for supporting the immune system. Elderberries are small, dark purple berries known for their potent antioxidant properties and have been traditionally used to combat colds, flu, and other respiratory infections.

Elderberry Immune Syrup

Among the various ways elderberries can be consumed, elderberry immune syrup stands out as a particularly effective and accessible form. This syrup not only captures the healing benefits of elderberries but also includes additional immune-boosting ingredients like honey, ginger, and cinnamon, creating a holistic approach to strengthening the body's defenses.

This section explores the properties of elderberry syrup, its benefits, the science behind its immune-boosting capabilities, and a step-by-step guide to preparing it at home. Additionally, we'll delve into practical uses, storage tips, and best practices to incorporate elderberry syrup as a natural remedy in daily life, making it a staple for anyone looking to support their immune system naturally.

The Science Behind Elderberries and Immunity

Elderberries are rich in antioxidants, specifically flavonoids and anthocyanins, which help protect the body's cells from damage caused by free radicals. These antioxidants are crucial in combating oxidative stress, a condition that can weaken immune function and make the body more susceptible to illness. Elderberries are particularly effective because they also contain vitamins A, B, and C, which play essential roles in maintaining immune health.

One of the primary components that make elderberries effective against viral infections is their ability to inhibit the replication of viruses. Studies have shown that elderberries can interfere with the way viruses enter and infect cells, essentially halting their progress in the body. This antiviral effect is especially beneficial during cold and flu season, as elderberry syrup can be used both preventatively and as a response to symptoms.

Elderberries also stimulate the production of cytokines, proteins that signal the immune system to respond to infection. By increasing cytokine levels, elderberries help the body mount a faster and more efficient immune response, which can reduce the duration and severity of illnesses. This immune-stimulating effect makes elderberry syrup a popular choice for families and individuals looking for natural ways to stay healthy during flu season.

Benefits of Elderberry Immune Syrup

Elderberry immune syrup is more than just a remedy for colds and flu. It offers a wide range of health benefits, particularly for the respiratory and immune systems. Regular use of elderberry syrup can provide the body with a boost of antioxidants, vitamins, and other nutrients that support overall wellness.

1. **Shortening Cold and Flu Duration**: Research indicates that elderberry syrup can reduce the duration of cold and flu symptoms when taken at the onset of illness. By preventing viruses from multiplying, elderberries help the body recover more quickly, alleviating symptoms like congestion, sore throat, and fatigue.

2. **Natural Cough Suppressant**: Elderberry syrup, especially when prepared with honey, acts as a natural cough suppressant. Honey has soothing properties for sore throats and, combined with elderberry's antiviral benefits, creates a powerful, gentle remedy for respiratory irritation.

3. **Antioxidant Protection**: The antioxidants in elderberries protect cells from damage, which is crucial for maintaining immune strength. Antioxidants support the body's detoxification processes, ensuring that cells function optimally and resist damage from environmental toxins.

4. **Safe for Most Age Groups**: Unlike many over-the-counter cold and flu medications, elderberry syrup is safe for most age groups, including children (over one year due to the honey content) and older adults. This makes it an ideal household remedy for families looking to avoid pharmaceuticals.

5. **Anti-inflammatory Properties**: Elderberries contain compounds that help reduce inflammation in the body, which can be particularly beneficial for individuals with chronic inflammatory conditions. This anti-inflammatory effect can help alleviate joint pain, reduce respiratory inflammation, and support heart health.

Ingredients and How They Enhance Elderberry Syrup

Elderberry syrup often includes additional natural ingredients like honey, ginger, cinnamon, and cloves, each contributing unique benefits that enhance the syrup's effectiveness.

- **Honey**: A natural sweetener, honey also has antimicrobial properties. It soothes sore throats, reduces cough, and provides additional antioxidants. Raw, unprocessed honey is ideal for its higher nutrient content.
- **Ginger**: Known for its anti-inflammatory and antioxidant properties, ginger supports digestion and helps relieve nausea, making elderberry syrup easier on the stomach for those who may experience digestive issues with illness.
- **Cinnamon**: Cinnamon adds warmth and flavor but also provides antimicrobial and anti-inflammatory benefits. It supports respiratory health and enhances the syrup's overall effectiveness.
- **Cloves**: Cloves have a high antioxidant content and contribute to immune health by fighting bacteria and supporting respiratory wellness. They add a slight numbing effect, which can be soothing for sore throats.

Step-by-Step Guide to Making Elderberry Immune Syrup at Home

Making elderberry syrup at home is a simple, cost-effective process. Here's a detailed recipe and preparation guide to creating this powerful remedy:

Ingredients:

- 1 cup dried elderberries (or 2 cups fresh elderberries)
- 4 cups filtered water
- 1 tablespoon fresh grated ginger (or 1 teaspoon dried ginger)
- 1 cinnamon stick (or 1 teaspoon ground cinnamon)
- 5-6 whole cloves (or 1/2 teaspoon ground cloves)
- 1 cup raw honey (adjust to taste)

Instructions:

1. **Combine Elderberries and Spices**: In a medium saucepan, combine the elderberries, water, ginger, cinnamon, and cloves. Stir the mixture to distribute the spices evenly.
2. **Simmer the Mixture**: Place the saucepan over medium heat and bring the mixture to a gentle boil. Once it reaches a boil, reduce the heat and let it simmer for about 45 minutes to an hour. This allows the elderberries to release their beneficial compounds into the water.

3. **Strain the Liquid**: After simmering, remove the saucepan from heat and allow it to cool slightly. Using a fine-mesh strainer or cheesecloth, strain the mixture into a clean bowl, pressing the berries to extract as much liquid as possible. Discard the elderberries and spices.

4. **Add Honey**: Once the mixture has cooled to room temperature, add honey and stir well to combine. Avoid adding honey while the liquid is hot, as heat can reduce the honey's nutritional value.

5. **Store the Syrup**: Transfer the syrup to a glass jar with a tight-fitting lid and store it in the refrigerator. Properly stored, homemade elderberry syrup can last up to two months in the fridge.

Dosage and Usage

For preventive purposes, a standard adult dosage is 1 tablespoon of elderberry syrup daily, while children can take 1 teaspoon. During times of illness, such as when experiencing cold or flu symptoms, this dosage can be increased to every 2-3 hours. Elderberry syrup is generally safe for regular use, but it's always wise to consult a healthcare professional before starting a new regimen, especially for individuals with underlying health conditions.

For children under one year, it's crucial to avoid elderberry syrup containing honey due to the risk of botulism. For these children, elderberry syrup without honey can be used as an alternative, or a healthcare provider can provide guidance on suitable remedies.

Storage and Safety Considerations

Homemade elderberry syrup, when stored properly in the refrigerator, can last about two months. However, if there's any sign of mold or fermentation (such as bubbling or an unusual odor), it should be discarded immediately. It's best to label the jar with the preparation date and store it in a cool part of the fridge to maintain freshness.

For individuals who prefer not to make elderberry syrup at home, many commercial options are available. It's essential to choose syrups made from organic elderberries and free from artificial preservatives and sugars, as these can diminish the syrup's health benefits.

Practical Uses and Tips for Incorporating Elderberry Syrup

Elderberry syrup is versatile and can be incorporated into the diet in various ways beyond taking it directly by the spoonful. Here are some practical ideas for incorporating elderberry syrup:

- **In Warm Beverages**: Elderberry syrup can be added to warm (not boiling) water or herbal tea for a comforting immune-boosting drink. This is especially helpful during the colder months when the immune system may need extra support.
- **As a Topping**: Elderberry syrup makes a delicious and healthful topping for oatmeal, yogurt, or pancakes. This adds a natural sweetness along with immune-boosting benefits.
- **In Smoothies**: Adding a tablespoon of elderberry syrup to a morning smoothie can enhance flavor and provide an immune boost, combining well with fruits like blueberries, strawberries, and bananas.
- **Mixed with Applesauce or Jam**: For children, mixing elderberry syrup with applesauce or a small amount of jam can make it more appealing. This is a great option for fussy eaters who may resist taking the syrup alone.

By making elderberry syrup part of one's daily routine, especially during cold and flu season, individuals can naturally support their immune system and enjoy the many benefits this powerful remedy provides.

Fire Cider Tonic

Fire Cider Tonic is a popular herbal remedy in the realm of natural health, known for its potent blend of spicy, tangy, and warming ingredients that stimulate the immune system, improve digestion, and provide natural relief from seasonal ailments. This traditional tonic is made by infusing apple cider vinegar with a variety of pungent herbs, roots, and vegetables, creating a powerful elixir that can be taken as a daily preventative or a natural treatment for colds and flu. The warming spices and herbs used in Fire Cider give it a "fiery" kick, which is why it is highly valued for its ability to invigorate the body and support overall vitality.

The popularity of Fire Cider has surged in recent years as more people turn to natural remedies to support their immune system and prevent illness. This tonic's combination of ingredients not only tastes bold but also carries a range of health benefits, making it a versatile and potent remedy in any wellness routine. By understanding the components and benefits of Fire Cider, individuals can learn to make this tonic at home and incorporate it into their self-care routine.

The Origins and Tradition of Fire Cider

Fire Cider is rooted in herbal medicine traditions, particularly within American folk medicine. Herbalist Rosemary Gladstar is credited with popularizing Fire Cider in the 1970s, although similar vinegar-based tonics have been used for centuries to stimulate circulation, aid digestion, and combat respiratory ailments. Gladstar developed Fire Cider as a way to make herbal remedies more accessible and enjoyable, blending powerful herbs and spices with apple cider vinegar to create a tonic that is as delicious as it is effective.

The name "Fire Cider" reflects the warming, spicy nature of the ingredients. Traditional recipes often include horseradish, garlic, ginger, hot peppers, and onions, which are known for their immune-boosting and anti-inflammatory properties. Over the years, herbalists and wellness enthusiasts have added their own twists to the recipe, incorporating additional herbs like turmeric, cinnamon, and rosemary to enhance both the flavor and health benefits of the tonic.

Key Ingredients in Fire Cider and Their Benefits

The strength of Fire Cider lies in its combination of ingredients, each of which brings its own unique set of health benefits. Together, these ingredients create a synergistic effect, boosting immunity, enhancing digestion, and reducing inflammation. Let's take a closer look at the key components of Fire Cider and how each contributes to its effectiveness:

1. **Apple Cider Vinegar**: The base of Fire Cider, apple cider vinegar (ACV) is a natural tonic on its own. ACV contains acetic acid, which aids digestion and supports gut health by promoting the growth of beneficial bacteria. It also helps balance blood sugar levels and may aid in weight management. The acidic nature of ACV helps extract and preserve the beneficial compounds from the herbs and spices, creating a potent infusion.

2. **Horseradish**: Known for its strong, pungent flavor, horseradish is a powerful decongestant and expectorant. It helps to clear mucus from the sinuses and respiratory tract, making it especially useful during cold and flu season. Horseradish is also rich in antioxidants and has anti-inflammatory properties that support immune health.

3. **Garlic**: Garlic is a well-known immune booster, thanks to its high allicin content, a compound with strong antimicrobial and antiviral properties. Garlic supports the

body's ability to fight infections and reduces inflammation, making it an invaluable addition to Fire Cider.

4. **Ginger**: With its warming and soothing effects, ginger helps improve circulation, ease digestive discomfort, and reduce nausea. Ginger is also anti-inflammatory and has been shown to help reduce muscle pain and soreness. Its spicy flavor adds a pleasant warmth to the Fire Cider, enhancing both its taste and its health benefits.

5. **Onion**: Onions contain quercetin, a potent antioxidant that supports the immune system and helps reduce inflammation. They also have expectorant properties, which can help relieve respiratory symptoms. Onions work synergistically with garlic to boost the tonic's immune-enhancing effects.

6. **Hot Peppers**: Often in the form of cayenne or jalapeño peppers, hot peppers add a spicy kick to Fire Cider and stimulate circulation. Capsaicin, the active compound in peppers, has pain-relieving properties and helps open nasal passages, making it easier to breathe. The heat from peppers also induces a slight sweating effect, which can help the body eliminate toxins.

7. **Turmeric**: This bright yellow spice is known for its powerful anti-inflammatory and antioxidant properties, largely due to its active compound, curcumin. Turmeric supports joint health, reduces inflammation, and strengthens the immune system. It also adds a distinct color and subtle flavor to the Fire Cider.

8. **Honey**: Raw honey is often added to Fire Cider after it has been strained to balance the acidity of the vinegar and add a touch of sweetness. Honey has natural antibacterial and antiviral properties and can soothe a sore throat. Additionally, it acts as a natural preservative, extending the shelf life of the tonic.

By combining these ingredients, Fire Cider provides a comprehensive blend of immune-supporting, anti-inflammatory, and digestive-enhancing benefits. Each ingredient plays a role in creating a balanced and potent tonic that can be taken as a daily preventative or used at the onset of illness.

Health Benefits of Fire Cider

Fire Cider offers a range of health benefits, making it a valuable addition to a natural health regimen. Some of the primary benefits include:

- **Immune System Support**: Fire Cider's ingredients work together to strengthen the immune system, helping the body defend itself against infections. The antimicrobial properties of garlic, ginger, and horseradish help fight off bacteria and viruses, while the antioxidants in onion and turmeric protect cells from oxidative stress.

- **Respiratory Health**: The warming and decongestant effects of horseradish, hot peppers, and garlic make Fire Cider an effective remedy for clearing mucus and relieving sinus congestion. It can be particularly helpful during cold and flu season when respiratory infections are common.

- **Digestive Aid**: The acetic acid in apple cider vinegar, combined with the digestive benefits of ginger, helps stimulate digestive enzymes and supports gut health. Fire Cider can improve digestion, reduce bloating, and promote the growth of beneficial gut bacteria.

- **Anti-Inflammatory Properties**: Ingredients like turmeric, ginger, and garlic have anti-inflammatory effects that can help reduce inflammation throughout the body. Regular consumption of Fire Cider may support joint health and alleviate symptoms of chronic inflammatory conditions.

- **Circulation and Detoxification**: The warming spices in Fire Cider stimulate circulation, which helps deliver nutrients and oxygen to cells and aids in the removal of waste products. This tonic can support the body's natural detoxification processes, helping to eliminate toxins and promote overall vitality.

How to Make Fire Cider at Home

Making Fire Cider at home is a simple process that allows individuals to tailor the recipe to their personal preferences. The following is a traditional recipe, but feel free to experiment by adding or adjusting ingredients to suit your taste.

Ingredients:
- 1-quart apple cider vinegar (preferably raw, unfiltered)
- 1/2 cup grated horseradish root
- 1/2 cup chopped onion
- 1/4 cup minced garlic
- 1/4 cup grated ginger root
- 1-2 hot peppers, sliced (adjust based on spice preference)
- 1/4 cup turmeric root, grated (or 1 tablespoon turmeric powder)
- Raw honey to taste (added after straining)

Instructions:
1. **Prepare the Ingredients**: Chop or grate all ingredients finely. The more surface area, the more potent the infusion will be.
2. **Combine and Cover**: Place all ingredients (except honey) in a clean, quart-sized glass jar. Pour apple cider vinegar over the ingredients until they are completely submerged. Cover the jar with a plastic lid or wax paper under a metal lid to prevent corrosion.
3. **Infuse**: Store the jar in a cool, dark place for 4-6 weeks. Shake the jar daily to help the ingredients infuse.
4. **Strain and Sweeten**: After 4-6 weeks, strain the mixture through a fine mesh strainer or cheesecloth into a clean jar. Add honey to taste, stirring well to combine.
5. **Store**: Store the finished Fire Cider in the refrigerator or a cool, dark place. It should last for several months, especially if kept refrigerated.

How to Use Fire Cider Tonic

Fire Cider is a versatile tonic that can be used in various ways depending on one's health goals and personal taste. The following are some common methods of incorporating Fire Cider into daily routines:

- **Daily Tonic**: Many people take 1-2 tablespoons of Fire Cider daily as a preventative measure. It can be taken on its own or diluted in a glass of water or juice.
- **At the Onset of Illness**: When feeling the first signs of a cold or sore throat, take a tablespoon of Fire Cider every few hours to boost immunity and reduce symptoms.
- **In Cooking**: Fire Cider's tangy flavor makes it a delicious addition to salad dressings, marinades, and sauces. Use it in place of vinegar in recipes to add both flavor and health benefits.
- **As a Shot**: For a quick and invigorating boost, take a small "shot" of Fire Cider first thing in the morning. The warming spices can help wake up the body and stimulate digestion.

Precautions and Considerations

While Fire Cider is generally safe for most people, it is highly acidic and should be consumed mindfully to avoid digestive discomfort. Some individuals

Peppermint, scientifically known as *Mentha piperita*, has been valued for centuries for its versatile healing properties. Known for its cooling and calming effects, peppermint is widely used in traditional and modern herbal medicine to address a range of ailments, from digestive issues to tension headaches and respiratory discomfort. One of the most effective ways to capture peppermint's medicinal benefits is through a tincture—a concentrated liquid extract that preserves the potency of peppermint and allows for easy use.

Peppermint tincture offers a fast-acting, portable remedy that can be used to relieve digestive discomfort, ease headaches, and provide respiratory relief. This section explores the various benefits of peppermint tincture, the science behind its soothing effects, a step-by-step guide to making it at home, and practical ways to incorporate it into daily routines to support wellness.

The Science Behind Peppermint's Healing Properties

Peppermint contains several active compounds, the most notable being menthol, menthone, and limonene, which contribute to its distinctive aroma and cooling sensation. Menthol, in particular, is responsible for the majority of peppermint's therapeutic effects, providing analgesic (pain-relieving), anti-inflammatory, and antispasmodic properties.

Menthol interacts with receptors in the skin and mucous membranes, producing a cooling effect that can help reduce pain and inflammation. It works by activating the body's cold-sensitive TRPM8 receptors, which are part of the sensory system that responds to temperature. This is why peppermint provides a soothing sensation on contact, making it effective for conditions that benefit from a cooling and calming action, such as muscle aches, skin irritation, and digestive cramps.

Additionally, peppermint has antimicrobial and antiviral properties, which make it useful for treating respiratory symptoms related to colds and flu. Its aromatic compounds can help clear nasal passages, relieve sinus congestion, and improve breathing, providing a natural option for respiratory support.

Benefits of Peppermint Soothing Tincture

Peppermint tincture is an effective remedy with numerous applications due to its diverse therapeutic benefits. Here are some of the primary benefits associated with peppermint tincture:

1. **Digestive Support**: Peppermint is well-known for its ability to relax the muscles in the gastrointestinal tract, making it useful for relieving symptoms of indigestion, bloating, and gas. Peppermint tincture can be taken after meals to ease discomfort and support healthy digestion.

2. **Headache Relief**: Peppermint's analgesic and cooling properties make it an effective natural remedy for headaches, particularly tension headaches. Applying a few drops of diluted peppermint tincture to the temples or massaging it into the scalp can provide relief from headache pain.

3. **Respiratory Relief**: Peppermint's menthol content helps to open up airways and relieve sinus congestion. Adding peppermint tincture to a steam inhalation can aid in clearing nasal passages and provide relief from respiratory discomfort.

4. **Muscle and Joint Relief**: Peppermint's anti-inflammatory and analgesic effects can help reduce muscle tension and soreness. Applying diluted peppermint tincture to sore muscles or joints can provide temporary pain relief.

5. **Energy and Mental Clarity**: Peppermint is also known for its invigorating properties, which can help improve focus and reduce mental fatigue. Inhaling the scent of peppermint tincture or taking a few drops internally can help enhance concentration and energy levels.

How to Make Peppermint Soothing Tincture at Home

Creating a peppermint tincture at home is a simple and cost-effective way to ensure you always have access to this powerful remedy. The following guide outlines the ingredients, equipment, and steps needed to make a high-quality peppermint tincture.

Ingredients:

- Fresh or dried peppermint leaves (approximately 1 cup for dried or 2 cups for fresh)
- High-proof alcohol, such as vodka (at least 80 proof; for a non-alcoholic option, use vegetable glycerin as a base)
- Clean glass jar with a tight-fitting lid
- Dark glass tincture bottles for storage

Instructions:

1. **Prepare the Peppermint Leaves**: If you're using fresh peppermint leaves, rinse them thoroughly and pat them dry. Lightly crush or chop the leaves to release their oils, as this will enhance the potency of the tincture. For dried leaves, simply place them in the jar.

2. **Fill the Jar with Alcohol**: Place the peppermint leaves in a clean glass jar, then pour the alcohol over the leaves, ensuring that they are fully submerged. Leave about an inch of space at the top of the jar to allow for any expansion.

3. **Seal and Shake**: Close the jar tightly and shake it well to mix the alcohol with the peppermint leaves. Store the jar in a cool, dark place for at least two weeks, shaking it once a day to help extract the beneficial compounds from the leaves. The tincture can be left to infuse for up to six weeks for a stronger extract.

4. **Strain the Tincture**: After the infusion period, strain the liquid through a fine-mesh strainer or cheesecloth into a clean bowl. Be sure to press down on the peppermint leaves to extract as much liquid as possible.

5. **Bottle the Tincture**: Transfer the liquid into dark glass tincture bottles to protect it from light, which can degrade the potency of the tincture over time. Label the bottles with the date and contents for reference.

6. **Storage**: Store the peppermint tincture in a cool, dark place. Properly stored, it can last up to one year.

Dosage and Usage of Peppermint Tincture

The recommended dosage of peppermint tincture varies depending on the intended use, but a general guideline is 10-15 drops in a glass of water, taken up to three times a day for digestive support. For headaches, 2-3 drops of tincture can be diluted with a carrier oil and massaged onto the temples. For respiratory relief, a few drops can be added to steam inhalation to help clear nasal passages.

It's important to note that peppermint tincture is highly concentrated, and it should always be diluted before internal or topical use. Pregnant women, breastfeeding mothers, and children under the age of six should avoid using peppermint tincture without consulting a healthcare provider.

Practical Applications and Tips for Using Peppermint Tincture

Peppermint tincture is highly versatile and can be used in various ways depending on individual needs. Here are some practical applications and tips for incorporating peppermint tincture into your daily routine:

- **For Digestive Comfort**: Add 10-15 drops of peppermint tincture to a glass of water and drink it after meals to relieve indigestion, bloating, or gas. The tincture helps to relax the muscles in the digestive tract, reducing spasms and discomfort. This can be particularly helpful after heavy or rich meals.
- **For Headache Relief**: Dilute 2-3 drops of peppermint tincture in a carrier oil, such as coconut or jojoba oil, and apply it to the temples or back of the neck for tension headache relief. The cooling effect of menthol provides a soothing sensation that can ease headache pain within minutes.
- **Steam Inhalation for Sinus Relief**: To relieve nasal congestion, add a few drops of peppermint tincture to a bowl of hot water, cover your head with a towel, and inhale the steam. This method can help clear nasal passages, reduce sinus pressure, and make breathing easier during colds or allergies.
- **Topical Application for Muscle Soreness**: For sore muscles or joints, dilute a few drops of peppermint tincture in a carrier oil and massage it into the affected area. The cooling sensation provides temporary pain relief, making it a great option after physical activity or for general muscle tension.
- **For Mental Clarity and Focus**: Inhaling peppermint tincture can help improve focus and concentration. Simply place a drop of tincture on a tissue and inhale deeply or add a few drops to a diffuser. This can be particularly useful during long study sessions, work hours, or when mental fatigue sets in.

Safety Considerations and Storage Tips

While peppermint tincture is generally safe, there are a few precautions to keep in mind. The tincture is highly concentrated, and it should be diluted before applying to the skin to avoid irritation. People with sensitive skin should perform a patch test before using it more widely, as peppermint can cause tingling or irritation in some individuals.

For internal use, it's important to avoid excessive consumption, as too much peppermint can cause side effects like heartburn or gastrointestinal discomfort. Sticking to recommended dosages and consulting with a healthcare provider if unsure can help ensure safe usage.

Peppermint tincture should be stored in a dark glass bottle in a cool, dark place to maintain its potency. Properly stored, it has a shelf life of about a year. Keeping tinctures away from direct sunlight and heat helps prevent degradation of the active compounds, ensuring that the tincture remains effective.

Incorporating Peppermint Tincture into a Holistic Wellness Routine

Peppermint tincture is a valuable addition to a holistic wellness routine, offering a natural, versatile remedy that can be used for a variety of health needs. As part of a self-care routine, it can be used in combination with other natural remedies, like chamomile for calming the digestive system or lavender for additional relaxation.

For those new to natural remedies, starting with peppermint tincture provides an accessible introduction to herbal wellness. It can be easily integrated into daily life, whether for occasional digestive relief, headache management, or mental refreshment. By keeping a small bottle of peppermint tincture on hand, individuals can enjoy its benefits at home, work, or even while traveling.

Creating a soothing peppermint tincture at home not only empowers individuals to take charge of their health but also fosters a deeper connection to the natural world. With regular use, peppermint tincture can become a trusted remedy in times of discomfort, providing a gentle yet effective way to support physical and mental well-being.

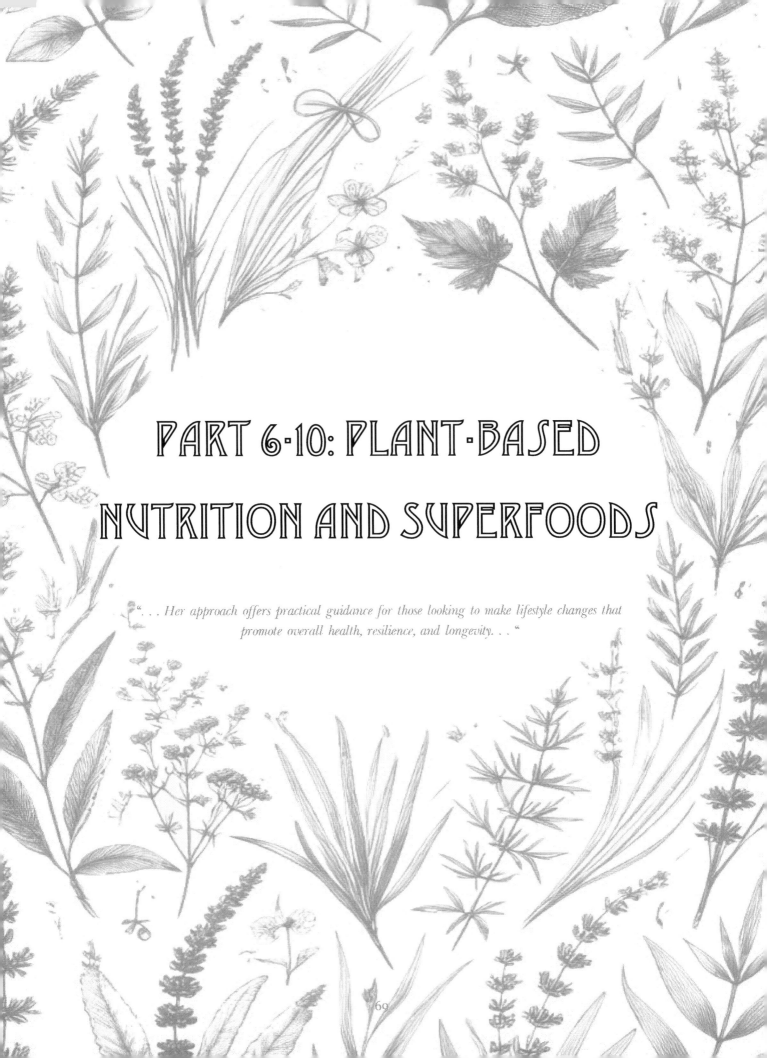

PART 6-10: PLANT-BASED NUTRITION AND SUPERFOODS

". . . Her approach offers practical guidance for those looking to make lifestyle changes that promote overall health, resilience, and longevity. . . "

Chapter 1: Plant-Based Eating Essentials

Barbara O'Neill's nutritional approach is grounded in the philosophy that food is one of the most powerful tools for achieving health and wellness. Through years of research, clinical practice, and public education, O'Neill has developed a comprehensive approach to nutrition that emphasizes whole, unprocessed foods, balanced meals, and strategic supplementation to support the body's natural healing mechanisms. Her philosophy goes beyond simply eating for survival; it focuses on choosing foods that nourish, restore, and empower the body's innate abilities to resist disease, maintain energy, and sustain mental clarity.

Barbara O'Neill's Nutritional Approach

O'Neill's nutritional recommendations are built upon a few foundational principles: the importance of nutrient density, the power of plant-based foods, the avoidance of processed and refined items, and the inclusion of foods that support gut health and the immune system. Her approach offers practical guidance for those looking to make lifestyle changes that promote overall health, resilience, and longevity.

The Foundation: Nutrient-Dense Whole Foods

A key element in O'Neill's nutritional philosophy is the emphasis on nutrient-dense foods. Nutrient density refers to the concentration of essential vitamins, minerals, and antioxidants per calorie. Foods with high nutrient density include vegetables, fruits, whole grains, nuts, and seeds, as well as lean proteins. By focusing on nutrient-dense foods, individuals can obtain the nutrients they need without consuming excessive calories, which is beneficial for maintaining a healthy weight and avoiding chronic conditions associated with obesity and poor diet.

For O'Neill, nutrient-dense foods are the basis of a healthy diet because they provide the essential building blocks for cellular function, energy production, immune response, and mental clarity. Vegetables, particularly leafy greens, are among her top recommendations, as they are rich in vitamins like A, C, K, and folate, and contain fiber that supports digestive health. Fruits, especially berries, provide antioxidants that protect cells from oxidative stress, a condition that contributes to aging and chronic diseases.

Whole grains, like quinoa, brown rice, and oats, are another staple in O'Neill's approach. These grains offer a complex source of carbohydrates that help stabilize blood sugar levels, providing sustained energy without causing the spikes and crashes associated with refined grains. Additionally, whole grains are high in fiber, which supports gut health, aids in satiety, and reduces the risk of conditions like diabetes and heart disease.

The Role of Plant-Based Foods and Phytochemicals

Barbara O'Neill strongly advocates for the inclusion of plant-based foods, which are rich in phytochemicals—natural compounds that provide health benefits beyond basic nutrition. Phytochemicals include flavonoids, carotenoids, and polyphenols, all of which have been shown to have antioxidant, anti-inflammatory, and immune-boosting properties. These compounds, found abundantly in fruits, vegetables, herbs, and spices, support the body's defenses against a range of diseases, including cancer, heart disease, and neurodegenerative disorders.

For example, O'Neill often recommends cruciferous vegetables like broccoli, cauliflower, and Brussels sprouts for their high levels of sulforaphane, a phytochemical with potent anti-cancer effects. Sulforaphane has been shown to stimulate enzymes that detoxify the body and reduce inflammation, making these vegetables a valuable component of a disease-preventive diet. Similarly, foods like garlic and onions contain allicin, a compound with antimicrobial properties that helps protect the body from infections.

O'Neill also promotes the use of fresh herbs and spices, such as turmeric, ginger, and rosemary, for their high antioxidant content. Turmeric, which contains curcumin, is particularly beneficial for reducing inflammation and supporting liver health. Adding these herbs and spices to daily meals enhances flavor while providing medicinal benefits that align with her philosophy of food as medicine.

Avoiding Processed Foods and Refined Sugars

A cornerstone of O'Neill's nutritional approach is the avoidance of processed foods and refined sugars. These foods are often stripped of nutrients and contain additives, preservatives, and artificial ingredients that can disrupt the body's natural processes. Refined sugars, in particular, are known to spike blood sugar levels, leading to insulin resistance over time. Chronic high blood sugar levels can contribute to a range of metabolic disorders, including diabetes, obesity, and heart disease.

O'Neill encourages individuals to eliminate refined sugars and instead choose natural sweeteners, such as raw honey or maple syrup, in moderation. These alternatives provide sweetness while also offering small amounts of vitamins and minerals, making them a healthier option than processed sugar. Additionally, avoiding refined sugar helps maintain stable energy levels, reduce cravings, and prevent the overgrowth of harmful bacteria and yeast in the gut, which can lead to digestive issues and weakened immunity.

Processed foods often contain unhealthy fats, such as trans fats and high levels of omega-6 fatty acids, which contribute to inflammation. O'Neill advocates for using healthy fats from sources like avocados, nuts, seeds, and cold-pressed olive oil. These fats support heart health, provide essential fatty acids, and help the body absorb fat-soluble vitamins like A, D, E, and K.

Supporting Gut Health and the Microbiome

Gut health is a central focus in Barbara O'Neill's nutritional approach, as a healthy digestive system is essential for nutrient absorption, immune function, and overall wellness. The gut microbiome, a community of trillions of microorganisms in the intestines, plays a crucial role in breaking down food, producing certain vitamins, and protecting against pathogens. An imbalanced microbiome, often caused by a diet high in processed foods and low in fiber, can lead to inflammation, poor digestion, and a weakened immune system.

O'Neill emphasizes the importance of consuming probiotic and prebiotic-rich foods to support a balanced microbiome. Probiotics, found in fermented foods like yogurt, kefir, sauerkraut, and kimchi, introduce beneficial bacteria to the gut, which can improve digestion and boost immune health. Prebiotics, found in foods like onions, garlic, bananas, and asparagus, feed these beneficial bacteria, helping them thrive and maintain a healthy balance.

For those who experience digestive discomfort or have had antibiotic treatments, which can disrupt the microbiome, O'Neill recommends gradually introducing fermented foods to rebuild gut health. She also advises limiting or avoiding foods that can irritate the gut lining, such as highly processed foods, excessive caffeine, and alcohol, which can contribute to inflammation and weaken the gut barrier.

The Importance of Hydration and Detoxification

Barbara O'Neill places significant emphasis on hydration as part of her nutritional approach. Proper hydration is essential for every bodily function, from digestion and detoxification to energy production and cognitive function. Water helps flush out toxins, lubricates joints, and supports cellular function. O'Neill recommends drinking filtered water throughout the day and avoiding sugary or artificially flavored beverages, which can dehydrate the body and introduce unnecessary additives.

In addition to water, O'Neill encourages the use of herbal teas as a way to support detoxification. Herbs like dandelion root, ginger, and nettle are known for their detoxifying effects and can aid in liver health and digestion. Drinking herbal teas not only provides hydration but also offers a gentle way to support the body's natural detoxification processes, which are essential for maintaining a clean, functioning system.

Balanced Meal Structure and Portion Awareness

Another aspect of Barbara O'Neill's approach is the emphasis on balanced meals and portion control. O'Neill recommends structuring meals to include a variety of macronutrients—proteins, healthy fats, and complex carbohydrates—to ensure steady energy and prevent blood sugar spikes. This balance supports sustained energy levels, mental focus, and satiety, helping individuals avoid the cycle of cravings and overeating.

Proteins are essential for building and repairing tissues, producing enzymes, and supporting immune health. O'Neill suggests including lean sources of protein, such as legumes, fish, and organic poultry, in meals. For individuals following a plant-based diet, she emphasizes the importance of combining different plant proteins, such as beans and rice, to obtain all essential amino acids.

Carbohydrates, particularly from whole grains and vegetables, are the body's primary source of energy. O'Neill encourages choosing complex carbohydrates over refined ones, as complex carbs break down slowly, providing a steady release of glucose into the bloodstream. This is especially important for maintaining focus and avoiding energy crashes throughout the day.

Strategic Supplementation

While Barbara O'Neill advocates for obtaining most nutrients from whole foods, she recognizes that some individuals may benefit from targeted supplementation. Factors such as age, lifestyle, and specific health conditions can create unique nutritional needs that are difficult to meet through diet alone. For example, vitamin D is often recommended for individuals with limited sun exposure, as it plays a critical role in immune health and bone strength.

O'Neill's approach to supplementation is highly individualized. She recommends consulting with a healthcare professional to determine specific deficiencies or needs. Common supplements in her approach include probiotics for gut health, omega-3 fatty acids for heart and brain health, magnesium for muscle and nerve function, and B vitamins for energy and stress support.

When selecting supplements, O'Neill advises choosing high-quality products from reputable brands and focusing on forms that are bioavailable, meaning they are easily absorbed by the body. For instance, magnesium glycinate is often preferred over other forms for its higher absorption rate and lower likelihood of causing digestive upset.

Practical Strategies for Incorporating Barbara O'Neill's Nutritional Approach

Implementing O'Neill's nutritional principles in daily life can begin with small, manageable changes that build healthier habits over time. She suggests starting by gradually increasing the intake of fresh fruits and vegetables, aiming for a variety of colors to ensure a broad spectrum of nutrients.

For those who are new to reducing processed foods, replacing one processed item with a whole-food alternative each week can make the transition less overwhelming. For example, swapping sugary breakfast cereals with a homemade oatmeal topped with berries and nuts introduces nutrient density and reduces added sugars.

Preparing meals at home is another effective strategy. Cooking at home allows individuals to control ingredients, avoid additives, and experiment with fresh herbs and spices. Meal planning and batch cooking on weekends can help make whole-food meals more accessible during busy weekdays.

Barbara O'Neill's nutritional approach isn't just about dietary changes; it's a lifestyle shift that emphasizes mindfulness, awareness, and intentional choices. Through balanced meals, hydration, the inclusion of nutrient-dense foods, and the avoidance of processed items, individuals can create a solid foundation for long-term health and vitality.

Macronutrients in a Plant-Based Diet

In a plant-based diet, macronutrients—carbohydrates, proteins, and fats—are essential for energy, growth, and maintaining overall health. While plant-based eating provides abundant vitamins, minerals, and antioxidants, understanding how to balance these macronutrients is key to achieving optimal nutrition. Each macronutrient plays a unique role in supporting bodily functions, and when combined in the right proportions, they contribute to a balanced and fulfilling diet that promotes long-term wellness.

Adopting a plant-based diet means paying attention to the quality and variety of these macronutrients. Plant-based foods, such as grains, legumes, nuts, seeds, fruits, and vegetables, offer all three macronutrients, though each varies in its content. The goal of a well-planned plant-based diet is to ensure that these macronutrients are included in adequate amounts and from diverse sources to meet the body's needs for energy, muscle repair, brain function, and hormone balance.

Carbohydrates: The Body's Primary Energy Source

Carbohydrates are the primary source of energy for the body, providing the fuel needed for daily activities, brain function, and cellular processes. In a plant-based diet, carbohydrates are mainly derived from whole grains, fruits, vegetables, and legumes. Unlike simple carbohydrates, such as refined sugars that cause rapid spikes in blood glucose, complex carbohydrates provide sustained energy, fiber, and essential nutrients.

Carbohydrates in plant-based diets also support gut health due to their fiber content. Fiber is a type of carbohydrate that the body cannot fully digest, allowing it to move through the digestive system and support a healthy microbiome. Fiber aids in digestion, prevents constipation, regulates blood sugar levels, and lowers cholesterol. Plant-based diets are naturally high in fiber, which is beneficial for overall health and longevity.

Sources of Carbohydrates in a Plant-Based Diet:

- **Whole Grains**: Brown rice, quinoa, oats, barley, and farro are rich in complex carbohydrates, fiber, and B vitamins. Whole grains release energy slowly, providing steady fuel throughout the day.
- **Fruits and Vegetables**: Apples, berries, carrots, and sweet potatoes offer both carbohydrates and a wealth of vitamins, minerals, and antioxidants. They also contain water and fiber, which help maintain hydration and satiety.

- **Legumes**: Beans, lentils, chickpeas, and peas provide not only carbohydrates but also protein and fiber, making them highly nutritious additions to a plant-based diet.

The fiber in these foods slows down digestion, preventing rapid spikes in blood sugar and helping to regulate hunger. For individuals with energy-intensive lifestyles, including whole grains and legumes can ensure that carbohydrate intake supports endurance, strength, and mental clarity.

Protein: Essential for Growth, Repair, and Immune Function

Proteins are vital macronutrients that serve as the building blocks for muscle tissue, enzymes, hormones, and antibodies. They are composed of amino acids, which the body needs to repair tissues, produce enzymes, and support immune health. There are 20 amino acids, nine of which are essential, meaning they must be obtained through diet because the body cannot synthesize them on its own.

Contrary to common misconceptions, plant-based diets can provide adequate protein when diverse protein sources are included. While animal proteins are considered "complete" because they contain all nine essential amino acids, many plant proteins are incomplete. However, by combining different protein sources, such as grains and legumes, individuals can consume all essential amino acids over the course of a day.

Sources of Protein in a Plant-Based Diet:

- **Legumes**: Black beans, lentils, chickpeas, and soybeans are excellent sources of protein. Soy-based foods like tofu, tempeh, and edamame provide all essential amino acids, making them complete protein sources.
- **Nuts and Seeds**: Almonds, chia seeds, hemp seeds, and pumpkin seeds contribute protein, healthy fats, and minerals. Hemp seeds are particularly beneficial because they contain all essential amino acids.
- **Whole Grains**: While not as protein-dense as legumes or nuts, whole grains like quinoa, farro, and bulgur contain protein and complement other protein sources to provide a complete amino acid profile.

The body's protein needs vary based on factors such as age, activity level, and health goals. Active individuals and those aiming to build muscle may require higher protein intake, which can be met through thoughtful combinations of plant-based sources. For example, pairing rice with beans or hummus with whole-grain pita provides a balanced amino acid profile and ensures a sufficient intake of essential proteins.

Fats: Supporting Brain Function, Hormone Production, and Cell Health

Fats are an essential macronutrient in a plant-based diet, providing energy, supporting brain function, aiding in hormone production, and helping absorb fat-soluble vitamins (A, D, E, and K). Healthy fats are vital for cellular health, as they form the structure of cell membranes and protect organs.

In plant-based diets, fats come from sources like nuts, seeds, avocados, olives, and plant oils. These sources provide unsaturated fats, which are beneficial for heart health. Omega-3 and omega-6 fatty acids, essential polyunsaturated fats, play significant roles in reducing inflammation, supporting cognitive function, and promoting cardiovascular health. Because the body cannot produce these essential fatty acids, they must be consumed through food.

Sources of Fats in a Plant-Based Diet:

- **Nuts and Seeds**: Walnuts, flaxseeds, chia seeds, and hemp seeds are rich in omega-3 fatty acids, which support brain and heart health. Chia and flaxseeds also provide fiber, enhancing their nutritional value.
- **Avocado**: Avocado is a source of monounsaturated fats, which are heart-healthy and anti-inflammatory. It also contains potassium and fiber, making it a highly nutritious choice.
- **Olive Oil**: Extra virgin olive oil is rich in monounsaturated fats and antioxidants. It is commonly used in Mediterranean diets and is known to support heart health.

Incorporating healthy fats in a plant-based diet helps maintain energy levels, improves cognitive function, and supports hormonal balance. Balancing fats with protein and carbohydrates ensures a well-rounded, satisfying meal.

Balancing Macronutrients for Optimal Health

The key to a balanced plant-based diet lies in combining macronutrients in appropriate proportions. While individual needs vary, a common macronutrient breakdown includes approximately 45-65% carbohydrates, 10-35% protein, and 20-35% fats. This balance can support energy levels, muscle maintenance, and overall health.

For example, a typical day might include:

- **Breakfast**: Oatmeal with chia seeds, topped with fresh berries and a handful of nuts, provides a blend of carbohydrates, protein, and fats.
- **Lunch**: A quinoa and black bean salad with mixed greens, avocado, and a drizzle of olive oil balances all three macronutrients.
- **Dinner**: Stir-fried vegetables with tofu and brown rice, cooked in a small amount of sesame oil, completes the day with a nutrient-dense meal.

Ensuring that each meal includes a combination of carbohydrates, protein, and fats helps prevent blood sugar spikes, supports sustained energy, and promotes satiety. By diversifying food choices, individuals can meet their nutritional needs without relying on animal products.

Common Challenges and Solutions for Macronutrient Balance

Transitioning to a plant-based diet may present some challenges, particularly when it comes to meeting protein needs or balancing omega-3 and omega-6 fatty acids. However, these challenges can be managed with mindful planning and food choices.

1. **Protein Intake**: Those new to plant-based eating may worry about getting enough protein. By including a variety of protein sources, such as beans, lentils, nuts, seeds, and whole grains, individuals can meet their protein needs. Incorporating high-protein plant foods like tofu, tempeh, and edamame can also boost protein intake.
2. **Omega-3 Fatty Acids**: Omega-3s are essential for health, but they are less abundant in plant foods compared to omega-6s. Including flaxseeds, chia seeds, walnuts, and algae-based supplements can help maintain a healthy omega-3 to omega-6 ratio.
3. **Sufficient Caloric Intake**: Plant-based diets are often high in fiber, which can make meals feel more filling with fewer calories. For those needing to maintain or gain weight, including calorie-dense foods like nuts, seeds, avocados, and whole grains can help meet energy needs without compromising nutrient quality.

With proper planning, individuals can successfully balance macronutrients and ensure that their plant-based diet supports their health and lifestyle goals.

Macronutrient Timing for Energy and Recovery

For those with active lifestyles or specific fitness goals, timing macronutrient intake can further enhance the benefits of a plant-based diet. Consuming carbohydrates before exercise provides readily available energy, while protein intake after exercise supports muscle recovery and growth.

1. **Pre-Workout Nutrition**: A combination of complex carbohydrates and a small amount of protein can fuel a workout. Options like a banana with almond butter or a smoothie with oats and protein powder provide energy for sustained performance.

2. **Post-Workout Nutrition**: After physical activity, consuming protein along with some carbohydrates helps replenish glycogen stores and supports muscle repair. A post-workout meal might include a smoothie with plant-based protein powder, berries, and a handful of spinach.

3. **Daily Snacking for Steady Energy**: Balanced snacks throughout the day, such as apple slices with peanut butter or hummus with carrot sticks, maintain energy levels and prevent hunger between meals.

By aligning macronutrient intake with activity levels, individuals can optimize their energy, improve recovery, and support fitness goals on a plant-based diet.

The Benefits of Macronutrient Diversity in Plant-Based Eating

A diverse diet that includes a variety of macronutrient sources is essential for both nutritional completeness and enjoyment. Eating a wide range of foods not only ensures that all nutrient needs are met but also supports a healthy microbiome, enhances digestion, and provides a satisfying culinary experience.

For instance, varying sources of protein, such as lentils, chickpeas, quinoa, and hemp seeds, introduces different amino acids and micronutrients. Including a mix of healthy fats from sources like avocados, olive oil, and nuts supplies the body with essential fatty acids while adding flavor to meals. Whole grains and starchy vegetables offer complex carbohydrates that fuel the body and contribute to satiety.

By embracing the diversity of plant-based foods, individuals can enjoy balanced and delicious meals that fulfill their macronutrient needs. This approach fosters a sustainable and satisfying way of eating that supports both health and well-being.

Protein Sources in Plants

As more individuals turn to plant-based diets for health, environmental, or ethical reasons, understanding plant-based protein sources has become increasingly important. Protein, a macronutrient essential for building and repairing tissues, producing enzymes and hormones, and supporting immune function, can be obtained from a wide range of plants. While traditionally associated with animal products, protein is abundant in legumes, grains, seeds, nuts, and vegetables, making a well-planned plant-based diet highly nutritious and sufficient in protein content.

This section explores the diverse sources of plant protein, the amino acid profiles of different plant foods, and how to incorporate these sources into a balanced diet. For those concerned about meeting their protein needs without animal products, this guide offers practical strategies and insights into harnessing the full potential of plant proteins.

Understanding Protein and Amino Acids

Proteins are made up of amino acids, which are often referred to as the building blocks of life. There are 20 amino acids, nine of which are considered essential because the body cannot produce them; they must be obtained through diet. Complete proteins contain all nine essential amino acids, and traditionally, animal products have been viewed as complete protein sources. However, various plant foods also contain complete proteins or can be combined to provide a complete amino acid profile.

For example, quinoa and soy are plant-based sources that offer all essential amino acids, making them complete proteins. Other plants, like beans and rice, may lack one or more essential amino acids individually, but when combined, they create a complete protein. This concept of protein complementation—pairing different plant foods to achieve a complete amino acid profile—is fundamental to a balanced plant-based diet.

Plant-based protein sources provide not only protein but also a variety of vitamins, minerals, fiber, and antioxidants that are beneficial for overall health. They are typically low in saturated fats and free of cholesterol, which is advantageous for heart health. Understanding the specific properties of plant-based proteins allows individuals to build balanced, nutrient-dense meals that support muscle function, energy production, and immune health.

Legumes: Powerhouses of Plant Protein

Legumes are among the richest sources of plant-based protein, and they offer additional nutrients like fiber, iron, potassium, and magnesium. Common legumes include lentils, chickpeas, black beans, kidney beans, and peas. Lentils, for instance, contain about 18 grams of protein per cooked cup and are an excellent source of folate and iron, both essential nutrients for energy and immune function.

Beans are versatile and can be used in a variety of dishes. Black beans, with 15 grams of protein per cooked cup, are particularly popular in Latin American cuisine and can be included in salads, stews, and burritos. Chickpeas, or garbanzo beans, contain around 14 grams of protein per cup and are rich in fiber and manganese, supporting digestion and bone health.

Edamame, young soybeans, are another high-protein legume option, with approximately 17 grams of protein per cup. Soybeans are one of the few plant-based sources that offer a complete amino acid profile, making them an ideal protein choice for vegetarians and vegans. Tofu and tempeh, both made from soybeans, are protein-rich and highly adaptable, allowing them to be used in various cuisines as a meat substitute.

Grains: An Overlooked Source of Protein

While grains are often considered a source of carbohydrates, certain grains provide a significant amount of protein as well. Quinoa, a pseudo-grain, contains about 8 grams of complete protein per cooked cup, offering all essential amino acids. It is also rich in fiber, magnesium, and manganese, making it an excellent choice for those on a plant-based diet. Quinoa can be used as a base for salads, added to soups, or served as a side dish.

Other grains, such as farro, amaranth, and barley, also offer considerable protein. Amaranth, like quinoa, is a complete protein and provides around 9 grams of protein per cooked cup. This ancient grain is also high in iron and calcium, supporting bone health and energy production. Barley, while not a complete protein, offers about 3.5 grams of protein per half-cup cooked and is particularly high in fiber, aiding digestion and promoting a feeling of fullness.

Oats are another grain that contributes protein, with approximately 6 grams per cup of cooked oats. Oats are particularly popular for breakfast and can be combined with nuts and seeds to increase protein content. For example, a bowl of oatmeal topped with chia seeds, almond butter, and berries provides a protein-packed, nutrient-dense breakfast.

Nuts and Seeds: Protein and Healthy Fats

Nuts and seeds are not only excellent sources of protein but also provide healthy fats, fiber, and essential vitamins and minerals. Almonds, for example, contain about 6 grams of protein per ounce and are high in vitamin E, an antioxidant that supports skin and immune health. Walnuts, while slightly lower in protein, are rich in omega-3 fatty acids, which are beneficial for heart and brain health.

Chia seeds and flaxseeds are notable for their protein content and high levels of omega-3 fatty acids and fiber. Chia seeds contain about 5 grams of protein per ounce, and their ability to absorb liquid makes them ideal for chia pudding, a popular breakfast or snack option. Flaxseeds, with about 1.5 grams of protein per tablespoon, can be ground and added to smoothies, oatmeal, or baked goods to boost protein and fiber intake.

Pumpkin seeds, also known as pepitas, are another protein-rich option, providing around 9 grams of protein per ounce. They are high in magnesium, which is essential for muscle function and energy production. Pumpkin seeds can be added to salads, granola, or eaten as a snack, offering both protein and a satisfying crunch.

Vegetables: Protein from Unexpected Sources

Certain vegetables also contribute a surprising amount of protein, making them valuable additions to a plant-based diet. For example, broccoli contains about 4 grams of protein per cup and is high in fiber, vitamin C, and vitamin K. Spinach offers approximately 5 grams of protein per cooked cup and provides iron, calcium, and folate, which are essential for energy production and bone health.

Brussels sprouts, asparagus, and artichokes are additional vegetables that contain protein, along with a variety of vitamins, minerals, and antioxidants. While vegetables alone may not provide sufficient protein for those with higher protein needs, they complement other protein sources and contribute to a balanced diet. Including a variety of protein-containing vegetables enhances nutrient diversity and ensures adequate intake of essential micronutrients.

Protein Complementation: Building Complete Proteins

While some plant-based foods, like quinoa and soy, are complete proteins, most plant proteins are incomplete, meaning they lack one or more essential amino acids. However, by combining different plant-based foods, individuals can achieve a complete amino acid profile. This is known as protein complementation, and it is easily achieved by consuming a variety of protein sources throughout the day.

For example, beans and rice are often paired together because they complement each other's amino acid profiles, forming a complete protein when eaten together. Similarly, combining lentils with whole grains, such as brown rice or whole wheat, provides all essential amino acids. It's not necessary to consume these combinations in the same meal; eating a variety of protein sources throughout the day will ensure that the body receives all necessary amino acids.

Another effective combination is pairing nuts or seeds with grains. For instance, a peanut butter sandwich on whole-grain bread provides a complete protein profile. Similarly, hummus, made from chickpeas and tahini (sesame seeds), is another example of a complete protein source in plant-based diets. These combinations not only provide complete proteins but also offer diverse flavors and textures, making meals more enjoyable and satisfying.

Practical Strategies for Incorporating Plant-Based Proteins

Incorporating a variety of plant-based proteins into daily meals can be simple and enjoyable. For those new to plant-based diets, starting with familiar ingredients like beans, lentils, and nuts can make the transition smoother. Here are a few practical strategies for adding more plant-based protein to meals:

- **Meal Preparation**: Preparing a batch of beans, quinoa, or lentils at the beginning of the week provides a base for quick meals. These ingredients can be added to salads, soups, or stir-fries, making it easier to include protein in every meal.

- **Smoothies with Seeds and Nut Butter**: Adding chia seeds, flaxseeds, or a tablespoon of almond or peanut butter to smoothies can increase protein content while also providing healthy fats. Smoothies are a versatile option for breakfast or snacks and can be customized with various fruits, greens, and protein sources.

- **Mixing Grains and Legumes**: Combining grains like brown rice or quinoa with lentils or chickpeas in a dish provides a balanced meal with a complete protein. This combination is ideal for hearty salads, stews, and casseroles.

- **Snacks with Nuts and Seeds**: Keeping nuts, seeds, or nut-based snacks on hand can help increase protein intake throughout the day. Almonds, pumpkin seeds, and trail mix are convenient options for boosting protein and energy.

Benefits Beyond Protein: Additional Nutrients in Plant Protein Sources

Plant-based protein sources offer a range of additional nutrients that contribute to overall health. For instance, legumes are high in fiber, which supports digestive health and helps regulate blood sugar levels. Fiber-rich foods also promote satiety, making them beneficial for weight management.

Nuts and seeds are not only protein-rich but also provide healthy fats, particularly omega-3 and omega-6 fatty acids, which support heart and brain health. The minerals found in nuts and seeds, such as magnesium, zinc, and calcium, are essential for bone health, immune function, and energy production.

Plant-based protein sources also contain antioxidants, which protect cells from oxidative damage and reduce inflammation. For example, lentils and chickpeas are high in polyphenols, compounds that have antioxidant effects and may lower the risk of chronic diseases.

Overcoming Common Concerns About Plant-Based Proteins

Some individuals worry that plant-based diets may lack sufficient protein or require complicated food combinations to meet protein needs. However, with a balanced and varied diet, it's entirely possible to meet protein requirements with plant-based foods. Including a mix of legumes, grains, nuts, seeds, and vegetables throughout the day ensures that all essential amino acids are obtained, supporting muscle health, energy levels, and overall wellness.

Fiber-Rich Foods

Fiber is a crucial component of a balanced diet, especially within a plant-based lifestyle. This nutrient, often overlooked, plays an essential role in digestive health, blood sugar control, and heart health. Found primarily in plant foods, fiber contributes to overall wellness by supporting the gut microbiome, aiding in the absorption of nutrients, and promoting a feeling of fullness. In a diet centered on natural and herbal remedies, incorporating fiber-rich foods becomes foundational, not only for physical health but also for sustained energy, mental clarity, and metabolic stability.

Fiber-rich foods are available in various forms, each offering unique health benefits. Consuming a range of these foods ensures the body receives both soluble and insoluble fiber, which work together to maintain digestive health and regulate other bodily functions.

Soluble fiber dissolves in water, forming a gel-like substance that can lower blood cholesterol and control blood sugar. Insoluble fiber, on the other hand, adds bulk to the stool, promoting regular bowel movements and preventing constipation. Together, these fibers support a healthy body and mind, which is why they are indispensable in any plant-based, holistic diet.

Understanding the Health Benefits of Fiber

Fiber contributes to multiple aspects of health, from digestion to immunity. This nutrient is unique because it passes through the digestive system mostly intact, meaning it doesn't get broken down or absorbed like other nutrients. Instead, fiber acts like a broom, sweeping through the digestive tract, feeding beneficial bacteria, and aiding in the removal of toxins and waste.

One of fiber's primary roles is to promote **gut health**. A diet high in fiber supports a diverse gut microbiome, which is crucial for immunity, mood regulation, and overall well-being. The gut is home to trillions of microorganisms that play a role in breaking down food, producing vitamins, and protecting against pathogens. Fiber serves as a prebiotic, feeding these beneficial bacteria and allowing them to thrive. In turn, these bacteria produce short-chain fatty acids (SCFAs) like butyrate, which help reduce inflammation in the gut lining, protect against digestive diseases, and support immune function.

Fiber is also instrumental in **blood sugar regulation**. Soluble fiber, found in foods like oats, beans, and apples, slows down the absorption of sugar, helping to prevent spikes in blood glucose. This can be particularly beneficial for individuals with diabetes or insulin resistance, as fiber helps maintain steady blood sugar levels and reduces the need for insulin. In addition, high-fiber foods tend to have a lower glycemic index, meaning they cause a slower and smaller rise in blood sugar compared to refined carbohydrates.

Furthermore, fiber plays a crucial role in **cardiovascular health**. Soluble fiber binds to cholesterol particles and removes them from the body, which can help lower overall cholesterol levels and reduce the risk of heart disease. Studies have shown that individuals who consume a diet rich in fiber have a lower risk of developing cardiovascular conditions, as fiber helps keep arteries clear and supports healthy blood pressure levels.

Types of Fiber and Their Functions

Fiber comes in two main types—soluble and insoluble—each offering different health benefits. A balanced diet should include both types of fiber, as they support the digestive system and overall health in complementary ways.

1. **Soluble Fiber**: This type of fiber dissolves in water and forms a gel-like consistency in the digestive tract. Soluble fiber is known for its ability to lower blood cholesterol and regulate blood sugar levels. Common sources include oats, apples, carrots, and beans. When consumed, soluble fiber slows down digestion, which allows for better nutrient absorption and contributes to a feeling of fullness.

2. **Insoluble Fiber**: Unlike soluble fiber, insoluble fiber does not dissolve in water. It adds bulk to the stool, which helps food pass more quickly through the stomach and intestines. This type of fiber is crucial for maintaining regular bowel movements and preventing constipation. Sources of insoluble fiber include whole grains, nuts, and vegetables like cauliflower and potatoes.

A well-rounded plant-based diet includes a balance of both soluble and insoluble fibers, ensuring optimal gut health, blood sugar stability, and digestive regularity.

Top Fiber-Rich Foods to Include in a Plant-Based Diet

Incorporating fiber-rich foods into a daily routine can be both easy and delicious. Here are some of the top plant-based foods that provide significant amounts of fiber, along with additional health benefits:

- **Lentils**: Lentils are incredibly versatile and rich in both protein and fiber, with about 15 grams of fiber per cup. They contain soluble fiber that aids in heart health and blood sugar regulation, making them an excellent choice for soups, stews, and salads.

- **Chia Seeds**: Known for their high fiber content, chia seeds offer around 10 grams of fiber per ounce. They absorb water and form a gel-like substance, making them ideal for puddings, smoothies, and as an egg replacement in baking. Chia seeds are also rich in omega-3 fatty acids, supporting heart and brain health.

- **Avocado**: Avocados are unique among fruits as they contain both soluble and insoluble fiber, with about 10 grams per medium avocado. They also provide healthy monounsaturated fats, which are beneficial for heart health. Avocados can be added to salads, smoothies, or eaten on their own.

- **Broccoli**: This cruciferous vegetable provides about 5 grams of fiber per cup and contains both soluble and insoluble fiber. Broccoli is also high in antioxidants, vitamins C and K, and has anti-inflammatory properties, making it a powerful addition to a fiber-rich diet.

- **Apples**: Apples offer around 4 grams of fiber per medium fruit, primarily in the form of soluble fiber called pectin. Pectin supports gut health and may lower cholesterol levels. Eating apples with the skin on maximizes fiber content and offers a range of vitamins and antioxidants.

- **Quinoa**: As a whole grain, quinoa provides approximately 5 grams of fiber per cup when cooked. It is a complete protein, containing all nine essential amino acids, and is a fantastic option for those looking to increase their fiber and protein intake simultaneously.

- **Almonds**: Almonds contain around 3.5 grams of fiber per ounce and provide healthy fats, protein, and magnesium. They make for a nutritious snack and can be added to salads, oatmeal, or yogurt.

- **Sweet Potatoes**: Sweet potatoes are rich in fiber, especially when eaten with the skin on, providing about 4 grams per medium potato. They are also high in beta-carotene, which the body converts to vitamin A, supporting eye health and immune function.

Including these fiber-rich foods in a plant-based diet can support digestion, boost heart health, and provide a steady source of energy throughout the day.

Practical Ways to Increase Fiber Intake

For those looking to increase their fiber intake, practical strategies can make the transition smooth and enjoyable. A gradual approach helps the body adjust, as a sudden increase in fiber can lead to digestive discomfort.

1. **Start with Breakfast**: Begin the day with a fiber-rich breakfast, such as oatmeal topped with berries and chia seeds. Adding fruits, nuts, and seeds to breakfast meals provides both fiber and a range of essential nutrients.

2. **Include Vegetables in Every Meal**: Adding leafy greens, carrots, bell peppers, and broccoli to meals is an easy way to boost fiber intake. These vegetables can be included in salads, stir-fries, and side dishes, enhancing both flavor and nutritional value.

3. **Snack on Nuts and Fruits**: Choosing high-fiber snacks like apples, almonds, and oranges is a convenient way to increase fiber intake without needing to prepare complex meals. These snacks also offer vitamins and minerals that support overall health.

4. **Switch to Whole Grains**: Replacing refined grains with whole grains like brown rice, quinoa, and whole wheat bread can significantly increase daily fiber intake. Whole grains are not only higher in fiber but also contain more nutrients than their refined counterparts.

5. **Incorporate Legumes**: Adding beans, lentils, and chickpeas to meals provides a substantial fiber boost. Legumes can be used in soups, salads, and even as meat substitutes in dishes like tacos and burgers.

Increasing fiber intake gradually and drinking plenty of water throughout the day helps the body process fiber more effectively, reducing the likelihood of bloating and discomfort.

Fiber's Role in Weight Management and Satiety

One of fiber's most valuable benefits is its role in promoting satiety, which can be helpful for weight management. High-fiber foods are more filling than low-fiber foods, as they absorb water and expand in the stomach. This can help reduce overall calorie intake by promoting a feeling of fullness, which may prevent overeating.

For individuals aiming to maintain or achieve a healthy weight, a diet rich in fiber can support these goals by stabilizing blood sugar and reducing hunger. By slowing down the absorption of sugars and increasing satiety, fiber helps prevent cravings and supports balanced energy levels.

Additionally, high-fiber foods tend to be lower in calories but high in volume, which means they can be eaten in larger quantities without leading to weight gain. For example, a salad with leafy greens, bell peppers, and a handful of chickpeas is nutrient-dense and filling, making it an ideal choice for those looking to manage their weight while maintaining a balanced, nutritious diet.

Fiber and Detoxification

Fiber plays an essential role in the body's natural detoxification processes. Soluble fiber binds to bile acids and cholesterol in the digestive tract, helping to remove these substances from the body. This process can reduce cholesterol levels and lower the risk of heart disease.

Insoluble fiber, meanwhile, promotes regular bowel movements, which are crucial for eliminating waste and toxins. When waste remains in the colon for too long, harmful substances can be reabsorbed into the bloodstream. By adding bulk to the stool and speeding up transit time, fiber ensures that toxins are efficiently removed from the body.

Moreover, fiber helps maintain a healthy gut microbiome by providing nourishment for beneficial bacteria. A balanced microbiome supports the liver, kidneys, and other detoxifying organs, enhancing the body's overall ability to manage and eliminate toxins.

Incorporating fiber-rich foods into a plant-based diet not only supports digestion and gut health but also aids the body's natural detoxification mechanisms, providing a foundation for long-term wellness and vitality.

Chapter 2: Exploring Superfoods

In the world of natural health, herbal remedies are renowned for their ability to support wellness and address specific health concerns. But to fully appreciate their potential, it's essential to understand exactly what these remedies entail and how they benefit the body. Herbal remedies encompass a wide variety of products derived from plants, including teas, tinctures, extracts, essential oils, and supplements.

Definition and Benefits

These natural solutions harness the therapeutic properties of plants, which have been used for centuries across different cultures for their healing and restorative effects. The benefits of herbal remedies are extensive, providing gentle yet effective support for the immune system, digestive health, mental well-being, and more.

This section explores the definition and advantages of herbal remedies, with a focus on their holistic benefits, how they function in harmony with the body's natural processes, and why they are increasingly valued as part of a balanced approach to health and wellness.

What Are Herbal Remedies?

Herbal remedies are plant-based solutions that utilize different parts of herbs—such as leaves, roots, flowers, seeds, and bark—to promote healing and wellness. They are created through various extraction processes, depending on the desired potency and application. Common forms include teas, which involve steeping herbs in hot water to release their active ingredients; tinctures, which use alcohol or glycerin to extract concentrated compounds; and essential oils, which are highly potent extracts used primarily in aromatherapy and topical applications.

The key difference between herbal remedies and synthetic medications is that herbs work in harmony with the body, often producing fewer side effects due to their natural composition. Plants contain complex compounds like flavonoids, alkaloids, and terpenes that interact with the body in unique ways, supporting not only symptom relief but also the body's innate healing processes. For example, an herb like peppermint, used in both tinctures and teas, contains menthol, which has antispasmodic properties that relax muscles and alleviate digestive discomfort. Similarly, chamomile contains flavonoids with anti-inflammatory and calming effects, making it ideal for anxiety and sleep support.

Because herbal remedies are derived from plants, they are part of a holistic health philosophy that focuses on treating the whole person rather than just the symptoms. This approach aligns well with the idea of "food as medicine," as many herbal remedies are simply concentrated forms of the beneficial compounds found in whole foods.

Holistic Benefits of Herbal Remedies

One of the primary benefits of herbal remedies is their holistic nature, which allows them to support multiple body systems simultaneously. Unlike pharmaceuticals that typically target a single symptom or system, herbs often have a broader range of actions. For example, turmeric is widely used for its anti-inflammatory properties, but it also supports liver health, enhances digestion, and provides antioxidant protection. This multi-faceted approach makes herbal remedies a valuable addition to wellness routines, addressing various aspects of health with fewer products.

Herbal remedies are also particularly beneficial for preventive care, strengthening the body's natural defenses before illness arises. Adaptogenic herbs like ashwagandha and rhodiola are excellent examples; they help the body adapt to stress, which can prevent immune suppression and reduce the risk of stress-related conditions. By supporting resilience, these herbs act as preventive allies, reducing the likelihood of illnesses linked to chronic stress, such as cardiovascular disease and fatigue.

Herbs also support mental and emotional well-being. For instance, herbs like lavender, lemon balm, and valerian root are known for their calming effects and are frequently used to manage anxiety, insomnia, and stress. Unlike conventional sleep aids or anti-anxiety medications, which often have sedative effects, these herbs offer gentle, non-addictive support for relaxation and improved sleep without grogginess or dependency.

How Herbal Remedies Work with the Body's Natural Processes

Herbal remedies are unique in that they work synergistically with the body's natural processes rather than overriding them. This synergy is possible because plants contain complex compounds that are structurally similar to certain chemicals in the human body, allowing them to interact naturally with bodily functions. For example, plants that contain phytoestrogens, such as red clover and soy, can help balance hormone levels by mimicking the effects of estrogen. This can be particularly beneficial for women experiencing menopause, providing relief from symptoms like hot flashes and mood swings without the need for synthetic hormone therapy.

Furthermore, many herbs contain compounds that act as antioxidants, neutralizing free radicals and protecting cells from oxidative damage. Herbs such as green tea, rosemary, and elderberry are rich in antioxidants, which play a critical role in reducing inflammation, slowing the aging process, and preventing chronic diseases. By providing antioxidant support, these herbs not only promote immediate health but also long-term vitality, helping the body stay resilient against environmental and lifestyle-related stressors.

Another way herbs work with the body is through adaptogenic effects. Adaptogens are a unique class of herbs, including ashwagandha, ginseng, and holy basil, that help the body adapt to stress and restore balance. These herbs work by modulating the stress response, reducing the impact of cortisol, the stress hormone, and enhancing the body's resilience. Unlike stimulants, which can lead to energy crashes, adaptogens provide a sustained boost in energy and mental clarity, supporting productivity and reducing the risk of burnout.

Specific Benefits of Common Herbal Remedies

1. **Digestive Health**: Many herbal remedies support digestive health by promoting bile flow, reducing inflammation, and alleviating discomfort. For instance, ginger is known for its ability to relieve nausea, stimulate digestion, and reduce bloating. Peppermint, with its antispasmodic effects, helps soothe irritable bowel syndrome (IBS) symptoms by relaxing the muscles in the gastrointestinal tract. Dandelion root, traditionally used as a digestive tonic, supports liver function and enhances detoxification, promoting a healthy digestive system.

2. **Immune System Support**: Herbal remedies play a significant role in strengthening the immune system, making them popular choices during cold and flu season. Elderberry is particularly renowned for its antiviral properties and ability to shorten the duration of colds and flu. Echinacea is another immune-boosting herb that stimulates white blood cell production, helping the body fight off infections. Adaptogenic herbs like astragalus are also used for immune support, enhancing the body's defenses and promoting resilience against seasonal illnesses.

3. **Mental Health and Stress Relief**: Herbal remedies are frequently used to support mental health and alleviate symptoms of anxiety and stress. Lavender and chamomile,

both calming herbs, are commonly used in teas and tinctures to reduce tension and promote relaxation. Passionflower, another popular herb, has been shown to reduce symptoms of anxiety without sedative effects, making it a natural option for those seeking relief from stress. Adaptogens like ashwagandha help balance stress hormones, allowing the body to handle stress more effectively.

4. **Anti-Inflammatory and Pain Relief**: Inflammation is at the root of many chronic diseases, and herbal remedies can provide natural anti-inflammatory benefits. Turmeric, containing the active compound curcumin, is widely recognized for its ability to reduce inflammation and pain, making it useful for arthritis and joint discomfort. Willow bark, which contains salicin (a compound similar to aspirin), has long been used for pain relief and can help alleviate headaches, muscle pain, and inflammation.

5. **Respiratory Health**: For those with respiratory issues, herbs like eucalyptus, thyme, and licorice root provide natural support. Eucalyptus, with its high menthol content, opens the airways and alleviates congestion, making it effective for colds and sinus infections. Licorice root has expectorant properties that help clear mucus and soothe irritated airways, while thyme provides antimicrobial benefits, helping to fight respiratory infections.

The Safety and Accessibility of Herbal Remedies

One of the notable advantages of herbal remedies is their safety profile. While they are potent, they generally cause fewer side effects than synthetic medications when used appropriately. However, it's essential to remember that "natural" does not always mean "safe." Some herbs can interact with medications or cause side effects in specific populations. For example, St. John's Wort, commonly used for depression, can interact with certain medications, reducing their effectiveness. This highlights the importance of consulting a healthcare provider before starting any herbal regimen, particularly for individuals with pre-existing health conditions or those taking medications.

The accessibility of herbal remedies makes them a practical choice for many people. Herbs can be grown in a garden, purchased as teas or supplements, or found in health food stores. This accessibility allows individuals to take an active role in their health, incorporating natural remedies into daily routines without the need for prescriptions or complex treatments. For example, incorporating ginger tea or chamomile tea as a nightly ritual is a simple yet effective way to support digestion and relaxation.

Herbal Remedies as Part of a Holistic Lifestyle

Incorporating herbal remedies into one's life aligns well with holistic health practices, which focus on achieving balance in all areas of health—physical, mental, and emotional. Herbs can be used alongside practices such as meditation, exercise, and a nutritious diet, enhancing their effectiveness and creating a well-rounded approach to wellness. This holistic synergy, where herbal remedies complement other health practices, enables individuals to address the root causes of health issues rather than merely treating symptoms.

For instance, using adaptogenic herbs like ashwagandha or rhodiola during stressful periods can enhance resilience, allowing individuals to manage stress better when combined with mindfulness practices or regular physical activity. Similarly, incorporating turmeric into meals not only adds flavor but also provides anti-inflammatory benefits that support joint health, especially when paired with exercise. This integration of herbal remedies with lifestyle practices represents a comprehensive approach to maintaining health and vitality.

Herbal remedies offer a versatile, effective, and natural way to support wellness, addressing a wide range of health concerns through gentle yet powerful means. Their ability to work harmoniously with the body, combined with their accessibility and holistic benefits, makes them an invaluable component of natural health.

Top Superfoods

Superfoods are nutrient-rich foods considered particularly beneficial for health and wellness. These foods contain high levels of vitamins, minerals, antioxidants, and other compounds that support the body in fighting disease, reducing inflammation, and enhancing energy and longevity. As the foundation of a natural, plant-based diet, superfoods offer targeted health benefits and can be easily incorporated into everyday meals to create a balanced, vibrant diet that supports both physical and mental health.

Superfoods are unique because they are naturally concentrated sources of nutrients, allowing even small servings to have a significant impact on health. Many of these foods have been used for centuries in traditional medicine for their healing properties, from boosting the immune system to improving cognitive function. By understanding the benefits and uses of these top superfoods, individuals can make informed choices that align with their health goals and enhance their overall wellness.

1. Blueberries: The Antioxidant Powerhouse

Blueberries are well-known for their high antioxidant content, particularly anthocyanins, which give them their deep blue color. These antioxidants protect cells from oxidative damage caused by free radicals, unstable molecules that can accelerate aging and contribute to various diseases, including cancer and heart disease. Additionally, blueberries contain vitamin C, vitamin K, and fiber, making them a well-rounded choice for overall health.

Research shows that consuming blueberries may improve cognitive function and memory, making them particularly beneficial for brain health. The antioxidants in blueberries reduce inflammation in the brain, which can help prevent age-related cognitive decline. Regular consumption of blueberries has also been linked to a reduced risk of heart disease, as they help to lower blood pressure and reduce cholesterol levels.

How to Use: Blueberries are versatile and can be added to smoothies, oatmeal, yogurt, and salads. They can also be enjoyed on their own as a nutritious snack.

2. Kale: The King of Leafy Greens

Kale is a leafy green vegetable rich in vitamins A, C, and K, as well as calcium, potassium, and fiber. It is also one of the most nutrient-dense foods, offering a high concentration of vitamins and minerals in very few calories. Kale's high levels of antioxidants, including quercetin and kaempferol, protect cells from inflammation and oxidative stress.

In addition to its antioxidant properties, kale is a great source of calcium, supporting bone health, and vitamin K, which plays a role in blood clotting and bone metabolism. The fiber content in kale supports digestive health, making it an excellent addition to a diet focused on gut health.

How to Use: Kale can be eaten raw in salads, added to smoothies, or cooked into soups and stews. Massaging raw kale with olive oil and lemon juice helps to soften its texture, making it more palatable in salads.

3. Chia Seeds: A Tiny but Mighty Source of Fiber and Omega-3s

Chia seeds are packed with fiber, protein, omega-3 fatty acids, and various micronutrients, including calcium, magnesium, and phosphorus. These tiny seeds absorb water and form a gel-like consistency, which helps to keep the digestive system functioning smoothly and promotes satiety, reducing overeating.

The omega-3 fatty acids in chia seeds, particularly alpha-linolenic acid (ALA), support heart health by reducing inflammation and lowering cholesterol. They also contain antioxidants that protect cells from damage and support skin health. Chia seeds are a great choice for anyone looking to increase their fiber intake while also benefiting from healthy fats.

How to Use: Chia seeds can be added to smoothies, oatmeal, and yogurt, or used to make chia pudding by soaking them in plant-based milk. They can also be used as an egg substitute in baking by mixing one tablespoon of chia seeds with three tablespoons of water.

4. Spirulina: The Protein-Rich Algae

Spirulina, a type of blue-green algae, is one of the most nutrient-dense foods on the planet. It is particularly high in protein, containing all essential amino acids, which makes it a complete protein source. Spirulina is also rich in B vitamins, iron, magnesium, and potassium, all of which support energy levels and immune health.

The pigments in spirulina, such as phycocyanin, provide powerful antioxidant and anti-inflammatory properties. Studies suggest that spirulina may help reduce blood pressure, lower cholesterol levels, and improve muscle endurance. Its iron content also makes it a good choice for those looking to boost their intake of this essential mineral, especially in plant-based diets.

How to Use: Spirulina is often available in powder form and can be added to smoothies, juices, or water. Its strong taste is best balanced with other flavors, such as citrus or sweet fruits.

5. Turmeric: The Golden Anti-Inflammatory Spice

Turmeric has been used in traditional medicine for centuries, particularly in Ayurvedic and Chinese medicine, for its anti-inflammatory and antioxidant properties. Its active compound, curcumin, is a powerful anti-inflammatory agent that helps reduce pain, improve joint health, and may even protect against cancer.

Curcumin is also known to support brain health, as it can cross the blood-brain barrier and reduce inflammation in the brain. This may help prevent neurodegenerative diseases such as Alzheimer's. Turmeric's antioxidant properties also benefit skin health by reducing oxidative stress and promoting a radiant complexion.

How to Use: Turmeric can be added to curries, soups, and smoothies. For better absorption, it is recommended to consume turmeric with black pepper, as piperine (a compound in black pepper) enhances curcumin absorption.

6. Quinoa: The Complete Protein Grain

Quinoa is a unique grain because it contains all nine essential amino acids, making it a complete protein source. This makes quinoa particularly valuable for those on a plant-based diet, as complete protein sources are less common in the plant kingdom. In addition to protein, quinoa is high in fiber, magnesium, B vitamins, iron, potassium, calcium, phosphorus, and vitamin E.

The fiber in quinoa supports digestive health, while its high magnesium content aids in muscle relaxation, nerve function, and heart health. Quinoa is also a source of antioxidants, which help to reduce inflammation and protect cells from damage.

How to Use: Quinoa can be used as a base for salads, added to soups, or served as a side dish. It can also be used as a breakfast cereal by cooking it with plant-based milk and adding fruits and nuts.

7. Ginger: A Root for Digestive and Immune Health

Ginger is a root with a long history of use for its medicinal properties. It is especially known for its ability to soothe nausea and improve digestion. Ginger contains compounds called gingerols and shogaols, which have anti-inflammatory and antioxidant effects. These compounds help reduce pain, boost immunity, and protect against chronic diseases.

Ginger's warming properties support circulation and metabolism, making it beneficial for cold hands and feet in winter months. It also acts as an anti-inflammatory agent, which can help alleviate symptoms of arthritis and muscle pain.

How to Use: Fresh ginger can be added to teas, smoothies, stir-fries, and soups. It can also be used in baking for a spicy, warming flavor.

8. Almonds: Nutrient-Dense Nuts for Heart Health

Almonds are a nutrient-dense nut high in healthy monounsaturated fats, fiber, protein, vitamin E, and magnesium. They are beneficial for heart health, as their healthy fats help reduce LDL cholesterol levels and improve overall cholesterol profiles. Almonds also provide antioxidants, particularly vitamin E, which helps protect cells from oxidative stress.

Regular almond consumption has been linked to improved blood sugar control, weight management, and better cognitive function. Almonds are also a good source of magnesium, which supports muscle and nerve function and helps maintain stable blood pressure.

How to Use: Almonds can be eaten as a snack, added to salads, oatmeal, and yogurt, or used in almond butter form as a spread or smoothie ingredient.

9. Sweet Potatoes: A Root Vegetable Rich in Beta-Carotene

Sweet potatoes are a nutritious root vegetable rich in beta-carotene, an antioxidant that the body converts into vitamin A. This vitamin supports immune function, vision, and skin health. Sweet potatoes are also high in fiber, which promotes digestive health, and contain vitamins C and B6, as well as potassium and manganese.

Sweet potatoes' complex carbohydrates provide steady energy, making them an ideal food for maintaining stable blood sugar levels. Their high fiber content aids in satiety, making them an excellent choice for weight management.

How to Use: Sweet potatoes can be roasted, mashed, or baked. They can also be added to soups, stews, and salads for a naturally sweet, nutritious boost.

10. Avocado: The Creamy Superfood

Avocado is a unique superfood because it is rich in healthy monounsaturated fats, fiber, vitamins, and minerals. The healthy fats in avocados support heart health, reduce inflammation, and improve cholesterol levels. Avocados are also a good source of potassium, which helps balance electrolytes and supports muscle function.

In addition to heart health, avocados are beneficial for skin health due to their high levels of antioxidants, including vitamins C and E. These vitamins help reduce inflammation and protect the skin from oxidative damage, promoting a healthy complexion.

How to Use: Avocado can be added to salads, sandwiches, smoothies, or eaten on its own. It can also be blended into dressings or used as a spread on toast.

Incorporating these superfoods into a daily diet not only enhances nutrient intake but also provides a wide range of health benefits that support holistic wellness. These nutrient-dense foods allow individuals to maximize their health potential through natural, plant-based nutrition.

Spirulina and Seaweed

Spirulina and seaweed have garnered significant attention for their exceptional nutritional profiles and numerous health benefits. Both are types of algae that have been used for centuries in various cultures as potent natural remedies and nutritional supplements. Rich in proteins, vitamins, minerals, and antioxidants, spirulina and seaweed offer a variety of health benefits, supporting immune function, detoxification, and overall wellness. This section delves into the unique properties of spirulina and seaweed, their benefits, practical ways to incorporate them into daily life, and why they have become increasingly popular in modern health and wellness practices.

Understanding Spirulina: The Superfood Algae

Spirulina is a blue-green algae, scientifically classified as *Arthrospira platensis* or *Arthrospira maxima*. It grows in both fresh and saltwater environments and is considered one of the most nutrient-dense foods on the planet. Spirulina has a long history of use; it was consumed by the Aztecs in ancient Mexico and has been cultivated in other parts of the world for its powerful health benefits.

One of spirulina's defining characteristics is its high protein content—approximately 60-70% of its dry weight is protein, which is remarkably high compared to most other plant-based sources. This makes spirulina an excellent option for individuals looking to increase their protein intake, especially vegetarians and vegans. Beyond protein, spirulina is packed with essential amino acids, vitamins B1, B2, and B3, iron, copper, and magnesium, as well as antioxidants such as phycocyanin and chlorophyll.

Nutritional Benefits of Spirulina

1. **High-Quality Protein Source**: Spirulina is often referred to as a "complete protein" because it contains all nine essential amino acids, similar to animal-based protein sources. This makes it an invaluable addition to plant-based diets where

complete proteins can be harder to obtain. Additionally, the protein in spirulina is highly digestible, allowing the body to absorb and utilize it efficiently.

2. **Rich in Antioxidants**: Spirulina is known for its high levels of antioxidants, particularly phycocyanin, which gives it a distinct blue-green color. Phycocyanin fights free radicals and reduces inflammation, supporting cellular health and protecting the body from oxidative stress. Spirulina also contains chlorophyll, a powerful antioxidant that helps detoxify the body by binding to toxins and removing them from the system.

3. **Supports Immune Function**: Studies have shown that spirulina can enhance immune function by increasing the production of antibodies and cytokines, proteins that play a crucial role in immune response. Additionally, spirulina's antiviral properties make it beneficial for protecting the body against certain infections.

4. **Detoxification and Heavy Metal Removal**: Spirulina is highly effective at binding to heavy metals, such as arsenic and mercury, and removing them from the body. This detoxifying effect is attributed to the chlorophyll content, which helps flush toxins from the bloodstream and liver. Regular consumption of spirulina can support liver health and enhance the body's natural detoxification processes.

5. **Promotes Cardiovascular Health**: Spirulina has been shown to lower cholesterol levels, reduce blood pressure, and decrease inflammation, all of which are beneficial for cardiovascular health. Its high antioxidant content also protects blood vessels from oxidative damage, reducing the risk of heart disease over time.

Seaweed: A Treasure Trove of Marine Nutrients

Seaweed, a type of marine algae, includes various edible species like nori, kelp, wakame, and dulse, each with its own unique nutritional profile and health benefits. Seaweed has been a dietary staple in many Asian cultures for centuries and is valued for its high iodine content, an essential mineral for thyroid health. In addition to iodine, seaweed is rich in calcium, magnesium, potassium, iron, and vitamins A, C, E, and K.

Seaweed also contains polysaccharides like fucoidan and alginate, which have been linked to health benefits such as enhanced immune function, reduced inflammation, and support for gut health. The nutrient density and variety in seaweed make it an excellent addition to a balanced diet, offering a broad spectrum of vitamins, minerals, and bioactive compounds that support wellness on multiple levels.

Nutritional Benefits of Seaweed

1. **Rich Source of Iodine**: Iodine is crucial for thyroid function, as it is needed to produce thyroid hormones that regulate metabolism. Seaweed is one of the few plant-based sources of iodine, making it especially valuable for individuals who do not consume dairy or seafood, which are other common sources of iodine.

2. **High Mineral Content**: Seaweed contains an impressive array of essential minerals, including calcium, magnesium, potassium, and iron, which support bone health, energy production, and muscle function. The high bioavailability of these minerals in seaweed means that the body can absorb and utilize them effectively.

3. **Supports Digestive Health**: Seaweed contains fiber and prebiotics, which are beneficial for gut health. The polysaccharides in seaweed, such as alginate, help feed beneficial gut bacteria, promoting a balanced microbiome and supporting digestive health. Additionally, the fiber content in seaweed aids in regular bowel movements and helps prevent constipation.

4. **Antioxidant and Anti-Inflammatory Properties**: Seaweed is rich in antioxidants like vitamins C and E, as well as unique compounds like fucoxanthin, which has been shown to have anti-inflammatory effects. These antioxidants protect cells from damage and help reduce chronic inflammation, which is a risk factor for various diseases.

5. **Potential for Weight Management**: Certain compounds in seaweed, such as alginate, may help with weight management by inhibiting the absorption of dietary fat. Additionally, seaweed's fiber content promotes satiety, reducing overall calorie intake and supporting weight control.

Spirulina vs. Seaweed: Similarities and Differences

While both spirulina and seaweed offer impressive health benefits, they are distinct in their nutrient profiles and applications. Spirulina is known for its exceptionally high protein content and specific antioxidants like phycocyanin, making it an ideal supplement for those needing a concentrated protein source and anti-inflammatory support. Seaweed, on the other hand, is a better source of iodine and a wider variety of minerals, which are essential for thyroid health, bone strength, and electrolyte balance.

Spirulina is often available in powder or tablet form, making it easy to incorporate into smoothies, juices, or supplements. Seaweed is commonly consumed in its natural form, such as nori sheets for sushi or dried seaweed snacks, allowing for more versatile culinary uses. For those looking to harness the benefits of both, incorporating a combination of spirulina and seaweed into their diets can provide comprehensive nutritional support.

Practical Ways to Incorporate Spirulina and Seaweed into Your Diet

Adding spirulina and seaweed to daily meals can be simple and enjoyable with the right recipes and preparation methods.

1. **Smoothies with Spirulina**: Spirulina powder can easily be added to smoothies for a nutrient boost. Combining it with fruits like bananas, berries, and a base like almond milk can create a tasty and energizing drink that provides protein, antioxidants, and minerals.

2. **Seaweed in Soups and Salads**: Seaweed like wakame and kelp can be added to soups, salads, and rice bowls for extra flavor and nutrients. Miso soup with wakame is a classic example that highlights seaweed's natural umami flavor while providing iodine, calcium, and fiber.

3. **Spirulina Energy Balls**: Spirulina powder can be incorporated into homemade energy balls along with ingredients like dates, nuts, and seeds. This snack offers a convenient way to consume spirulina while providing sustained energy from healthy fats and protein.

4. **Nori as a Snack or Wrap**: Nori sheets, commonly used in sushi, can also be enjoyed as a healthy snack. Nori is high in iodine and makes for a low-calorie, nutrient-dense alternative to processed snacks. It can also be used as a wrap for vegetables, hummus, or other fillings.

5. **Seaweed Seasoning**: Seaweed flakes or powder can be used as a seasoning on salads, roasted vegetables, or popcorn. This is an easy way to incorporate the minerals and antioxidants in seaweed without significantly altering the flavor of a dish.

Safety Considerations and Quality Selection

When incorporating spirulina and seaweed into your diet, quality is essential. Spirulina should be sourced from reputable suppliers to ensure it is free of contaminants, as some sources of spirulina can contain heavy metals or harmful bacteria. Seaweed, while highly nutritious, should be consumed in moderation due to its iodine content. Excessive iodine intake can lead to thyroid imbalances, so it's best to limit seaweed intake to recommended amounts, especially for individuals with pre-existing thyroid conditions.

When selecting seaweed products, it's advisable to choose certified organic or sustainably sourced options, as seaweed can absorb pollutants from its environment. Reading labels and choosing trusted brands can help ensure that the seaweed is pure and free from contaminants.

The Unique Health Potential of Spirulina and Seaweed

The combination of spirulina and seaweed provides a comprehensive array of nutrients that support many aspects of health. From immune function and energy levels to heart health and detoxification, these algae-based superfoods offer benefits that are difficult to find in other plant-based foods. Spirulina's high protein and antioxidant content make it ideal for those looking to enhance their diet with a concentrated source of nutrients. Seaweed's mineral richness and iodine content, meanwhile, make it indispensable for thyroid health and overall mineral balance.

Incorporating spirulina and seaweed into a wellness routine can yield substantial health benefits, particularly for individuals seeking natural ways to support vitality, resilience, and holistic health. As research continues to explore the applications of these superfoods, spirulina and seaweed are likely to remain central components of natural health practices, offering solutions grounded in the power of the ocean and earth.

Nuts and Seeds for Vitality

Nuts and seeds are some of nature's most nutrient-dense foods, packed with essential fats, proteins, vitamins, and minerals that support energy, brain function, heart health, and overall vitality. Including a variety of nuts and seeds in a plant-based diet provides a wealth of nutrients that are crucial for maintaining physical health and mental clarity. These small but mighty foods offer sustained energy, help in balancing hormones, and are rich in antioxidants that protect the body from oxidative stress.

Nuts and seeds are especially valuable in a plant-based diet because they provide a rich source of protein and healthy fats, including omega-3 and omega-6 fatty acids. The unique combination of macronutrients and micronutrients found in these foods makes them ideal for boosting daily energy levels and supporting a wide range of bodily functions. By understanding the specific health benefits of different nuts and seeds, individuals can incorporate these powerful foods into their diets in ways that best support their wellness goals.

The Health Benefits of Nuts

Nuts are known for their high-fat content, but these fats are primarily unsaturated fats that benefit heart health and cognitive function. They also contain plant-based protein, fiber, and essential nutrients like magnesium, vitamin E, and B vitamins. Eating nuts has been linked to a reduced risk of chronic diseases, including heart disease, type 2 diabetes, and certain cancers. Here are some of the top nuts to include in a vitality-boosting diet:

1. **Almonds**: Almonds are high in monounsaturated fats, vitamin E, and magnesium. Vitamin E is a powerful antioxidant that protects cells from oxidative damage, supports skin health, and helps reduce inflammation. Magnesium in almonds aids in muscle relaxation, nerve function, and blood sugar control, making them a particularly good choice for those with active lifestyles or concerns about blood sugar stability. Almonds are also high in fiber, which promotes satiety and digestive health.

How to Use: Almonds can be eaten raw as a snack, added to salads, or used as almond butter on toast or in smoothies.

2. **Walnuts**: Walnuts are an excellent source of omega-3 fatty acids, specifically alpha-linolenic acid (ALA), which supports brain health and reduces inflammation. Walnuts also contain polyphenols, compounds with antioxidant properties that protect the brain and cardiovascular system. Studies have shown that regular walnut consumption may improve cognitive function and reduce the risk of heart disease.

How to Use: Walnuts can be added to oatmeal, salads, and baked goods. They pair well with both sweet and savory dishes, making them a versatile addition to meals.

3. **Pistachios**: Pistachios are lower in calories than many other nuts and are rich in protein, potassium, and vitamin B6. Vitamin B6 is essential for brain development, immune health, and mood regulation. Pistachios are also a good source of antioxidants, including lutein and zeaxanthin, which support eye health.

How to Use: Enjoy pistachios as a snack, sprinkle them over yogurt, or blend them into pesto for a unique twist.

4. **Cashews**: Cashews are creamy and rich in monounsaturated fats, iron, zinc, and magnesium. They are also high in copper, which supports collagen production and

immune function. The healthy fats in cashews make them satisfying and beneficial for skin health.

How to Use: Cashews can be eaten on their own, used in dairy-free sauces and creams, or added to stir-fries and salads.

5. **Brazil Nuts**: Brazil nuts are one of the best natural sources of selenium, a mineral with antioxidant properties that supports thyroid function and immune health. Selenium is essential for reproductive health, and just one or two Brazil nuts a day can provide the recommended daily intake of this mineral.

How to Use: Due to their high selenium content, Brazil nuts should be eaten in moderation. Add one or two to a daily nut mix or enjoy them as a standalone snack.

The Health Benefits of Seeds

Seeds may be small, but they are loaded with essential nutrients that support energy, digestion, and overall health. Like nuts, seeds provide plant-based protein, fiber, and healthy fats, as well as minerals such as magnesium, zinc, and iron. Seeds are particularly beneficial for those on plant-based diets, as they offer a concentrated source of omega-3 fatty acids and amino acids. Here are some of the most nutrient-dense seeds to include in a vitality-focused diet:

1. **Chia Seeds**: Chia seeds are high in fiber, omega-3 fatty acids, and antioxidants. Their high fiber content supports digestive health, promotes satiety, and can help regulate blood sugar levels. Chia seeds absorb water and form a gel-like consistency, making them ideal for supporting hydration and promoting a feeling of fullness.

How to Use: Add chia seeds to smoothies, yogurt, and oatmeal, or use them to make chia pudding by soaking them in plant-based milk.

2. **Flaxseeds**: Flaxseeds are rich in omega-3 fatty acids and lignans, plant compounds with antioxidant and estrogen-like properties. Lignans may help balance hormones, making flaxseeds beneficial for hormonal health. The fiber in flaxseeds supports heart health by lowering cholesterol levels and improving digestion.

How to Use: Ground flaxseeds are easier to digest and can be added to smoothies, oatmeal, or baked goods. They can also be mixed with water to create a vegan egg substitute for baking.

3. **Pumpkin Seeds**: Pumpkin seeds, also known as pepitas, are a great source of magnesium, zinc, and healthy fats. Magnesium supports muscle function, nerve

health, and blood pressure regulation, while zinc plays a role in immune function and wound healing. Pumpkin seeds are also high in tryptophan, an amino acid that the body converts into serotonin, supporting mood and relaxation.

How to Use: Pumpkin seeds can be eaten raw or roasted, sprinkled over salads, or added to granola for a nutrient boost.

4. **Hemp Seeds**: Hemp seeds are a complete protein source, containing all nine essential amino acids. They are also rich in omega-3 and omega-6 fatty acids in an ideal ratio, which supports heart health and reduces inflammation. Hemp seeds contain a high amount of magnesium and are easy to digest, making them an excellent protein source for those on plant-based diets.

How to Use: Add hemp seeds to smoothies, yogurt, and salads, or use them as a topping for avocado toast.

5. **Sesame Seeds**: Sesame seeds are high in calcium, magnesium, and zinc, supporting bone health and immune function. They also contain sesamin, a compound with antioxidant and anti-inflammatory properties. Sesame seeds are often used in traditional medicine to support joint health and skin hydration.

How to Use: Sprinkle sesame seeds on salads, stir-fries, and baked goods. Tahini, a paste made from sesame seeds, can be used as a spread or dressing for a creamy, nutritious addition.

Balancing Nuts and Seeds in a Daily Diet

Including a variety of nuts and seeds in a daily diet ensures a balanced intake of essential nutrients. Nuts and seeds can be enjoyed in many forms, making them a convenient addition to meals and snacks. A handful of mixed nuts or seeds provides a satisfying snack, while adding these foods to salads, oatmeal, or yogurt enhances both flavor and nutrition.

For those aiming to increase their omega-3 intake, a combination of chia, flax, and walnuts offers a substantial source of this essential fatty acid, which is especially important in plant-based diets. Additionally, rotating between different nuts and seeds allows individuals to benefit from the unique nutrients each type offers, from selenium in Brazil nuts to zinc in pumpkin seeds.

Practical Tips for Incorporating Nuts and Seeds

1. **Start with Breakfast**: Adding a tablespoon of chia seeds, flaxseeds, or a handful of almonds to oatmeal, smoothies, or yogurt can boost fiber, protein, and healthy fat intake first thing in the morning.

2. **Snack Smartly**: Keep a small bag of mixed nuts or seeds on hand for a quick, nutritious snack. A mix of almonds, walnuts, and pumpkin seeds provides a balance of fats, protein, and antioxidants.

3. **Add to Salads and Main Dishes**: Sprinkle hemp seeds or sesame seeds on salads, stir-fries, or roasted vegetables for added texture and nutrition. Nuts and seeds can also be incorporated into pesto or salad dressings for a creamy, nutrient-dense option.

4. **Use as a Topping**: Nuts and seeds make great toppings for smoothie bowls, soups, and even desserts. Their natural crunch and rich flavor enhance both sweet and savory dishes.

5. **Incorporate Nut and Seed Butters**: Nut butters, such as almond butter and tahini, offer all the benefits of whole nuts and seeds in a convenient form. Spread nut butters on toast, use them in smoothies, or mix them into sauces for a creamy texture and added nutrients.

The Role of Nuts and Seeds in Energy and Metabolism

The healthy fats and proteins found in nuts and seeds provide sustained energy, making them ideal for those with active lifestyles or for anyone looking to avoid energy crashes throughout the day. Unlike simple carbohydrates that cause quick spikes in blood sugar, the fats and proteins in nuts and seeds release energy slowly, helping to maintain stable blood sugar levels and reduce cravings.

Magnesium, found abundantly in almonds, pumpkin seeds, and chia seeds, plays a key role in energy production at the cellular level. This mineral supports the function of enzymes involved in the metabolism of food, ensuring that the body can effectively convert nutrients into energy. For those seeking to boost their vitality, adding magnesium-rich nuts and seeds can support both physical and mental energy.

The high fiber content in nuts and seeds also aids in satiety, which can support healthy weight management and prevent overeating. Fiber slows digestion, keeping blood sugar levels stable and helping individuals feel full longer. By incorporating nuts and seeds into meals and snacks, individuals can benefit from sustained energy and improved metabolic health.

Supporting Vitality with Antioxidants and Anti-Inflammatory Properties

Many nuts and seeds are rich in antioxidants, which protect the body from oxidative stress and reduce inflammation. Chronic inflammation is a contributing factor in many diseases, including heart disease, diabetes, and arthritis. By incorporating nuts and seeds with antioxidant properties—such as walnuts, almonds, and flaxseeds—individuals can support their body's natural defenses and promote long-term health.

Additionally, the omega-3 fatty acids in chia, flax, and walnuts have anti-inflammatory effects, which benefit the heart, brain, and joints. These healthy fats help balance the body's inflammatory response, reducing the risk of chronic inflammation and supporting overall vitality.

Nuts and seeds are not only convenient and versatile foods but also powerful allies in promoting energy, protecting against disease, and supporting a balanced and healthful diet. Incorporating these nutrient-dense foods into daily meals is a simple yet effective strategy for enhancing vitality and well-being.

Chapter 3: Detox Diets and Cleansing Routines

In today's environment, exposure to toxins is almost inevitable. From pollutants in the air to chemicals in household products and even in our food and water, our bodies are continually confronted with substances that can accumulate and potentially harm our health.

Safe Detox Techniques

Detoxification, or detox, is a process aimed at supporting the body in removing these unwanted compounds, enhancing our natural ability to heal, rejuvenate, and function optimally. However, a safe and effective detox requires careful planning, a focus on gentle methods, and support for the body's detox organs, such as the liver, kidneys, lungs, skin, and digestive system.

Detoxification is not about quick fixes or extreme diets; it is about fostering long-term health and reducing the toxic load on our body. This section provides an in-depth exploration of safe detox techniques, addressing how detoxification works, effective strategies for supporting detox naturally, and specific herbs and practices that aid in the detox process.

Understanding Detoxification and the Body's Natural Process

The body has an intricate system designed to process and eliminate toxins through various organs and pathways. The liver is the primary detox organ, as it breaks down toxins into less harmful compounds that can be excreted through the kidneys or bile. The kidneys filter the blood, removing waste products and excess substances through urine. The lungs expel volatile toxins with each breath, and the skin eliminates toxins through sweat. The digestive system also plays a critical role, as it removes waste and supports a healthy microbiome that prevents harmful bacteria and toxins from entering the bloodstream.

To maintain optimal function, these organs need support. When the body becomes overwhelmed by toxins, these systems can slow down, and symptoms like fatigue, bloating, headaches, and skin issues may arise. A safe detox focuses on enhancing these natural processes without placing undue stress on the body, fostering a balanced approach to long-term wellness.

Hydration: The Foundation of Any Detox

Water is essential for almost every bodily function, particularly in supporting the kidneys and liver in processing and eliminating toxins. Staying well-hydrated helps maintain blood flow to the kidneys, supporting their ability to filter waste products. For detox purposes, water can be consumed in various forms, including herbal teas and infused waters with detoxifying herbs such as lemon and mint, which add subtle flavor and additional nutrients.

A simple way to increase detoxification is by drinking warm lemon water in the morning. Lemon contains vitamin C and antioxidants, which support the liver, and warm water encourages digestion. Adding a slice of fresh ginger can further enhance this effect by stimulating digestive enzymes and promoting circulation.

To optimize hydration during a detox, aim for 8-10 glasses of water per day, adjusted based on activity level, climate, and individual needs. Coconut water is another excellent hydrating option, as it provides electrolytes, which help maintain mineral balance and support cellular health.

Nutrient-Dense Diet: Supporting Detox Through Food

A nutrient-dense diet is key to safe detoxification. Incorporating whole foods—particularly fruits, vegetables, whole grains, and healthy fats—provides the body with the vitamins, minerals, and antioxidants it needs to process and eliminate toxins. Cruciferous vegetables like broccoli, cauliflower, and Brussels sprouts are particularly beneficial, as they contain sulfur compounds that aid liver detoxification.

Leafy greens, such as kale, spinach, and dandelion greens, are also rich in chlorophyll, which helps bind toxins and removes them from the body. Beets are another valuable detox food due to their high fiber content and betaine, which supports liver function and bile flow. Including fiber-rich foods, like whole grains and legumes, is essential, as fiber binds toxins in the digestive tract and facilitates their removal through bowel movements.

Healthy fats, especially those found in avocados, nuts, seeds, and olive oil, are vital for cellular function and help transport fat-soluble toxins out of the body. Additionally, incorporating probiotic-rich foods like yogurt, sauerkraut, and kimchi supports gut health, promoting a balanced microbiome that prevents harmful bacteria from proliferating and producing toxins.

Herbal Support for Detoxification

Herbs can play a powerful role in supporting safe detoxification. Herbal remedies have been used for centuries to cleanse the body and enhance the functions of the liver, kidneys, and lymphatic system. Here are some key herbs known for their detoxifying properties:

1. **Milk Thistle**: One of the most well-known liver-supporting herbs, milk thistle contains silymarin, a compound that helps protect liver cells and regenerate liver tissue. Milk thistle can be taken in tincture or capsule form or added to teas. Studies show that milk thistle helps reduce liver inflammation and supports the liver's ability to process toxins.

2. **Dandelion Root**: Dandelion root acts as a gentle diuretic, helping the kidneys eliminate toxins through urine. It also supports liver function and bile production, making it effective for digestion and detoxification. Dandelion root tea is a popular choice for daily detox support.

3. **Burdock Root**: Burdock root has a long history in herbal medicine as a blood purifier and liver tonic. It promotes lymphatic drainage, which helps the body remove waste products more efficiently. Burdock root can be consumed as a tea or taken in capsule form.

4. **Ginger**: Ginger supports digestion, circulation, and lymphatic flow, all of which are beneficial during detox. It stimulates digestive enzymes and promotes warmth in the body, which can enhance the effectiveness of other detox practices. Fresh ginger can be added to hot water or used as a spice in meals.

5. **Turmeric**: Known for its anti-inflammatory and antioxidant properties, turmeric supports liver health and helps the body combat oxidative stress. Curcumin, the active compound in turmeric, aids in the breakdown of toxins and enhances bile production. Consuming turmeric with black pepper improves its absorption.

Sweat It Out: Skin and Sweat Detoxification

The skin is the body's largest organ and plays a significant role in detoxification through sweat. Practices that promote sweating can help eliminate toxins, as well as improve circulation and boost metabolism. Saunas, particularly infrared saunas, are effective for encouraging sweat-based detox, as they heat the body from the inside out, promoting a deep sweat that reaches toxins stored in fat cells.

For those without access to a sauna, a hot bath with Epsom salts is another excellent way to encourage sweating. Epsom salts contain magnesium sulfate, which is absorbed through the skin and helps relax muscles, relieve tension, and promote circulation. Adding a few drops of detoxifying essential oils, such as eucalyptus or lavender, can enhance relaxation and support respiratory health.

Physical exercise is also essential for sweating and overall detox support. Activities that increase the heart rate, such as running, cycling, and yoga, promote circulation and lymphatic flow, supporting the body's ability to process and eliminate toxins.

The Importance of Restorative Sleep in Detox

Sleep is a crucial component of detoxification, as it provides the body with the time it needs to repair and regenerate. During sleep, the brain flushes out waste products through the glymphatic system, a network of channels that remove toxins from the central nervous system. This process is particularly important for mental clarity and cognitive health, as it helps prevent the buildup of toxins that may contribute to neurodegenerative diseases.

To support detox through sleep, aim for 7-9 hours of quality rest per night. Establishing a regular sleep routine, reducing screen time before bed, and creating a calm sleep environment can enhance sleep quality. Herbal teas with chamomile, valerian root, or passionflower are helpful for relaxation and preparing the body for restorative sleep.

Lymphatic Support: Dry Brushing and Rebounding

The lymphatic system plays a vital role in detoxification by transporting waste products from tissues to be filtered and eliminated. Unlike the circulatory system, the lymphatic system relies on muscle movement to keep lymph flowing. Practicing lymphatic support techniques, such as dry brushing and rebounding, can significantly enhance detox efforts.

Dry brushing involves using a natural bristle brush on dry skin before showering. This practice stimulates lymphatic flow, exfoliates dead skin cells, and promotes circulation. Begin brushing from the feet and move upward towards the heart in gentle, circular motions. Regular dry brushing not only supports detoxification but also improves skin health.

Rebounding, or jumping on a mini-trampoline, is another effective way to stimulate lymphatic flow. The up-and-down motion helps flush out toxins and improve lymphatic drainage. Even short sessions of rebounding, around 5-10 minutes a day, can be beneficial for detox support.

Reducing Toxin Exposure for Lasting Detoxification

Supporting the body's detoxification processes is essential, but reducing exposure to toxins is equally important. Making mindful choices in everyday life can minimize the toxic burden on the body and create a cleaner environment for long-term health. Here are some strategies for reducing toxin exposure:

1. **Choose Organic Foods**: Organic produce is free from synthetic pesticides, herbicides, and other chemicals that can accumulate in the body. Prioritizing organic options, especially for fruits and vegetables with thin skins, reduces pesticide exposure.

2. **Use Natural Cleaning Products**: Many conventional cleaning products contain harmful chemicals that contribute to indoor pollution. Switching to natural cleaning products made with ingredients like vinegar, baking soda, and essential oils can reduce toxin exposure.

3. **Avoid Plastics**: Plastics contain chemicals like BPA and phthalates that can leach into food and water. Opt for glass, stainless steel, or ceramic containers for food storage and avoid heating food in plastic containers.

4. **Filter Tap Water**: Tap water may contain contaminants like chlorine, heavy metals, and pharmaceutical residues. Using a high-quality water filter removes these impurities, ensuring cleaner, safer drinking water.

5. **Switch to Natural Personal Care Products**: Personal care items, such as lotions, shampoos, and cosmetics, can contain synthetic chemicals that are absorbed through the skin. Choosing natural and organic products reduces exposure to these toxins.

Mindful Breathing for Lung Detoxification

The lungs are continually exposed to environmental pollutants, allergens, and toxins that can accumulate over time. Practicing deep, mindful breathing exercises promotes lung health and oxygenation, helping to expel pollutants. Techniques like diaphragmatic breathing, where the breath is drawn deep into the abdomen, strengthen the lungs and enhance oxygen flow. Spending time in clean, natural environments, such as parks or forests, provides fresh air and reduces exposure to pollutants, supporting lung detoxification.

Practices like steam inhalation with eucalyptus or peppermint essential oil can further clear the respiratory system, open airways, and provide relief from respiratory irritants.

How Detox Supports Health

Detoxification, or detox, is the body's natural process of removing harmful substances or toxins that can accumulate due to external sources like pollution, food additives, and chemicals, as well as internal sources from metabolic waste. A well-functioning detoxification system is essential for maintaining optimal health, as it supports the liver, kidneys, digestive system, and skin in processing and eliminating these toxins. In a world where exposure to pollutants and artificial ingredients is increasingly common, understanding how detox works and supporting it with natural methods can play a crucial role in promoting vitality and preventing illness.

Detoxification not only impacts physical health but also influences mental clarity and emotional well-being. When the body is overloaded with toxins, individuals may experience symptoms such as fatigue, brain fog, digestive discomfort, and skin issues. By engaging in practices that support the body's detox pathways, people can improve energy levels, boost immunity, and enjoy a heightened sense of overall well-being.

The Body's Natural Detoxification System

The body has a built-in detoxification system composed of several organs and processes that work together to identify, neutralize, and eliminate toxins. The primary organs involved in detoxification are the liver, kidneys, lungs, digestive system, and skin. Each of these organs plays a unique role in filtering out harmful substances and maintaining internal balance.

1. **The Liver**: The liver is the primary detoxification organ. It processes toxins into forms that can be safely eliminated from the body. This process occurs in two main phases: in Phase I, the liver converts toxins into intermediate forms using enzymes, and in Phase II, these intermediates are further broken down and combined with other compounds, making them water-soluble for elimination through bile or urine.

The liver also metabolizes drugs, alcohol, and hormones, ensuring that harmful substances do not accumulate.

2. **The Kidneys**: The kidneys filter waste and excess fluids from the bloodstream, eliminating them through urine. They also play a role in regulating electrolytes, balancing pH levels, and filtering out byproducts of protein metabolism, which are essential for maintaining blood health and hydration.

3. **The Lungs**: The lungs remove carbon dioxide, a byproduct of metabolism, and can also help expel airborne toxins through exhalation. Deep breathing techniques can enhance lung capacity and aid in the release of toxins, providing benefits for respiratory health.

4. **The Digestive System**: The gastrointestinal tract plays a critical role in detoxification by breaking down food and absorbing nutrients, while eliminating waste products. A healthy gut microbiome also supports detox by assisting in the breakdown of toxic substances and producing short-chain fatty acids that reduce inflammation in the gut lining.

5. **The Skin**: As the largest organ, the skin aids detoxification by releasing waste through sweat. Sweat glands expel toxins, particularly heavy metals, making exercise and sweating a valuable part of a detox regimen.

Each of these organs functions to keep the body free from harmful substances, but supporting these systems can improve their efficiency, especially in a world where toxic exposure is difficult to avoid.

Benefits of Detox for Overall Health

Detoxification offers a wide range of health benefits, as it allows the body to eliminate toxins that can otherwise interfere with cellular function, energy production, and immune response. Here are some of the ways that a well-functioning detoxification system supports health:

- **Increased Energy**: Toxins place a burden on the liver, kidneys, and digestive system, leading to fatigue and sluggishness. By reducing the toxic load, the body's organs can function more efficiently, providing a natural boost in energy levels.

- **Enhanced Immunity**: A buildup of toxins can compromise the immune system, making the body more susceptible to illness. Detoxification helps by reducing inflammation, supporting gut health, and providing nutrients that are essential for immune cell production.

- **Mental Clarity and Focus**: Many toxins, especially those found in processed foods and environmental pollutants, can impact cognitive function and mood. By reducing toxic exposure and supporting detox pathways, individuals often experience improved mental clarity and reduced brain fog.

- **Skin Health**: The skin reflects internal health, and toxin buildup can lead to skin issues such as acne, rashes, and dullness. Detoxing can support clearer, brighter skin by improving liver function and encouraging elimination through sweat.

- **Hormonal Balance**: Many toxins mimic hormones, particularly estrogen, leading to hormonal imbalances. By reducing the load of hormone-disrupting chemicals, the body can maintain a more balanced hormonal state, benefiting mood, metabolism, and reproductive health

Natural Ways to Support Detoxification

There are several ways to support the body's natural detox processes through dietary choices, lifestyle habits, and specific practices that enhance the function of detox organs. Incorporating these practices can help reduce the accumulation of toxins and improve overall health.

1. **Increase Hydration**: Drinking enough water is essential for kidney health and for flushing out toxins through urine. Water also aids in digestion and helps the liver metabolize waste products. Herbal teas, especially those with detoxifying properties like dandelion and milk thistle, can also support hydration and liver function.

2. **Eat Fiber-Rich Foods**: Fiber binds to toxins in the digestive tract and promotes regular bowel movements, which is essential for eliminating waste. Fiber-rich foods like fruits, vegetables, whole grains, and legumes support gut health and aid in detoxification by feeding beneficial bacteria that assist in the breakdown of harmful substances.

3. **Incorporate Antioxidant-Rich Foods**: Antioxidants neutralize free radicals and reduce oxidative stress, protecting cells from damage. Berries, green leafy vegetables, and nuts are excellent sources of antioxidants, and they help support liver function during detoxification.

4. **Include Detoxifying Herbs**: Certain herbs, such as dandelion root, milk thistle, and turmeric, have long been used to support liver health. Dandelion root acts as a diuretic, encouraging urine production and the elimination of toxins. Milk thistle is known for its protective effects on liver cells, while turmeric has anti-inflammatory and antioxidant properties that aid in liver function.

5. **Practice Deep Breathing and Exercise**: Deep breathing techniques improve lung function, aiding in the release of airborne toxins. Exercise promotes sweating, which helps eliminate toxins through the skin. Engaging in activities like yoga or brisk walking can also improve circulation and support lymphatic drainage, which removes waste from cells.

6. **Avoid Processed Foods and Sugar**: Processed foods contain additives, preservatives, and artificial ingredients that burden the liver and digestive system. Reducing the intake of processed foods, refined sugars, and unhealthy fats can alleviate stress on detox organs and improve metabolic health.

Common Signs of Toxin Overload

When the body's natural detoxification system becomes overwhelmed, it can lead to various symptoms that signal the need for detox support. Recognizing these signs can help individuals take action to alleviate their toxic load and restore balance:

- **Persistent Fatigue**: When the liver and kidneys are overworked, energy levels can drop, leading to chronic tiredness that doesn't improve with rest.
- **Digestive Issues**: Bloating, constipation, and gas may indicate that the digestive system is struggling to process and eliminate toxins.
- **Brain Fog and Poor Concentration**: Toxins can impair brain function, leading to difficulties with focus, memory, and mental clarity.
- **Skin Problems**: Acne, rashes, and dull skin often reflect internal toxicity, as the skin is one of the body's primary detox organs.
- **Body Odor and Bad Breath**: Excess toxins can lead to unpleasant body odor and bad breath, as the body attempts to eliminate waste through sweat and the digestive system.

These symptoms may be temporary, but addressing them through detox support can help restore energy and improve overall well-being.

Using Natural Remedies for Detoxification

Natural remedies can provide gentle yet effective support for detoxification. Herbal teas, juices, and plant-based foods are often recommended to encourage the elimination of toxins and provide essential nutrients that support detox organs.

- **Lemon Water**: Drinking lemon water first thing in the morning stimulates liver function and aids in digestion. Lemon contains vitamin C and antioxidants that support detox, and its acidic properties help balance pH levels.
- **Green Tea**: Green tea contains catechins, antioxidants that support liver function and reduce inflammation. Drinking green tea daily can provide gentle detox support and promote metabolic health.
- **Ginger and Turmeric Tea**: Both ginger and turmeric have anti-inflammatory properties and support liver health. A warm ginger-turmeric tea can improve digestion, enhance circulation, and provide antioxidant support for detoxification.
- **Beetroot Juice**: Beets contain betaine, a compound that supports liver function and bile flow, which is essential for processing fats and toxins. Beet juice is a potent liver cleanser that also provides vitamins and minerals to support detox.
- **Cilantro and Parsley**: These herbs help chelate heavy metals and support kidney function. Adding fresh cilantro and parsley to salads, smoothies, or soups can provide gentle detox support.

Creating a Sustainable Detox Routine

Detox should not be an occasional event but rather a sustainable routine that supports the body's natural detoxification processes. By making simple lifestyle changes and incorporating natural remedies into daily habits, individuals can maintain an ongoing detoxification regimen that benefits long-term health.

1. **Start the Day with Hydration**: Begin each morning with a glass of water, possibly infused with lemon or a dash of apple cider vinegar, to jumpstart liver and kidney function.
2. **Focus on a Balanced Diet**: Emphasize whole foods, including vegetables, fruits, lean proteins, and healthy fats. Avoid artificial ingredients, preservatives, and added sugars, which add to the body's toxic burden.

3. **Incorporate Physical Activity**: Regular exercise, especially activities that encourage sweating, supports detoxification through the skin and improves circulation, which enhances lymphatic drainage and the elimination of waste.

4. **Prioritize Sleep and Stress Management**: Quality sleep allows the body to repair and reset, while stress management techniques reduce cortisol, a hormone that can contribute to toxin buildup.

A balanced, consistent detox routine is not about deprivation but about providing the body with the tools it needs to cleanse itself naturally. Supporting detoxification through whole foods, hydration, and healthy lifestyle choices creates a foundation for optimal health, energy, and resilience.

Chapter 4: Detoxifying Herbal Recipes

D andelion root tea is an herbal remedy that has gained popularity as a natural, gentle detoxifying agent with a wide array of health benefits. Made from the roots of the common dandelion plant (*Taraxacum officinale*), this tea has been used for centuries in traditional medicine to support liver health, improve digestion, and promote overall wellness.

Dandelion Root Tea

The unique compounds found in dandelion root, including inulin, taraxasterol, and various antioxidants, make it a powerful ally in natural health practices, especially for those seeking a safe and effective way to support the body's natural detoxification processes.

In this section, we will explore the benefits of dandelion root tea, its active components, the role it plays in detoxification, practical ways to incorporate it into daily life, and some safety considerations. With a long history of use and a promising profile of health benefits, dandelion root tea offers a nourishing and accessible option for individuals looking to enhance their wellness routines naturally.

Understanding Dandelion Root and Its Active Compounds

Dandelion root is rich in bioactive compounds that contribute to its therapeutic properties. Some of the most significant components include:

1. **Inulin**: A type of prebiotic fiber that supports gut health by nourishing beneficial bacteria. Inulin also aids in digestion, promoting regular bowel movements and reducing the risk of constipation. Prebiotics like inulin can enhance gut health, which plays a critical role in overall immunity and detoxification.

2. **Taraxasterol**: This compound, specific to dandelion, has anti-inflammatory properties that help reduce inflammation in the body, particularly in the liver. Taraxasterol supports liver health by aiding bile production, which is essential for the digestion of fats and the removal of waste products.

3. **Antioxidants**: Dandelion root contains powerful antioxidants, including beta-carotene, flavonoids, and polyphenols. These antioxidants combat oxidative stress, protecting cells from damage caused by free radicals. By reducing oxidative stress, dandelion root may help prevent chronic diseases and support healthy aging.

4. **Minerals and Vitamins**: Dandelion root is a source of essential minerals such as potassium, magnesium, and calcium, which play a role in muscle function, heart health, and bone strength. These nutrients add to the overall health benefits of dandelion root tea, making it a nourishing addition to the diet.

Health Benefits of Dandelion Root Tea

1. **Liver Detoxification and Support**: Dandelion root tea is particularly known for its liver-supporting properties. The liver is responsible for filtering toxins from the blood, producing bile, and processing nutrients. Dandelion root stimulates bile production, which assists in the digestion and breakdown of fats, promoting liver function. The anti-inflammatory and antioxidant properties of dandelion root further protect liver cells from damage, supporting its ability to process and remove toxins.

2. **Digestive Health**: The inulin content in dandelion root acts as a prebiotic, promoting the growth of beneficial gut bacteria that are crucial for digestion and immune health. Regular consumption of dandelion root tea can improve digestion by encouraging bile flow, reducing bloating, and preventing constipation. Enhanced digestion also means that the body is better equipped to absorb nutrients and eliminate waste products effectively.

3. **Kidney Health and Diuretic Effect**: Dandelion root has a mild diuretic effect, meaning it encourages the kidneys to excrete excess water and waste products through urine. This action can help reduce water retention and support kidney health. By promoting urination, dandelion root tea assists in flushing out toxins, making it a gentle and safe way to support the body's natural detoxification processes.

4. **Anti-Inflammatory Properties**: Chronic inflammation is linked to numerous health conditions, including heart disease, diabetes, and arthritis. Dandelion root contains compounds that help reduce inflammation, such as taraxasterol. By consuming dandelion root tea regularly, individuals may experience relief from minor inflammatory conditions, such as joint discomfort or digestive inflammation.

5. **Antioxidant Support for Cellular Health**: Antioxidants in dandelion root, such as beta-carotene and polyphenols, combat oxidative stress, a factor that contributes to aging and various diseases. These antioxidants protect cells from free radical damage, which is particularly beneficial for organs involved in detoxification, such as the liver and kidneys.

How to Make Dandelion Root Tea

Dandelion root tea can be made using either fresh or dried dandelion roots, and it is available in pre-made tea bags at health food stores. Making the tea at home is simple and allows for control over the strength and flavor. Here is a basic recipe for preparing dandelion root tea from scratch:

Ingredients:

- 1-2 teaspoons of dried dandelion root (or 1 tablespoon if using fresh root)
- 1 cup of water
- Optional: honey or lemon to taste

Instructions:

1. **Prepare the Root**: If using fresh dandelion root, wash it thoroughly and chop it into small pieces. For dried root, use it as is.
2. **Simmer the Root**: Place the root in a small pot with water. Bring the mixture to a boil, then reduce the heat and let it simmer for about 10-15 minutes.
3. **Strain and Serve**: Remove from heat, strain the tea into a mug, and let it cool slightly before drinking. Add honey or lemon for taste if desired.

For a more robust flavor and enhanced benefits, some people allow the tea to steep for an additional 5-10 minutes after simmering.

Practical Applications and Usage Tips for Dandelion Root Tea

Dandelion root tea can be enjoyed daily as part of a balanced wellness routine. For those new to detox teas, starting with one cup per day is advisable, as it allows the body to adjust to the mild diuretic and detoxifying effects. Over time, individuals can increase their intake to two to three cups per day, depending on personal preference and health goals.

For optimal liver support, drinking a cup of dandelion root tea in the morning before breakfast can stimulate bile production and prepare the digestive system for the day.

Additionally, sipping dandelion root tea in the evening can aid digestion and relaxation, supporting the liver's nighttime detox processes.

Combining Dandelion Root Tea with Other Herbal Remedies

Dandelion root tea can be combined with other detoxifying herbs to enhance its benefits. For example, blending dandelion root with milk thistle seeds can provide additional liver support, as milk thistle is known for its ability to protect liver cells and regenerate liver tissue. Adding ginger to dandelion root tea introduces anti-inflammatory and digestive benefits, creating a soothing tea that is ideal for cold days or after meals.

Another popular combination is dandelion root with nettle leaves. Nettle is rich in vitamins and minerals and has diuretic properties that complement dandelion's detox effects, supporting kidney health. Together, these herbs create a well-rounded detox tea that can be enjoyed regularly as part of a natural wellness routine.

Safety and Considerations

While dandelion root tea is generally safe for most people, there are a few precautions to keep in mind. Due to its diuretic effect, those with kidney conditions or on diuretic medications should consult a healthcare provider before consuming dandelion root tea regularly. The tea may also interact with certain medications, such as lithium and antibiotics, so individuals on prescription medications should seek medical advice.

People with allergies to ragweed or related plants should use caution, as dandelion may cause allergic reactions in sensitive individuals. Starting with a small amount and monitoring for adverse reactions is a safe approach.

Dandelion Root Tea for Detox and Beyond

Dandelion root tea is more than just a detox tea; it is a nourishing beverage that supports multiple aspects of health, from digestion to liver function and inflammation reduction. For those looking to incorporate a natural detox method into their wellness routine, dandelion root tea offers a gentle, accessible, and effective solution. By aiding the body's detoxification organs, dandelion root tea provides a foundation for long-term health, supporting vitality and resilience against daily environmental stressors.

Ginger and Turmeric Detox Drink

The combination of ginger and turmeric is one of the most powerful and well-known blends in natural medicine, celebrated for its anti-inflammatory, antioxidant, and detoxifying properties. A detox drink featuring ginger and turmeric can be a potent addition to a daily wellness routine, supporting the body's natural detoxification processes and providing a range of health benefits. Ginger and turmeric are both rhizomes, or underground stems, used for centuries in traditional medicine, especially in Ayurvedic and Chinese practices, for their healing and cleansing effects. Together, they form a drink that is not only deeply nourishing but also easy to incorporate into a balanced, natural lifestyle.

The ginger and turmeric detox drink is particularly beneficial for supporting liver health, aiding digestion, reducing inflammation, and boosting immune function. Regular consumption of this drink can help enhance the body's ability to process and eliminate toxins, improve circulation, and promote overall vitality.

Health Benefits of Ginger

Ginger, scientifically known as *Zingiber officinale*, is a versatile herb renowned for its numerous health benefits. It contains bioactive compounds like gingerols and shogaols, which have powerful anti-inflammatory and antioxidant effects. These compounds help reduce oxidative stress in the body, combat inflammation, and support a wide range of bodily functions.

1. **Digestive Health**: Ginger is highly effective for soothing the digestive system. It helps stimulate saliva, bile, and gastric enzymes, which facilitate digestion and prevent bloating, nausea, and indigestion. Ginger is often used to alleviate nausea associated with pregnancy, motion sickness, or chemotherapy, making it a beneficial herb for anyone experiencing digestive discomfort.

2. **Anti-Inflammatory Properties**: The anti-inflammatory effects of ginger make it a valuable natural remedy for joint and muscle pain. By inhibiting pro-inflammatory enzymes and cytokines, ginger reduces inflammation in the body, which is particularly beneficial for those with arthritis or chronic inflammation.

3. **Immune Support**: Ginger has antimicrobial and antiviral properties, which help the immune system defend against pathogens. It's especially useful during cold and flu season, as it helps clear congestion, warms the body, and soothes a sore throat.

4. **Blood Sugar Regulation**: Research suggests that ginger can help improve insulin sensitivity and lower blood sugar levels, making it a helpful herb for individuals

managing diabetes or metabolic syndrome. By supporting stable blood sugar, ginger helps prevent energy dips and enhances overall metabolic health.

Health Benefits of Turmeric

Turmeric, or *Curcuma longa*, is often called the "golden spice" due to its vibrant color and wide array of health benefits. Its active compound, curcumin, is responsible for turmeric's therapeutic effects, offering antioxidant, anti-inflammatory, and detoxifying properties.

1. **Liver Health**: Turmeric is one of the best natural herbs for supporting liver detoxification. Curcumin enhances the liver's ability to produce bile, which helps in the digestion and breakdown of fats. By promoting bile flow, turmeric aids in the removal of toxins from the body, making it an essential herb for anyone focused on liver health and overall detoxification.

2. **Anti-Inflammatory and Antioxidant Effects**: Curcumin is a powerful antioxidant that neutralizes free radicals and reduces oxidative stress. Its anti-inflammatory properties make it effective for managing chronic inflammation and reducing symptoms of inflammatory diseases, such as arthritis and digestive disorders.

3. **Cognitive Health**: Curcumin can cross the blood-brain barrier, providing neuroprotective effects that may help prevent neurodegenerative diseases like Alzheimer's. Regular consumption of turmeric can support mental clarity and reduce brain fog, benefiting individuals looking to enhance cognitive function.

4. **Heart Health**: Turmeric has been shown to reduce the oxidation of LDL cholesterol and improve endothelial function, which is the health of the blood vessels' lining. These effects can help lower the risk of heart disease by promoting circulation and reducing the buildup of plaque in the arteries.

How Ginger and Turmeric Work Together in a Detox Drink

When ginger and turmeric are combined, they create a synergistic effect that enhances each other's benefits. Ginger's warming properties improve circulation, which helps distribute the anti-inflammatory and antioxidant effects of turmeric throughout the body. Together, these ingredients support the body's detox pathways, promoting digestion, liver function, and immune health.

The ginger and turmeric detox drink also aids in hydration, which is essential for detoxification. When the body is well-hydrated, the kidneys can effectively filter out waste and the liver can perform its detox functions more efficiently. This drink is easy to prepare and can be customized with additional ingredients like lemon, black pepper, and honey to further enhance its health benefits.

How to Make a Ginger and Turmeric Detox Drink

Here is a basic recipe for making a ginger and turmeric detox drink:

Ingredients:

- 1-2 inches of fresh ginger root, peeled and grated
- 1-2 inches of fresh turmeric root, peeled and grated (or 1 teaspoon of ground turmeric)
- 2 cups of water
- Juice of half a lemon
- A pinch of black pepper (to enhance curcumin absorption)
- Honey or maple syrup (optional, to taste)

Instructions:

1. Bring the water to a gentle boil in a saucepan.
2. Add the grated ginger and turmeric to the water and let it simmer for about 10-15 minutes.
3. Strain the liquid into a mug.
4. Add the lemon juice, black pepper, and honey or maple syrup if desired.
5. Stir well and enjoy warm.

This drink can be enjoyed in the morning to kickstart the digestive system and liver function, or in the evening for its calming and anti-inflammatory effects.

Enhancing Detox with Additional Ingredients

The basic ginger and turmeric detox drink can be customized with additional ingredients to enhance its detoxifying effects. Some common additions include:

1. **Lemon**: Lemon is rich in vitamin C, a powerful antioxidant that supports liver function and boosts the immune system. The acidity of lemon also aids in digestion and helps maintain the body's pH balance.

2. **Black Pepper**: Adding a pinch of black pepper to the drink increases the bioavailability of curcumin in turmeric, allowing the body to absorb and utilize it more effectively.

3. **Honey**: Raw honey provides natural sweetness and adds antibacterial properties to the drink. Honey can soothe the throat and support immune health, especially when consumed in the colder months.

4. **Cayenne Pepper**: For those who enjoy a bit of spice, a small pinch of cayenne pepper can be added. Cayenne improves circulation and stimulates metabolism, making it a valuable addition to any detox drink.

5. **Cinnamon**: Cinnamon adds warmth and flavor while providing its own antioxidant and anti-inflammatory benefits. It may also help regulate blood sugar levels and improve digestion.

Practical Tips for Incorporating the Ginger and Turmeric Detox Drink

1. **Drink It Regularly**: For optimal benefits, consistency is key. Try drinking the ginger and turmeric detox drink daily or several times a week to support ongoing detoxification and reduce inflammation.

2. **Use Fresh Ingredients When Possible**: Fresh ginger and turmeric roots provide the highest concentration of beneficial compounds. If fresh roots are unavailable, powdered ginger and turmeric can be used, but it's best to select organic powders to avoid additives.

3. **Pair with Hydration**: Detoxification relies heavily on hydration. Drinking plenty of water throughout the day supports the kidneys and helps flush out toxins, enhancing the effects of the detox drink.

4. **Consider Fasting Periods**: Consuming the detox drink on an empty stomach can maximize absorption and allow the body to focus on detoxification. Drinking it first thing in the morning or in the evening before bed can be particularly beneficial.

Potential Health Benefits and Outcomes

By incorporating the ginger and turmeric detox drink into a daily routine, individuals may experience a variety of health benefits, such as:

- **Improved Digestion**: Ginger and turmeric stimulate digestive enzymes, reduce bloating, and promote regular bowel movements, which are crucial for eliminating waste.

- **Reduced Inflammation**: Both ginger and turmeric have strong anti-inflammatory effects, which can alleviate joint and muscle pain, improve flexibility, and support recovery from physical activity.

- **Enhanced Immune Function**: The antimicrobial properties of ginger combined with the immune-boosting effects of turmeric and lemon make this drink ideal for supporting immunity, particularly during cold and flu season.

- **Clearer Skin**: The detoxifying properties of ginger and turmeric help eliminate toxins that contribute to skin issues, resulting in a clearer, healthier complexion.

- **Mental Clarity and Mood Improvement**: Turmeric's effects on brain health, combined with ginger's ability to enhance circulation, may improve mental clarity, reduce brain fog, and support a positive mood.

Safety and Considerations

While the ginger and turmeric detox drink is generally safe for most people, certain individuals should consult a healthcare provider before consuming it regularly, especially those with specific health conditions or sensitivities. For example:

- **Pregnancy and Breastfeeding**: While ginger is commonly used to alleviate pregnancy-related nausea, large amounts of ginger and turmeric should be consumed with caution during pregnancy and breastfeeding.

- **Gallbladder Issues**: Turmeric can stimulate bile production, which may exacerbate symptoms in people with gallbladder problems or bile duct obstruction.

- **Blood Thinners**: Both ginger and turmeric have mild blood-thinning effects. Individuals taking anticoagulant medications should use this drink with caution to avoid potential interactions.

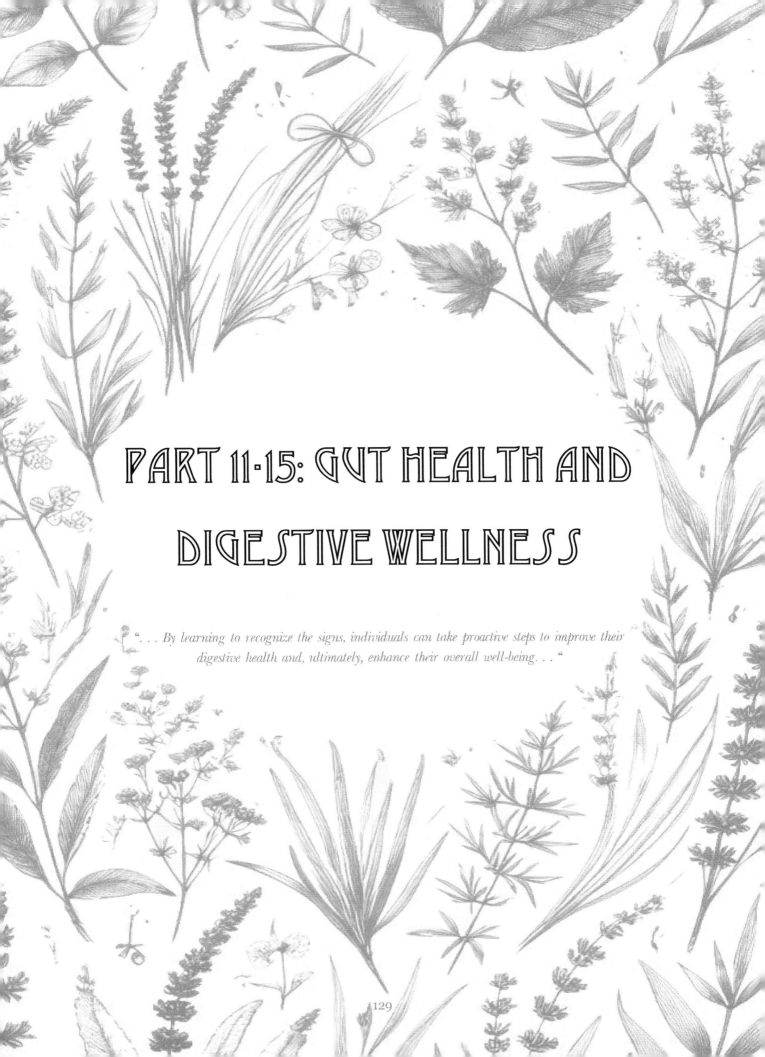

PART 11-15: GUT HEALTH AND DIGESTIVE WELLNESS

"... By learning to recognize the signs, individuals can take proactive steps to improve their digestive health and, ultimately, enhance their overall well-being..."

Chapter 1: Understanding Gut Health

The health of our gut, often referred to as the "second brain," has a profound impact on overall wellness. The digestive system is not only responsible for processing food and absorbing nutrients, but it also plays a key role in immune function, mood regulation, and the prevention of chronic disease.

Signs of Poor Gut Health

When gut health is compromised, a range of physical and mental symptoms can arise, often in subtle ways that are easy to overlook. Understanding the signs of poor gut health is essential for identifying issues early on and taking steps toward restoring balance.

In this section, we'll explore the indicators of poor gut health, the underlying mechanisms that contribute to these issues, and practical strategies for identifying and addressing these symptoms. By learning to recognize the signs, individuals can take proactive steps to improve their digestive health and, ultimately, enhance their overall well-being.

Digestive Discomfort: Bloating, Gas, and Indigestion

One of the most common signs of poor gut health is frequent digestive discomfort, including bloating, gas, and indigestion. While occasional digestive upset is normal, experiencing these symptoms regularly may indicate an imbalance in the gut microbiome or issues with digestive enzyme production.

Bloating often occurs when there is an excess of gas in the digestive tract, which can be caused by an imbalance of gut bacteria, known as dysbiosis. When harmful bacteria or yeast overgrow, they can produce gas as a byproduct, leading to discomfort and visible bloating. This imbalance can also interfere with proper digestion, causing food to ferment rather than break down efficiently.

Indigestion, characterized by a burning sensation in the upper abdomen, can be a result of low stomach acid, which prevents food from being adequately broken down. Without sufficient stomach acid, proteins and fats are not fully digested, leading to discomfort and sometimes acid reflux. Low stomach acid can also affect the absorption of essential nutrients, leading to deficiencies over time.

Irregular Bowel Movements: Constipation and Diarrhea

The frequency and consistency of bowel movements can be a clear indicator of gut health. Regular, well-formed stools are a sign of a balanced gut, while constipation or diarrhea can indicate problems within the digestive system.

Constipation may occur when there is not enough fiber or hydration to support regular bowel movements, but it can also be a result of slow gut motility, often related to an imbalance in the gut microbiome. An overgrowth of certain bacteria can slow down the movement of the digestive tract, causing stool to become hard and difficult to pass.

On the other hand, diarrhea is often a sign of inflammation or irritation in the gut lining, which can result from infections, food sensitivities, or an overgrowth of harmful bacteria. Diarrhea can lead to dehydration and nutrient loss, as the body is unable to absorb essential vitamins and minerals effectively. Chronic or recurring diarrhea may be indicative of underlying issues such as irritable bowel syndrome (IBS) or small intestinal bacterial overgrowth (SIBO).

Food Sensitivities and Intolerances

Another common sign of poor gut health is the development of food sensitivities or intolerances. While food allergies are an immune response to specific proteins, food sensitivities often involve a more subtle reaction within the gut, leading to symptoms like bloating, gas, cramping, and diarrhea.

Poor gut health can compromise the integrity of the gut lining, leading to a condition known as "leaky gut" or increased intestinal permeability. When the gut lining becomes permeable, undigested food particles and toxins can pass into the bloodstream, triggering an immune response. This can result in sensitivities to foods that were previously well-tolerated, such as gluten, dairy, or certain carbohydrates.

Over time, these sensitivities can further disrupt the gut microbiome, as they create a cycle of inflammation and irritation in the digestive system. Identifying and addressing food sensitivities is essential for restoring gut health and preventing further issues.

Frequent Fatigue and Low Energy

The gut plays a crucial role in energy production, as it is responsible for breaking down food and absorbing nutrients that fuel the body. When gut health is compromised, the body may struggle to absorb essential vitamins and minerals, leading to fatigue and low energy.

Chronic fatigue may also be related to inflammation within the gut. When the gut lining is inflamed or irritated, the immune system may become overactive, causing the body to expend more energy fighting off perceived threats. This constant state of immune activation can drain the body's energy resources, leading to feelings of tiredness even after a full night's sleep.

The gut also influences neurotransmitter production, including serotonin, which regulates mood and energy levels. Poor gut health can disrupt this process, further contributing to fatigue and reduced mental clarity. Individuals experiencing persistent fatigue, despite a healthy diet and adequate sleep, may need to consider gut health as a potential underlying factor.

Skin Issues: Acne, Eczema, and Rashes

The connection between gut health and skin health is well-established. Conditions such as acne, eczema, and other skin rashes are often linked to imbalances in the gut microbiome and inflammation within the digestive system. When the gut is unable to properly process and eliminate toxins, these substances may be expelled through the skin, leading to breakouts and irritation.

Dysbiosis, or an imbalance of gut bacteria, can also trigger inflammation throughout the body, including the skin. For example, an overgrowth of harmful bacteria can lead to systemic inflammation, which is associated with acne and other skin issues. Additionally, a compromised gut lining can lead to leaky gut, allowing toxins to enter the bloodstream and potentially triggering inflammatory skin conditions like eczema.

Many individuals notice improvements in their skin after addressing gut health through dietary changes, probiotics, and other gut-supportive practices. By focusing on the root cause, rather than solely treating the skin externally, it is often possible to achieve longer-lasting improvements.

Brain Fog, Anxiety, and Mood Swings

The gut-brain connection is a complex communication network linking the gut and brain through the vagus nerve and various signaling pathways. As a result, poor gut health can have a significant impact on mental well-being, contributing to symptoms such as brain fog, anxiety, and mood swings.

An imbalanced gut microbiome can disrupt the production of neurotransmitters like serotonin and dopamine, which play essential roles in mood regulation and cognitive function. Serotonin, often referred to as the "feel-good" neurotransmitter, is largely produced in the gut, making gut health critical for mental health. When the gut is out of balance, serotonin production may decrease, contributing to feelings of anxiety, irritability, and mood instability.

Brain fog, a condition characterized by confusion, forgetfulness, and difficulty concentrating, is also commonly linked to gut health. Chronic inflammation and the presence of toxins due to poor gut function can affect brain function, impairing mental clarity. Those who experience frequent mental fatigue and mood swings may benefit from exploring ways to support gut health to improve mental clarity and emotional stability.

Frequent Infections and Weakened Immunity

Approximately 70% of the immune system resides in the gut, where it interacts closely with gut bacteria to defend against pathogens. A healthy gut microbiome helps stimulate and regulate immune function, while an imbalanced gut can weaken the immune response, making the body more susceptible to infections.

When the gut lining is compromised, the body's defenses against harmful bacteria and viruses may be weakened, increasing the risk of illness. Individuals with poor gut health often experience frequent colds, respiratory infections, and other minor illnesses, as their immune system struggles to fend off threats effectively. Supporting gut health through probiotics, a nutrient-rich diet, and other natural remedies can help strengthen immunity and reduce the likelihood of infections.

Weight Fluctuations and Difficulty Managing Weight

Gut health plays a role in weight management, as the bacteria in the gut influence metabolism, energy storage, and the balance of hormones that regulate hunger and fullness.

Dysbiosis can affect the way the body processes and stores nutrients, leading to weight gain or loss that may be difficult to control.

For example, certain bacteria in the gut produce short-chain fatty acids, which regulate fat storage and energy expenditure. An imbalance in these bacteria can disrupt this process, leading to increased fat storage or reduced energy levels. Additionally, poor gut health can lead to cravings for sugar and processed foods, which further contribute to weight gain and blood sugar imbalances.

Addressing gut health through dietary changes, probiotics, and other natural methods can help restore balance and support healthy weight management. For those struggling with unexplained weight fluctuations, gut health may be an overlooked factor that can provide insights into their challenges.

Autoimmune Conditions and Chronic Inflammation

An unhealthy gut is often associated with chronic inflammation, which can contribute to the development of autoimmune conditions. When the gut lining becomes permeable, or "leaky," toxins and undigested food particles can enter the bloodstream, triggering an immune response. Over time, this immune activation can lead to chronic inflammation, which is a risk factor for autoimmune diseases such as rheumatoid arthritis, lupus, and multiple sclerosis.

Autoimmune conditions are characterized by the immune system attacking the body's own tissues, often due to a miscommunication caused by chronic inflammation. By improving gut health and reducing gut permeability, it may be possible to lower inflammation levels and reduce the risk of developing autoimmune conditions. For those with existing autoimmune disorders, supporting gut health can help alleviate symptoms and improve quality of life.

Poor Gut Health and Hormonal Imbalances

The gut plays an essential role in hormone regulation, including the processing of estrogen, cortisol, and insulin. Poor gut health can disrupt the delicate balance of these hormones, leading to issues such as insulin resistance, estrogen dominance, and adrenal fatigue.

For example, the gut microbiome is involved in the metabolism of estrogen. When the gut is imbalanced, estrogen may not be properly metabolized, leading to an excess of this hormone in the body. This condition, known as estrogen dominance, is associated with symptoms like weight gain, mood swings, and menstrual irregularities.

An unhealthy gut can also increase levels of cortisol, the body's stress hormone. Chronic stress and poor gut health often go hand-in-hand, creating a cycle that exacerbates hormonal imbalances and contributes to fatigue, weight gain, and mood disturbances.

Recognizing the signs of poor gut health is essential for taking proactive steps to restore balance and enhance overall wellness. By addressing these symptoms early and adopting gut-friendly practices, individuals can support their digestive system, immune function, mental clarity, and long-term health.

Chapter 2: Foods for Digestive Health

Probiotics are beneficial microorganisms that play a vital role in maintaining gut health, boosting immunity, and enhancing overall wellness. Probiotic-rich foods contain live cultures of these helpful bacteria and yeasts, which populate the gut and promote a balanced microbiome.

Probiotic-Rich Foods

This microbiome, consisting of trillions of microorganisms, affects digestion, mental health, immune response, and even weight management. Including probiotic-rich foods in a diet can be one of the most natural and effective ways to support gut health and improve overall well-being.

For those interested in natural healing, understanding the benefits and uses of probiotic-rich foods can be transformative. Incorporating these foods into daily meals not only supports the digestive system but also fosters resilience against illnesses and stress. In the American market, fermented foods have gained popularity as accessible sources of probiotics, allowing people to make health-conscious choices that align with a balanced lifestyle.

The Importance of Gut Health and Probiotics

The gut is often referred to as the "second brain" due to the extensive communication between the gut and brain through the gut-brain axis. The balance of bacteria in the gut microbiome influences everything from mental clarity to immune function, and disruptions in this balance can lead to digestive discomfort, inflammation, and mood disorders. Probiotics play a critical role in maintaining this balance by promoting beneficial bacteria, inhibiting harmful bacteria, and supporting the overall integrity of the gut lining.

A healthy microbiome contributes to nutrient absorption, production of certain vitamins (such as B vitamins and vitamin K), and the breakdown of dietary fibers into short-chain fatty acids (SCFAs) that provide energy to the cells lining the gut. This delicate ecosystem can be disrupted by factors like poor diet, antibiotics, stress, and environmental toxins, which is why maintaining a regular intake of probiotic-rich foods is essential for sustaining a resilient gut.

Types of Probiotic-Rich Foods and Their Benefits

Many traditional cultures have long included fermented foods in their diets, recognizing their health-promoting properties. These foods undergo a natural fermentation process that enhances both their flavor and nutrient profile, while also introducing beneficial bacteria. Here are some of the most well-known and widely available probiotic-rich foods:

1. **Yogurt**: Yogurt is one of the most popular and well-studied sources of probiotics. It is made by fermenting milk with bacterial cultures, typically *Lactobacillus bulgaricus* and *Streptococcus thermophilus*. These bacteria help improve lactose digestion, making yogurt a suitable option even for some people with lactose intolerance. Yogurt is particularly beneficial for gut health, as it can enhance the diversity of beneficial bacteria, support regular bowel movements, and prevent the overgrowth of harmful bacteria.

How to Use: Yogurt can be enjoyed on its own, with fruits, or added to smoothies. To ensure maximum probiotic benefits, choose plain, unsweetened yogurt with live and active cultures.

2. **Kefir**: Kefir is a fermented milk drink that is similar to yogurt but contains a more diverse range of bacterial and yeast strains. It has a slightly tangy taste and a thinner consistency than yogurt. Kefir provides a more potent dose of probiotics and has been shown to aid digestion, reduce inflammation, and improve bone health due to its high calcium content.

How to Use: Kefir can be consumed as a drink, added to smoothies, or used as a base for salad dressings. Like yogurt, it's best to choose unsweetened kefir with live cultures for maximum benefits.

3. **Sauerkraut**: Sauerkraut is made by fermenting finely chopped cabbage with salt, creating a sour and tangy food rich in probiotics and fiber. The fermentation process in sauerkraut encourages the growth of *Lactobacillus* bacteria, which support digestion and boost immune health. Sauerkraut is also high in vitamins C and K, contributing to its overall nutritional value.

How to Use: Sauerkraut can be enjoyed as a side dish, topping for sandwiches, or mixed into salads. To retain the probiotic benefits, look for raw, unpasteurized sauerkraut, as pasteurization kills beneficial bacteria.

4. **Kimchi**: Kimchi is a traditional Korean side dish made from fermented vegetables, typically napa cabbage and radishes, seasoned with chili pepper, garlic, ginger, and other spices. Kimchi is rich in *Lactobacillus* bacteria, as well as antioxidants and anti-inflammatory compounds from the vegetables and spices. It is known for supporting digestion, reducing inflammation, and enhancing immune health.

How to Use: Kimchi can be eaten on its own, added to rice and noodle dishes, or used as a flavorful topping for salads and tacos. As with sauerkraut, it's important to select unpasteurized kimchi to ensure live probiotics.

5. **Miso**: Miso is a fermented paste made from soybeans, rice, or barley. It is commonly used in Japanese cuisine, particularly in soups and sauces. Miso contains a variety of probiotic bacteria, including *Tetragenococcus halophilus*, which aids in digestion and supports immune function. Miso is also high in minerals such as manganese and zinc, adding to its nutritional profile.

How to Use: Miso can be added to soups, salad dressings, and marinades. It's best not to boil miso, as high temperatures can destroy the beneficial bacteria. Instead, add it to warm dishes just before serving.

6. **Tempeh**: Tempeh is a fermented soybean product originating from Indonesia. It has a firm texture and a nutty flavor and is rich in protein, fiber, and probiotics. Unlike tofu, which is unfermented, tempeh contains beneficial bacteria that support gut health and provide a range of nutrients, including B vitamins, magnesium, and iron.

How to Use: Tempeh can be sliced, marinated, and grilled, or added to stir-fries and salads. Its firm texture makes it a good meat substitute in plant-based diets.

7. **Kombucha**: Kombucha is a fermented tea drink made with black or green tea and a culture of bacteria and yeast known as a SCOBY (symbiotic culture of bacteria and yeast). This drink is lightly fizzy and slightly tangy, offering a variety of probiotics that support digestion and detoxification. Kombucha is also a source of antioxidants from the tea, which can provide additional health benefits.

How to Use: Kombucha is typically enjoyed as a beverage. It can be found in various flavors, though it's best to choose varieties with minimal added sugars.

8. **Pickles**: Pickled cucumbers, when fermented naturally with saltwater rather than vinegar, can be a source of probiotics. The fermentation process produces beneficial bacteria that support gut health. However, not all pickles are probiotic-rich, as many are made with vinegar, which doesn't encourage probiotic growth.

How to Use: Pickles can be eaten as a snack, added to sandwiches, or chopped into salads. To ensure probiotic content, select pickles labeled as fermented or raw.

Practical Tips for Incorporating Probiotic-Rich Foods

Including probiotic-rich foods in your daily diet doesn't have to be complicated. These foods can be easily integrated into meals to enhance both flavor and nutrition:

1. **Start Small**: For those new to probiotic-rich foods, it's best to start with small servings and gradually increase. This allows the body to adjust to the influx of beneficial bacteria, minimizing digestive discomfort.

2. **Include a Variety of Sources**: Different probiotic foods contain different strains of beneficial bacteria. Incorporating a variety of probiotic-rich foods ensures exposure to a broader range of bacterial strains, which supports a more diverse gut microbiome.

3. **Combine with Prebiotic Foods**: Prebiotics are fibers that feed beneficial bacteria in the gut, enhancing the effectiveness of probiotics. Foods rich in prebiotics include garlic, onions, asparagus, bananas, and oats. Combining probiotic-rich and prebiotic-rich foods helps create a supportive environment for gut health.

4. **Consume Probiotics Regularly**: To maintain a balanced microbiome, consistency is key. Regularly including probiotic-rich foods in your diet can help sustain the beneficial bacteria population and support long-term gut health.

5. **Pair with Hydration**: Drinking enough water helps the digestive system function smoothly and aids in the transport of probiotics throughout the gut.

Potential Health Benefits of Probiotic-Rich Foods

Regularly consuming probiotic-rich foods can offer a wide range of health benefits:

- **Enhanced Digestive Health**: Probiotics aid in breaking down food, absorbing nutrients, and supporting regular bowel movements. They can also reduce symptoms of irritable bowel syndrome (IBS), such as bloating, gas, and discomfort.

- **Improved Immunity**: A significant portion of the immune system is located in the gut. By supporting a healthy microbiome, probiotics can enhance immune response and reduce the risk of infections.
- **Mood and Mental Health Support**: The gut-brain axis links gut health to mental well-being. Probiotics can positively impact mood, reduce stress, and alleviate symptoms of anxiety and depression by supporting neurotransmitter production and reducing inflammation.
- **Weight Management**: Certain strains of probiotics have been associated with weight regulation. Probiotics can influence appetite, metabolism, and the storage of fat, which may support weight loss or maintenance.
- **Skin Health**: The gut-skin connection suggests that a healthy microbiome can improve skin conditions like acne, eczema, and rosacea. By reducing inflammation and promoting detoxification, probiotics contribute to clearer, healthier skin.

Choosing Quality Probiotic Foods

When selecting probiotic-rich foods, quality matters. Here are some tips for choosing the best options:

1. **Check for Live Cultures**: Look for products that specify "live and active cultures" on the label. This indicates that the food contains live probiotics, which are essential for gut health benefits.
2. **Avoid Added Sugars and Artificial Ingredients**: Many commercial probiotic products, particularly yogurts and kombucha, contain added sugars and artificial flavors. Choosing plain, unsweetened versions allows for a purer probiotic experience.
3. **Opt for Organic and Non-GMO**: Organic and non-GMO options help reduce exposure to pesticides and additives, which can interfere with gut health and reduce the effectiveness of probiotics.
4. **Choose Unpasteurized Varieties**: Pasteurization kills both harmful and beneficial bacteria, so fermented foods that are pasteurized may not contain live probiotics. Look for unpasteurized options to ensure maximum benefit.

Integrating Probiotics into a Holistic Health Routine

Incorporating probiotic-rich foods into a daily diet can be a cornerstone of holistic health. By supporting gut health, these foods enhance the body's resilience and foster a sense of vitality that extends beyond digestion. For those interested in natural herbal remedies and wellness, probiotic foods offer a simple yet powerful way to nourish the body from the inside out, contributing to a balanced and sustainable approach to health.

Fiber Sources

Fiber is an essential component of a healthy diet, playing a key role in digestive health, blood sugar regulation, and overall wellness. While often overlooked, fiber provides numerous benefits to the body by supporting gut health, preventing constipation, and aiding in weight management. There are two primary types of dietary fiber—soluble and insoluble—each with unique properties that contribute to health in different ways. Soluble fiber dissolves in water to form a gel-like substance, which helps regulate blood sugar and cholesterol levels, while insoluble fiber adds bulk to stool, promoting regular bowel movements and preventing constipation.

Understanding where to find fiber-rich foods and how to incorporate them into daily meals is crucial for those aiming to improve or maintain gut health. This section will explore the different types of fiber sources, their benefits, and practical ways to include them in a balanced diet.

The Role of Fiber in Gut Health

Fiber is vital for gut health because it supports a balanced microbiome, which consists of trillions of bacteria that reside in the digestive tract. These beneficial bacteria feed on fiber, particularly soluble fiber, and produce short-chain fatty acids (SCFAs) like butyrate, which play a crucial role in reducing inflammation, supporting immune function, and maintaining the integrity of the gut lining. A diet rich in fiber promotes the growth of these beneficial bacteria, while a low-fiber diet can lead to dysbiosis, or an imbalance in the microbiome, which is associated with digestive issues, inflammation, and an increased risk of chronic diseases.

Fiber also aids in regular bowel movements by adding bulk to stool, making it easier to pass through the digestive system. This process helps prevent constipation, reduce the risk of hemorrhoids, and eliminate waste products from the body efficiently. Regular elimination is essential for detoxification, as it prevents toxins from accumulating in the digestive tract.

Types of Fiber: Soluble and Insoluble

Soluble Fiber: Soluble fiber dissolves in water and forms a gel-like substance in the digestive tract. This gel slows down digestion, helping to stabilize blood sugar levels by slowing the absorption of glucose. It also binds to cholesterol in the gut, reducing its absorption and helping to lower cholesterol levels. Common sources of soluble fiber include oats, barley, chia seeds, flaxseeds, apples, and citrus fruits.

Insoluble Fiber: Insoluble fiber does not dissolve in water, and it adds bulk to stool, which helps promote regular bowel movements. This type of fiber acts as a natural laxative, moving waste through the intestines more efficiently and preventing constipation. Insoluble fiber is found in foods such as whole grains, nuts, seeds, and the skins of fruits and vegetables.

Both types of fiber are essential for a balanced diet, as they work together to support various aspects of health, from gut function to metabolic health. Including a variety of fiber sources ensures that the body receives both soluble and insoluble fibers, enhancing overall digestive health.

Top Sources of Fiber

1. **Fruits and Vegetables**

Fruits and vegetables are excellent sources of fiber, especially when consumed with their skins. Apples, pears, and berries are particularly high in fiber, with apples providing around 4 grams of fiber per medium fruit, primarily in the skin. Berries, such as raspberries and blackberries, offer about 8 grams of fiber per cup, making them one of the richest sources among fruits.

Vegetables like carrots, broccoli, and Brussels sprouts are also high in fiber. For example, one cup of cooked Brussels sprouts contains about 4 grams of fiber, while a medium carrot has roughly 2 grams. Leafy greens like spinach and kale contain fiber, though in smaller amounts, and can be paired with other vegetables to increase fiber intake.

Practical Tip: To maximize fiber intake, aim to include fruits and vegetables with every meal. Adding berries to breakfast, snacking on apples, or including a side salad with lunch or dinner are easy ways to boost fiber intake naturally.

2. **Whole Grains**

Whole grains are a rich source of insoluble fiber, especially when consumed in their unrefined form. Brown rice, quinoa, oats, barley, and bulgur are all high-fiber grains that support gut health and stabilize blood sugar levels. One cup of cooked oatmeal provides around 4 grams of fiber, while a cup of cooked quinoa contains about 5 grams.

Choosing whole grains over refined grains ensures that the outer bran layer, which is rich in fiber, remains intact. This layer also contains essential nutrients like B vitamins, iron, and magnesium, making whole grains a nutritious addition to any diet.

Practical Tip: Replace refined grains with whole grains whenever possible. Instead of white rice, choose brown rice or quinoa, and opt for whole-grain bread and pasta instead of white varieties. Including oats or whole-grain cereals at breakfast is another simple way to increase fiber intake.

3. Legumes

Legumes, including beans, lentils, chickpeas, and peas, are some of the most fiber-dense foods available. A cup of cooked lentils provides around 15 grams of fiber, while black beans contain about 15 grams per cup as well. These high levels make legumes an excellent choice for those aiming to boost fiber intake.

Legumes are also rich in protein, making them a valuable addition to plant-based diets. In addition to supporting gut health, legumes help maintain stable blood sugar levels, as their high fiber content slows digestion and prevents rapid glucose spikes.

Practical Tip: Incorporate legumes into meals by adding them to soups, stews, salads, and grain bowls. Hummus, made from chickpeas, is another fiber-rich option that can be enjoyed as a dip or spread.

4. Nuts and Seeds

Nuts and seeds are not only rich in healthy fats but also provide a good amount of fiber. For example, almonds contain around 3.5 grams of fiber per ounce (about 23 almonds), while chia seeds offer a whopping 10 grams of fiber per ounce (about 2 tablespoons). Flaxseeds are also high in fiber, with around 7 grams per ounce.

These nutrient-dense foods provide both soluble and insoluble fiber, along with protein, antioxidants, and essential fatty acids that support heart health and reduce inflammation.

Practical Tip: Add chia seeds or ground flaxseeds to smoothies, oatmeal, or yogurt. Nuts like almonds and walnuts make great fiber-rich snacks, while sunflower or pumpkin seeds can be sprinkled on salads for added fiber and crunch.

5. Root Vegetables and Tubers

Root vegetables like sweet potatoes, carrots, and beets are excellent sources of fiber. Sweet potatoes, for example, contain about 4 grams of fiber per medium-sized potato, primarily in the skin. Root vegetables are also high in essential vitamins and minerals, including vitamin A, potassium, and magnesium.

Tubers, such as potatoes and yams, also provide fiber, particularly if consumed with their skins. These starchy vegetables offer both soluble and insoluble fiber, supporting digestion and helping to regulate blood sugar.

Practical Tip: Incorporate root vegetables into meals by roasting them as a side dish or adding them to soups and stews. Leaving the skin on when possible maximizes fiber content.

Benefits of a High-Fiber Diet

1. **Supports Digestive Health**: Fiber adds bulk to stool, which promotes regular bowel movements and prevents constipation. A high-fiber diet also supports a balanced gut microbiome, as beneficial bacteria feed on fiber and produce SCFAs, which have anti-inflammatory effects and protect the gut lining.

2. **Regulates Blood Sugar Levels**: Soluble fiber slows the absorption of glucose, preventing rapid blood sugar spikes. This is particularly beneficial for individuals with diabetes or those at risk of developing the condition, as it helps maintain stable blood sugar levels and improves insulin sensitivity.

3. **Aids in Weight Management**: High-fiber foods are often more filling, as they require longer chewing and digest more slowly. This leads to increased satiety, which can reduce overall calorie intake and support weight management. Fiber also promotes the release of satiety hormones, helping individuals feel full longer.

4. **Lowers Cholesterol Levels**: Soluble fiber binds to cholesterol in the gut and prevents it from being absorbed into the bloodstream. This can help reduce total cholesterol levels, particularly LDL (low-density lipoprotein) cholesterol, which is linked to an increased risk of heart disease.

5. **Reduces Risk of Chronic Diseases**: Studies show that high-fiber diets are associated with a lower risk of various chronic diseases, including heart disease, type 2 diabetes, and certain cancers. The anti-inflammatory and blood sugar-stabilizing effects of fiber contribute to these protective benefits.

Fiber Supplements: When and How to Use Them

For individuals struggling to get enough fiber from food alone, fiber supplements can be a helpful addition. Common types include psyllium husk, methylcellulose, and inulin. Psyllium husk is a soluble fiber supplement that forms a gel in the digestive tract, supporting bowel regularity and reducing cholesterol levels.

While fiber supplements can be beneficial, they should be used with caution. It's important to increase fiber intake gradually to avoid digestive discomfort and to drink plenty of water, as fiber requires hydration to function effectively. Supplements should not replace whole-food sources of fiber, as whole foods provide additional nutrients and phytochemicals that contribute to health.

Increasing Fiber Intake Gradually

For those new to a high-fiber diet, it's essential to increase fiber intake gradually. A sudden increase can lead to bloating, gas, and digestive discomfort, as the gut microbiome adjusts to the higher fiber levels. Start by adding small portions of fiber-rich foods to meals and gradually increase the amount over several weeks.

Additionally, staying well-hydrated is crucial when consuming more fiber, as water helps move fiber through the digestive tract and prevents constipation.

Practical Strategies for a Fiber-Rich Diet

Incorporating fiber-rich foods into daily meals can be enjoyable and easy with a few practical strategies:

- **Start the Day with Fiber**: Choose whole-grain cereals, oatmeal with fruit, or a smoothie with chia or flaxseeds for breakfast to set a fiber-rich foundation for the day.
- **Make Vegetables the Star**: Add vegetables to every meal, whether in salads, stir-fries, or soups, and experiment with a variety of colors and textures.
- **Snack Smartly**: Nuts, seeds, and fruit make convenient fiber-rich snacks that can be enjoyed on the go.
- **Explore Legumes**: Include beans, lentils, and chickpeas in salads, stews, and even as spreads like hummus to increase fiber intake.

By following these strategies, individuals can enjoy the numerous health benefits of fiber while maintaining a balanced and nourishing diet.

Soluble Fiber and Its Benefits

Soluble fiber is a type of dietary fiber that dissolves in water to form a gel-like substance, which plays a significant role in supporting digestive health, regulating blood sugar, and maintaining heart health. Unlike insoluble fiber, which primarily aids in moving food through the digestive tract, soluble fiber slows digestion and offers a range of health benefits by binding to water in the digestive system. This type of fiber is found in a variety of plant-based foods, including oats, legumes, fruits, and certain vegetables, making it a valuable addition to a balanced diet.

Incorporating adequate amounts of soluble fiber into daily meals is essential for promoting long-term health, as it contributes to gut health, supports immune function, and helps maintain steady energy levels. For those interested in natural health and herbal remedies, understanding the benefits of soluble fiber and the best sources can empower them to make dietary choices that improve their overall well-being and support natural detoxification.

The Role of Soluble Fiber in Digestive Health

One of the primary functions of soluble fiber is its ability to support digestive health by slowing down the movement of food through the intestines. This slow movement allows for more complete nutrient absorption and helps prevent digestive issues such as constipation and diarrhea. The gel-like substance formed by soluble fiber creates a coating along the intestinal lining, protecting the gut wall and promoting the growth of beneficial bacteria.

A healthy digestive system is essential for effective detoxification, as it enables the body to process waste efficiently and remove toxins through regular bowel movements. Soluble fiber contributes to this process by feeding beneficial bacteria in the gut, particularly those that produce short-chain fatty acids (SCFAs), which help reduce inflammation and maintain the integrity of the gut barrier.

Additionally, soluble fiber helps prevent digestive discomfort by softening stools, making it easier for waste to pass through the colon. This action can reduce the risk of developing hemorrhoids and other digestive problems associated with irregular bowel movements.

Soluble Fiber and Blood Sugar Control

One of the most well-known benefits of soluble fiber is its role in regulating blood sugar levels. Soluble fiber slows down the absorption of glucose in the intestines, which helps prevent rapid spikes in blood sugar after meals. This effect is especially beneficial for individuals with diabetes or those at risk of developing diabetes, as it supports insulin sensitivity and reduces the likelihood of blood sugar fluctuations.

When soluble fiber forms a gel in the digestive tract, it traps sugars and slows their release into the bloodstream. This gradual release keeps blood sugar levels stable and provides sustained energy throughout the day. By including soluble fiber-rich foods in meals, individuals can better manage their blood sugar levels, avoid energy crashes, and reduce cravings for sugary snacks.

Soluble fiber has also been shown to improve insulin response by enhancing the body's ability to utilize glucose effectively. This improvement in insulin sensitivity is important not only for diabetes prevention but also for metabolic health, as it supports weight management and reduces the risk of cardiovascular diseases.

Heart Health Benefits of Soluble Fiber

Soluble fiber is particularly beneficial for heart health, as it has been shown to lower LDL (low-density lipoprotein) cholesterol levels, often referred to as "bad" cholesterol. High levels of LDL cholesterol contribute to the buildup of plaque in the arteries, which increases the risk of atherosclerosis, heart attacks, and strokes. Soluble fiber binds to cholesterol in the digestive tract, preventing it from being absorbed into the bloodstream and allowing it to be excreted from the body.

Studies have shown that individuals who consume high amounts of soluble fiber have lower cholesterol levels and a reduced risk of heart disease. In addition to lowering LDL cholesterol, soluble fiber may also help raise HDL (high-density lipoprotein) cholesterol, known as "good" cholesterol, which supports heart health by transporting cholesterol away from the arteries and back to the liver for removal.

Moreover, the anti-inflammatory properties of soluble fiber contribute to heart health by reducing inflammation in blood vessels. Chronic inflammation is a major risk factor for heart disease, and soluble fiber's ability to support a healthy inflammatory response is a valuable asset in a heart-healthy diet.

Sources of Soluble Fiber

Soluble fiber is found in a variety of plant-based foods, making it easy to incorporate into meals for a fiber-rich diet. Here are some of the best sources of soluble fiber:

1. **Oats**: Oats are one of the richest sources of soluble fiber, particularly in the form of beta-glucan, a type of fiber known for its cholesterol-lowering effects. Beta-glucan also helps stabilize blood sugar levels and supports immune function.

2. **Legumes**: Beans, lentils, and peas are high in soluble fiber and provide protein and complex carbohydrates. The fiber in legumes supports digestion and promotes satiety, making them ideal for weight management and blood sugar control.

3. **Fruits**: Fruits such as apples, oranges, pears, and berries are high in soluble fiber, especially in the skin and pulp. These fruits are also rich in antioxidants, vitamins, and minerals that support overall health.

4. **Vegetables**: Certain vegetables, like carrots, broccoli, and Brussels sprouts, contain soluble fiber along with a variety of essential nutrients. Including these vegetables in meals adds bulk to the diet, supporting digestive health and reducing cholesterol levels.

5. **Nuts and Seeds**: Nuts and seeds, particularly chia seeds and flaxseeds, are high in soluble fiber and healthy fats. They are an excellent addition to smoothies, yogurt, and oatmeal for a fiber boost.

6. **Barley**: Barley is another grain rich in beta-glucan, making it beneficial for heart health. It has a chewy texture and can be added to soups, stews, and salads for a nutritious fiber source.

By incorporating a variety of these foods into daily meals, individuals can ensure they are meeting their soluble fiber needs and reaping the health benefits associated with a fiber-rich diet.

Practical Tips for Increasing Soluble Fiber Intake

1. **Start Gradually**: For those new to a high-fiber diet, it's important to increase soluble fiber intake gradually to allow the digestive system to adjust. This can help prevent gas, bloating, and discomfort that sometimes accompany a sudden increase in fiber.

2. **Stay Hydrated**: Soluble fiber absorbs water to form a gel, so drinking enough water is essential for it to work effectively. Adequate hydration ensures that fiber moves smoothly through the digestive tract, preventing constipation.

3. **Combine Soluble and Insoluble Fiber**: A balance of both types of fiber is beneficial for digestive health. Insoluble fiber adds bulk to stools, while soluble fiber

softens them, creating a balanced digestive process. Including a variety of fiber-rich foods provides a mix of both types.

4. **Add Fiber-Rich Foods to Every Meal**: Incorporating soluble fiber-rich foods into each meal supports steady blood sugar levels and provides sustained energy. For example, adding oatmeal to breakfast, a salad with beans for lunch, and roasted vegetables for dinner ensures a steady intake of soluble fiber throughout the day.

5. **Opt for Whole Foods Over Processed Fiber Supplements**: While fiber supplements are available, whole foods provide additional nutrients and bioactive compounds that enhance fiber's health benefits. Eating a variety of fruits, vegetables, grains, and legumes offers a more comprehensive approach to fiber intake.

The Role of Soluble Fiber in Weight Management

Soluble fiber plays a role in weight management by promoting satiety and reducing overall calorie intake. When soluble fiber forms a gel in the stomach, it slows the emptying of food from the stomach into the small intestine, which creates a feeling of fullness that can reduce the urge to snack between meals. This effect can be beneficial for those aiming to manage their weight, as it helps regulate appetite and supports mindful eating.

Additionally, soluble fiber influences the release of appetite-regulating hormones, such as ghrelin, which signals hunger, and peptide YY (PYY), which signals fullness. By balancing these hormones, soluble fiber supports a healthy relationship with food and can contribute to long-term weight management.

Soluble fiber's impact on blood sugar regulation is also important for weight management, as stable blood sugar levels reduce cravings for sugary snacks and prevent energy crashes. By promoting balanced energy levels, soluble fiber supports individuals in making healthier food choices and avoiding overeating.

Soluble Fiber and Gut Health

The gel-like substance formed by soluble fiber in the digestive tract provides food for beneficial bacteria, particularly those that produce short-chain fatty acids (SCFAs) like butyrate, acetate, and propionate. These SCFAs play a critical role in maintaining gut health by reducing inflammation, strengthening the gut barrier, and promoting immune function. SCFAs also help regulate pH levels in the gut, creating an environment that discourages the growth of harmful bacteria.

A balanced gut microbiome is essential for nutrient absorption, immune defense, and even mood regulation, as the gut is closely connected to the brain through the gut-brain axis. By feeding beneficial bacteria, soluble fiber helps maintain this balance and supports a healthy, resilient gut microbiome.

For individuals with conditions like irritable bowel syndrome (IBS), soluble fiber can be especially beneficial, as it is often easier to tolerate than insoluble fiber and can help regulate bowel movements. Soluble fiber's gentle action on the digestive system makes it a suitable choice for those with sensitive digestion, as it reduces symptoms of constipation and diarrhea without causing irritation.

Soluble Fiber and Detoxification

Soluble fiber plays a role in detoxification by binding to waste products, toxins, and excess cholesterol in the digestive tract, facilitating their elimination from the body. This binding action prevents toxins from being reabsorbed into the bloodstream, reducing the body's toxic load and supporting liver health.

The liver relies on the digestive system to remove waste effectively, as it processes toxins into compounds that are excreted through bile. Soluble fiber helps bind to these compounds, promoting their removal through the digestive system and reducing the burden on the liver. This detoxifying effect of soluble fiber contributes to overall wellness by supporting the body's natural cleansing processes.

By understanding the diverse benefits of soluble fiber and incorporating it into daily meals, individuals can support their digestive health, heart health, and overall well-being. Soluble fiber is a powerful component of a balanced diet, offering practical and accessible ways to enhance health through natural, plant-based foods.

Insoluble Fiber for Regularity

Insoluble fiber is an essential component of a balanced diet, playing a critical role in maintaining digestive health and promoting regular bowel movements. Unlike soluble fiber, which dissolves in water to form a gel-like substance, insoluble fiber does not dissolve. Instead, it adds bulk to the stool, facilitating movement through the digestive tract. This unique property of insoluble fiber makes it an invaluable tool for preventing constipation and supporting gut health.

In this section, we will explore the specific benefits of insoluble fiber for regularity, its mechanisms of action in the digestive system, and the best dietary sources of this type of fiber. We will also provide practical tips for incorporating more insoluble fiber into your daily diet, ensuring you receive its full range of health benefits.

Understanding Insoluble Fiber and Its Role in Digestion

Insoluble fiber, often referred to as "roughage," is made up of plant-based compounds that the body cannot digest or absorb. This type of fiber passes through the digestive system largely intact, helping to move other food and waste along with it. The primary function of insoluble fiber is to add bulk to the stool, which aids in preventing constipation and promoting regular bowel movements.

The structure of insoluble fiber allows it to retain water, increasing the volume of stool and making it easier to pass. By doing so, it helps maintain a steady transit time through the intestines, preventing waste from lingering too long in the digestive tract, which could lead to discomfort and bloating. This mechanism also supports detoxification, as it helps expel waste products and toxins from the body more efficiently.

The Benefits of Insoluble Fiber for Digestive Regularity

1. **Prevention of Constipation**: Insoluble fiber is particularly effective at preventing constipation, as it adds bulk to stool and helps food pass more quickly through the stomach and intestines. Regular consumption of insoluble fiber can reduce the risk of developing chronic constipation, which can lead to other digestive issues such as hemorrhoids and diverticulitis.

2. **Promotes Healthy Gut Bacteria**: Although insoluble fiber is not digested by the body, it plays an indirect role in supporting gut health. By speeding up the passage of food, it prevents harmful bacteria from growing in the intestines, reducing the likelihood of gut-related issues and maintaining a balanced microbiome. Insoluble fiber also aids in the production of short-chain fatty acids by acting as a substrate for some beneficial bacteria.

3. **Supports Colon Health**: The faster transit time promoted by insoluble fiber helps reduce the amount of time waste spends in the colon, which may reduce the risk of certain digestive disorders, including colorectal cancer. By keeping the intestines

clean and free of waste buildup, insoluble fiber contributes to a healthier digestive tract overall.

4. **Prevents Bloating and Gas**: Slow-moving food in the digestive tract can ferment, leading to gas production and bloating. By promoting efficient digestion and regular bowel movements, insoluble fiber helps prevent these uncomfortable symptoms, allowing for smoother digestion and less discomfort.

Types of Insoluble Fiber

Insoluble fiber is found in various plant-based foods, primarily in the outer layers or skins of fruits and vegetables, as well as in whole grains, nuts, and seeds. There are several types of insoluble fiber, each with its own unique properties:

1. **Cellulose**: This is the most common type of insoluble fiber, found in the cell walls of plants. Cellulose helps retain water in the stool, promoting regularity. It is abundant in foods like whole grains, vegetables, and the skins of fruits.

2. **Hemicellulose**: Found in both the cell walls and the bran layers of grains, hemicellulose is another source of insoluble fiber that adds bulk to stool. It is commonly found in whole grains, legumes, and certain vegetables.

3. **Lignin**: Unlike other fibers, lignin is not a carbohydrate. It is a woody component of plant cell walls and provides structure and rigidity. Lignin is found in seeds, nuts, and the stems of vegetables. It contributes to stool bulk, enhancing regularity.

4. **Resistant Starch**: Although not traditionally classified as fiber, resistant starch behaves similarly by resisting digestion in the small intestine and moving into the colon, where it supports bowel regularity. Sources include green bananas, cooked and cooled potatoes, and certain whole grains.

Best Food Sources of Insoluble Fiber

1. Whole Grains

Whole grains are one of the richest sources of insoluble fiber, particularly when consumed in their unrefined form. Examples include wheat bran, brown rice, bulgur, and whole wheat. Wheat bran, in particular, is exceptionally high in insoluble fiber, with about 12 grams per cup. These grains are ideal for adding bulk to the diet, supporting regular bowel movements, and maintaining gut health.

Practical Tip: Replace refined grains with whole grains to maximize fiber intake. For instance, choose whole-grain bread over white bread, and opt for brown rice or bulgur instead of white rice. Adding a sprinkle of wheat bran to smoothies or oatmeal is another simple way to increase insoluble fiber intake.

2. Vegetables

Vegetables are an abundant source of insoluble fiber, especially those with skins or tough, fibrous parts. Leafy greens like kale and collard greens, root vegetables like carrots and beets, and cruciferous vegetables like broccoli all contain significant amounts of insoluble fiber. A medium-sized carrot provides around 2 grams of fiber, mostly insoluble.

Practical Tip: To increase fiber intake, include a variety of vegetables in your meals. Aim to fill half your plate with fiber-rich vegetables, and try to consume them in their raw or minimally cooked form to preserve their fiber content.

3. Nuts and Seeds

Nuts and seeds, particularly almonds, sunflower seeds, and flaxseeds, provide a good amount of insoluble fiber. For example, a handful of almonds (about 1 ounce) contains around 3 grams of fiber, mostly insoluble. These foods also offer healthy fats and protein, making them a nutritious addition to any meal or snack.

Practical Tip: Add a handful of nuts or a tablespoon of seeds to salads, yogurt, or oatmeal to increase fiber intake. Ground flaxseeds can also be added to smoothies for a boost in both fiber and omega-3 fatty acids.

4. Fruit Skins

The skins of fruits such as apples, pears, and plums are high in insoluble fiber. For instance, a medium apple with the skin on provides about 4 grams of fiber, much of which is insoluble. Fruit skins not only contribute to digestive regularity but also provide additional vitamins and antioxidants.

Practical Tip: Whenever possible, consume fruits with their skins intact to maximize fiber intake. Wash fruits thoroughly to remove any pesticides or wax coatings, or opt for organic produce to ensure safer consumption of the skins.

5. Legumes

Legumes like beans, lentils, and chickpeas are high in both soluble and insoluble fiber. A cup of cooked black beans, for example, contains around 15 grams of fiber, with a significant portion being insoluble. Legumes are also rich in protein, making them an excellent choice for those following plant-based diets.

Practical Tip: Include legumes in your diet by adding them to soups, salads, and stews. Canned beans are a convenient option, but be sure to rinse them thoroughly to reduce sodium content.

Practical Tips for Increasing Insoluble Fiber Intake

For those aiming to increase insoluble fiber intake, it's essential to do so gradually. A sudden increase in fiber can lead to gas, bloating, and digestive discomfort as the gut microbiome adjusts. Starting with small amounts and gradually incorporating more fiber-rich foods can help prevent these issues.

Additionally, hydration is critical when increasing fiber intake, as water helps fiber move through the digestive system smoothly. Without sufficient water, fiber can harden in the intestines, leading to constipation rather than alleviating it.

Here are some practical tips for boosting insoluble fiber intake:

- **Begin with Breakfast**: Choose high-fiber cereals, whole-grain bread, or oatmeal to start the day with a fiber-rich foundation. Add fruit with skins, like apples or berries, for an extra fiber boost.

- **Incorporate Vegetables in Every Meal**: Adding vegetables to every meal ensures a consistent intake of fiber throughout the day. Try including a side of roasted vegetables with lunch or dinner and adding raw vegetables as snacks.

- **Snack on Nuts and Seeds**: Nuts and seeds are easy to carry and can be enjoyed as snacks or sprinkled on salads, yogurt, or oatmeal for added fiber.

- **Experiment with Whole Grains**: Incorporate a variety of whole grains, such as quinoa, barley, and bulgur, into meals. These grains are versatile and can be used in salads, as a side dish, or as a base for main courses.

The Importance of Balance in Fiber Intake

While insoluble fiber is essential for regularity, it is most effective when consumed as part of a balanced diet that includes both soluble and insoluble fibers. Soluble fiber provides additional health benefits, such as stabilizing blood sugar and lowering cholesterol, while insoluble fiber primarily supports digestive health and regularity.

Achieving a balance between these two types of fiber allows for comprehensive support of gut health, weight management, and disease prevention.

Chapter 3: Remedies for Digestive Issues

Bloating is a common digestive issue characterized by a feeling of fullness, tightness, or swelling in the abdomen, often accompanied by discomfort or pain. While occasional bloating can be triggered by dietary habits or specific foods, chronic or frequent bloating may indicate digestive imbalances or sensitivities.

Herbal Remedies for Bloating

Many people experience bloating due to gas buildup, constipation, or the consumption of hard-to-digest foods. Herbal remedies offer a gentle, natural way to alleviate bloating, promote digestive comfort, and restore balance to the gut.

Herbs have been used for centuries to treat digestive issues, and modern science has confirmed the efficacy of many of these natural remedies. By incorporating specific herbs into one's daily routine, individuals can support digestion, reduce gas, and prevent bloating. These remedies are especially appealing for those seeking alternatives to over-the-counter medications, as they offer a holistic approach to digestive health that targets the root cause of bloating rather than just treating the symptoms.

Understanding the Causes of Bloating

Bloating can result from a variety of factors, including:

1. **Gas and Air Swallowing**: Swallowing air while eating or drinking, consuming carbonated beverages, or eating quickly can lead to the buildup of gas in the digestive tract, causing bloating and discomfort.

2. **Indigestion**: The consumption of fatty, spicy, or processed foods can slow digestion, leading to bloating. Indigestion, often marked by stomach pain and nausea, can contribute to feelings of fullness and tightness in the abdomen.

3. **Food Intolerances**: Many people experience bloating after consuming foods they are intolerant to, such as lactose or gluten. Food intolerances make it difficult for the digestive system to break down certain foods, resulting in gas production and bloating.

4. **Constipation**: Constipation can lead to bloating, as the buildup of stool in the intestines creates a feeling of fullness. When waste is not eliminated regularly, it can contribute to gas and digestive discomfort.

5. **Imbalance of Gut Bacteria**: An imbalance in the gut microbiome, also known as dysbiosis, can lead to excessive gas production and bloating. Certain bacterial strains in the gut are more likely to produce gas, which can contribute to bloating.

By understanding the root causes of bloating, individuals can select the herbal remedies that best address their specific digestive needs, helping to promote relief and support healthy digestion.

Effective Herbal Remedies for Bloating

Herbal remedies for bloating often work by stimulating digestion, reducing gas, and promoting the elimination of waste. Here are some of the most effective herbs for managing bloating:

1. **Peppermint**: Peppermint is one of the most well-known herbs for digestive relief. Its active compound, menthol, relaxes the muscles in the digestive tract, allowing trapped gas to pass more easily and reducing discomfort from bloating. Peppermint can also help relieve indigestion and improve the flow of bile, aiding in the breakdown of fats.

How to Use: Peppermint tea is a popular and gentle way to relieve bloating. Steep one teaspoon of dried peppermint leaves in hot water for 5-10 minutes, then strain and drink. Peppermint oil capsules are also available and can be effective for more intense relief.

2. **Ginger**: Ginger is a natural anti-inflammatory and digestive aid that helps stimulate saliva, bile, and gastric enzymes, promoting efficient digestion. Its compounds, gingerols and shogaols, reduce inflammation in the gut and ease the discomfort associated with bloating. Ginger is particularly effective for preventing bloating that results from indigestion and can reduce nausea as well.

How to Use: Fresh ginger root can be sliced and steeped in hot water to make ginger tea, or it can be added to meals. Ginger capsules and powders are also available for convenient use.

3. **Fennel**: Fennel seeds have carminative properties, meaning they help reduce gas in the digestive tract. They relax the muscles of the intestines, facilitating the release of trapped gas and easing bloating. Fennel seeds are commonly used in many cultures as a remedy for digestive discomfort.

How to Use: Chewing on a teaspoon of fennel seeds after meals can help reduce bloating. Fennel tea, made by steeping a teaspoon of crushed seeds in hot water for 10 minutes, is another effective option.

4. **Chamomile**: Chamomile has soothing and anti-inflammatory properties that calm the digestive system, making it beneficial for reducing bloating, gas, and indigestion. Chamomile also has mild antispasmodic effects, which help relax the muscles in the gut and promote a smoother digestion process.

How to Use: Chamomile tea is the most common way to enjoy this herb. Steep a tablespoon of dried chamomile flowers in hot water for 5-10 minutes, strain, and drink before or after meals to aid digestion.

5. **Caraway Seeds**: Caraway seeds contain compounds that help reduce gas production and support the smooth movement of food through the digestive tract. They are often used to alleviate bloating, gas, and cramps by encouraging the release of digestive enzymes.

How to Use: Caraway seeds can be chewed on their own or steeped in hot water to make a tea. Adding caraway seeds to meals, particularly beans and cruciferous vegetables, can also reduce gas production.

6. **Lemon Balm**: Lemon balm, a member of the mint family, has mild sedative and antispasmodic properties that help relieve digestive discomfort, including bloating and indigestion. Lemon balm relaxes the muscles in the stomach, reducing gas buildup and promoting smooth digestion.

How to Use: Lemon balm tea is a soothing way to enjoy this herb. Steep a tablespoon of dried lemon balm leaves in hot water for 5-10 minutes, then strain and drink.

7. **Dandelion Root**: Dandelion root is a natural diuretic and digestive stimulant, making it beneficial for reducing water retention and promoting bile production. By enhancing bile flow, dandelion root supports fat digestion, which can help reduce bloating caused by fatty foods.

How to Use: Dandelion root tea can be prepared by simmering a teaspoon of dried root in hot water for 10 minutes. Dandelion root supplements are also available.

8. **Coriander**: Coriander seeds have carminative and digestive-enhancing properties, helping to reduce gas and ease bloating. In traditional medicine, coriander is often used to alleviate digestive issues and support liver health.

How to Use: Coriander seeds can be brewed into tea or added to foods as a spice. For tea, steep one teaspoon of crushed seeds in hot water for 5-10 minutes.

Combining Herbal Remedies for Maximum Benefit

In many cases, combining multiple herbal remedies can provide greater relief from bloating, as different herbs work through various mechanisms. For example, a blend of peppermint, fennel, and ginger can provide a comprehensive approach to relieving bloating by addressing gas, inflammation, and digestive efficiency.

1. **Peppermint and Ginger Tea**: A combination of peppermint and ginger can be particularly effective for reducing bloating caused by indigestion. Both herbs aid in relaxing the digestive tract and improving digestion, while ginger adds anti-inflammatory benefits.

2. **Fennel and Chamomile**: This soothing combination is ideal for calming digestive distress and reducing gas. Fennel reduces gas production, while chamomile soothes and relaxes the digestive muscles.

3. **Lemon Balm and Dandelion Root**: For bloating associated with water retention or fatty foods, lemon balm and dandelion root work well together. Lemon balm reduces spasms and discomfort, while dandelion root promotes bile production and helps the body release excess water.

These combinations can be prepared as teas by adding equal parts of each herb to hot water, steeping, and straining before drinking. Using these blends regularly or after meals may help prevent bloating and promote overall digestive health.

Practical Tips for Using Herbal Remedies for Bloating

1. **Use After Meals**: Many herbal teas are most effective when taken after meals, as they help stimulate digestion and prevent gas buildup. Drinking tea after eating can aid in digestion and reduce the likelihood of bloating.

2. **Stay Consistent**: Herbal remedies can take time to show results, especially for those with chronic bloating. Consistency is key, and using these herbs regularly can help maintain a balanced digestive system and prevent bloating.

3. **Pair with Dietary Adjustments**: Herbal remedies are most effective when combined with a diet that minimizes bloating triggers. Reducing intake of processed

foods, carbonated beverages, and high-sugar foods can further support digestive health.

4. **Stay Hydrated**: Proper hydration supports digestion and prevents constipation, which can contribute to bloating. Herbal teas count toward daily water intake, making them a convenient way to stay hydrated.

Supporting Gut Health for Long-Term Relief

Herbal remedies can provide immediate relief from bloating, but supporting gut health over the long term is essential for preventing recurrent issues. Probiotics, prebiotics, and a fiber-rich diet are essential for maintaining a balanced microbiome and reducing the likelihood of bloating.

1. **Probiotics**: Including probiotic-rich foods such as yogurt, kefir, and fermented vegetables can help maintain a balanced gut microbiome, reducing gas and supporting regular digestion.

2. **Prebiotics**: Prebiotic fibers, found in foods like garlic, onions, and bananas, feed beneficial bacteria in the gut, helping to promote a healthy balance of microorganisms that support digestion.

3. **Soluble Fiber**: Soluble fiber from foods such as oats, apples, and chia seeds helps to regulate digestion

Natural Remedies for IBS

Irritable Bowel Syndrome (IBS) is a common gastrointestinal disorder that affects millions of people worldwide. Characterized by a range of symptoms including abdominal pain, bloating, gas, diarrhea, and constipation, IBS can significantly impact a person's quality of life. While the exact cause of IBS remains unknown, several factors, including stress, diet, and gut sensitivity, are believed to contribute to its onset. Managing IBS often requires a holistic approach that addresses these factors to reduce symptom severity and improve overall well-being.

In this section, we'll explore various natural remedies that may help manage IBS symptoms. From dietary adjustments to herbal supplements, these remedies offer a gentle and natural approach to alleviating the discomfort associated with IBS. Each remedy is supported by insights into its mechanisms, practical application, and safety considerations, providing a comprehensive guide for individuals seeking relief from this challenging condition.

Dietary Adjustments: The Foundation of IBS Management

Dietary changes are often the first line of defense for managing IBS symptoms. Many people with IBS find that certain foods trigger their symptoms, while others can provide relief. Implementing a diet that minimizes triggers while supporting digestive health is essential for long-term symptom management.

1. **Low-FODMAP Diet**

The low-FODMAP diet has gained popularity as an effective strategy for reducing IBS symptoms. FODMAPs (fermentable oligosaccharides, disaccharides, monosaccharides, and polyols) are a group of short-chain carbohydrates that are poorly absorbed in the small intestine. When these carbohydrates reach the colon, they can ferment, producing gas and causing bloating, pain, and diarrhea. The low-FODMAP diet involves eliminating high-FODMAP foods and gradually reintroducing them to identify which ones trigger symptoms.

Examples of High-FODMAP Foods to Avoid:

- Dairy products (lactose)
- Certain fruits (apples, pears, watermelon)
- Certain vegetables (onions, garlic, broccoli)
- Legumes (beans, lentils)
- Wheat products

Practical Tip: Working with a nutritionist or dietitian can be helpful when following a low-FODMAP diet, as it requires careful planning to ensure nutritional balance. Once triggers are identified, individuals can customize their diet to include low-FODMAP foods that support gut health without triggering symptoms.

2. **Increased Fiber Intake (with Caution)**

Fiber is essential for digestive health, but it can be tricky for people with IBS. While fiber can aid in regularity, it can also exacerbate symptoms in some individuals, particularly if it is introduced too quickly or in large amounts. Insoluble fiber, in particular, can cause irritation for some IBS sufferers, so it's important to choose fiber sources wisely.

Recommended Fiber Sources:

o Soluble fiber: Found in foods like oats, bananas, and sweet potatoes, soluble fiber absorbs water and forms a gel, which can help manage both diarrhea and constipation.

o Psyllium husk: This natural fiber supplement is often well-tolerated by people with IBS and can support regularity without causing excessive gas or bloating.

Practical Tip: Introduce fiber gradually and stay well-hydrated to minimize discomfort. Pay attention to your body's response to different types of fiber, as individual tolerance levels can vary.

3. Probiotics for Gut Balance

Probiotics are beneficial bacteria that can help support a healthy gut microbiome, which plays a crucial role in digestion and immune function. Research suggests that people with IBS often have an imbalance in their gut microbiota, and supplementing with probiotics may help restore this balance, reducing symptoms such as bloating, gas, and irregular bowel movements.

Common Probiotic Strains for IBS:

o *Bifidobacterium infantis*: Known for reducing bloating and abdominal pain.

o *Lactobacillus acidophilus*: May improve symptoms of diarrhea-predominant IBS.

o *Saccharomyces boulardii*: A beneficial yeast that can help reduce diarrhea and support gut health.

Practical Tip: Look for a high-quality probiotic supplement with clinically studied strains specific to IBS, or incorporate fermented foods like yogurt, kefir, and sauerkraut into your diet for a natural probiotic boost.

Herbal Remedies for IBS Symptom Relief

Several herbs have been traditionally used to soothe digestive discomfort and may provide relief for IBS symptoms. While these remedies do not cure IBS, they can be helpful in managing symptoms when used alongside dietary adjustments.

1. Peppermint Oil

Peppermint oil is one of the most studied herbal remedies for IBS and is known for its ability to relax the muscles of the gastrointestinal tract. The active compound in peppermint oil, menthol, has an antispasmodic effect, which can reduce cramping and alleviate pain associated with IBS.

How to Use Peppermint Oil:

- o Peppermint oil capsules are widely available and can be taken before meals to prevent cramping.
- o Enteric-coated capsules are recommended, as they release peppermint oil in the intestines rather than the stomach, reducing the risk of heartburn.

Safety Note: Peppermint oil may cause side effects like heartburn, especially if taken on an empty stomach or without an enteric coating. Consult a healthcare provider before using peppermint oil if you have acid reflux or GERD.

2. Ginger

Ginger has long been used to relieve digestive issues, including nausea, bloating, and indigestion. It contains compounds called gingerols and shogaols, which have anti-inflammatory and antispasmodic effects that may help relax the muscles of the digestive tract.

How to Use Ginger:

- o Fresh ginger can be added to tea, smoothies, or meals.
- o Ginger supplements are available in capsule form for a more concentrated dose.

Practical Tip: Drinking ginger tea after meals can aid digestion and reduce bloating. For those who find the flavor too strong, ginger can be paired with honey or lemon for a milder taste.

3. Chamomile

Chamomile is a calming herb often used to relieve anxiety and digestive issues. It has anti-inflammatory and antispasmodic properties that may help reduce bloating, gas, and cramping in people with IBS. Chamomile also promotes relaxation, which can be beneficial for stress-induced IBS symptoms.

How to Use Chamomile:

- o Chamomile tea is a popular option for those looking to relax and soothe their digestive system.
- o Chamomile supplements are available but should be used with caution, as some people may be allergic to chamomile, especially if they have a ragweed allergy.

4. **Fennel**

Fennel is commonly used to relieve gas, bloating, and digestive discomfort. It has carminative properties, meaning it helps expel gas from the intestines, making it beneficial for people with IBS who experience bloating and flatulence.

How to Use Fennel:

- o Fennel seeds can be chewed after meals to aid digestion and reduce gas.
- o Fennel tea is another option that can be enjoyed after meals to support digestion.

5. **Turmeric**

Turmeric is known for its anti-inflammatory properties and may benefit those with IBS by reducing inflammation in the gut. The active compound in turmeric, curcumin, has been shown to improve symptoms of abdominal pain and discomfort in some individuals with IBS.

How to Use Turmeric:

- o Turmeric can be added to meals or taken as a supplement for a concentrated dose of curcumin.
- o For optimal absorption, turmeric should be consumed with black pepper and a source of healthy fat.

Mind-Body Techniques for Stress Management

Stress is a significant trigger for many individuals with IBS, as the gut and brain are closely connected through the gut-brain axis. Managing stress is, therefore, an essential part of IBS symptom management. Various mind-body techniques can help reduce stress and improve gut health by calming the nervous system.

1. **Mindfulness Meditation**

Mindfulness meditation involves focusing on the present moment without judgment, which can help reduce stress and anxiety. Regular practice has been shown to improve IBS symptoms by reducing the gut's sensitivity to stress.

Practical Tip: Start with just 5-10 minutes of mindfulness meditation each day, gradually increasing the time as you become more comfortable with the practice.

2. **Yoga and Gentle Exercise**

Yoga and other gentle forms of exercise can help relax the muscles, reduce stress, and improve digestion. Certain yoga poses, such as twists and forward folds, are believed to stimulate the digestive organs and relieve bloating and discomfort.

Practical Tip: Incorporate yoga or light stretching into your daily routine to support relaxation and digestion. Even a few minutes of deep breathing and gentle movement can have a positive effect on IBS symptoms.

3. Cognitive Behavioral Therapy (CBT)

Cognitive Behavioral Therapy (CBT) is a type of therapy that focuses on changing negative thought patterns and behaviors. CBT has been shown to be effective for people with IBS, as it can help them develop healthier responses to stress and anxiety, which are often triggers for symptoms.

Practical Tip: Working with a trained therapist can provide personalized strategies for managing IBS-related stress. Some therapists specialize in gut-directed CBT, which is tailored specifically for people with gastrointestinal disorders.

The Importance of Lifestyle Adjustments

Lifestyle factors, such as sleep, hydration, and meal timing, can also impact IBS symptoms. Prioritizing these aspects of daily life is essential for managing IBS naturally.

1. Adequate Hydration

Drinking enough water is crucial for digestive health, as dehydration can lead to constipation and exacerbate IBS symptoms. Staying well-hydrated helps keep stool soft and easy to pass, supporting regularity.

2. Consistent Meal Timing

Eating meals at regular intervals can help regulate digestion and prevent overloading the digestive system. Skipping meals or eating too quickly can trigger IBS symptoms, as can consuming large meals in one sitting.

3. Prioritize Sleep

Quality sleep is essential for overall health and can impact digestion. Poor sleep can increase stress levels and trigger IBS symptoms. Aim for at least 7-8 hours of sleep each night to support both physical and mental well-being.

By adopting a holistic approach that combines dietary adjustments, herbal remedies, mind-body techniques, and lifestyle changes, individuals with IBS can find relief and regain control over their symptoms. Each person's experience with IBS is unique, so it may take time and experimentation to discover which combination of remedies works best.

Chapter 4: Herbal Recipes for Gut Health

Slippery elm, derived from the inner bark of the slippery elm tree (*Ulmus rubra*), is a natural remedy known for its soothing effects on the digestive and respiratory systems. Traditionally used by Native Americans and early American settlers, slippery elm is celebrated for its mucilaginous properties, which create a gel-like texture when mixed with water.

Slippery Elm Porridge

This soothing gel coats and protects mucous membranes, providing relief from irritation and inflammation. Slippery elm porridge is one of the most effective ways to harness the benefits of this remarkable herb, offering a gentle, nourishing meal that promotes digestive health and supports overall wellness.

For those interested in natural remedies, slippery elm porridge serves as a powerful tool for managing digestive discomforts, including acid reflux, irritable bowel syndrome (IBS), and constipation. This porridge is not only soothing but also rich in nutrients, making it an ideal choice for individuals with sensitive digestive systems or those seeking a restorative addition to their diet.

The Benefits of Slippery Elm for Digestive Health

Slippery elm contains mucilage, a soluble fiber that becomes thick and slippery when combined with water. This mucilage is responsible for its unique healing properties, as it coats and protects the lining of the stomach and intestines. Here's how slippery elm can benefit digestive health:

1. **Soothing Irritation**: The mucilage in slippery elm forms a protective barrier along the gastrointestinal tract, reducing inflammation and irritation. This effect is particularly beneficial for individuals with acid reflux, as the coating action can help protect the esophagus from stomach acid.

2. **Alleviating Constipation and Diarrhea**: Slippery elm's mucilage can normalize bowel movements by adding bulk to stool in cases of diarrhea and softening stool in

cases of constipation. This dual action makes it suitable for individuals with IBS or other digestive disorders marked by irregular bowel movements.

3. **Promoting Healthy Gut Flora**: Slippery elm is a prebiotic, which means it supports the growth of beneficial bacteria in the gut. A balanced gut microbiome is essential for overall health, as it plays a role in digestion, immunity, and mental well-being.

4. **Supporting Nutrient Absorption**: By soothing the digestive tract, slippery elm allows for more efficient nutrient absorption. A healthy gut lining is crucial for absorbing essential vitamins and minerals, and slippery elm's protective properties support this process.

5. **Reducing Stomach Acid and Heartburn**: Slippery elm's mucilage acts as a buffer, absorbing excess stomach acid and reducing the likelihood of heartburn. This quality makes it a gentle, natural remedy for individuals struggling with acid reflux.

How to Make Slippery Elm Porridge

Slippery elm porridge is simple to prepare and can be customized with various ingredients to suit individual tastes and nutritional needs. Here's a basic recipe to create a soothing and nutrient-rich slippery elm porridge.

Ingredients:

- 1 tablespoon slippery elm powder
- 1 cup water (or almond milk for a creamier texture)
- Honey, cinnamon, or ginger for flavor (optional)

Instructions:

1. In a small saucepan, bring the water or almond milk to a gentle simmer.
2. Gradually whisk in the slippery elm powder, stirring constantly to prevent lumps from forming.
3. Continue stirring for 2-3 minutes until the mixture thickens to a porridge-like consistency.
4. Remove from heat and let it cool slightly before adding honey, cinnamon, or ginger for flavor, if desired.
5. Enjoy the porridge warm. This recipe can be consumed once or twice daily, particularly when experiencing digestive discomfort.

This porridge can be adjusted with different flavorings to keep it varied and enjoyable. The gentle nature of slippery elm makes it suitable for regular use, providing ongoing support for digestive health.

Additional Ingredients to Enhance Slippery Elm Porridge

To create a well-rounded, nutrient-dense meal, additional ingredients can be added to slippery elm porridge. These ingredients complement the soothing properties of slippery elm and provide extra health benefits:

1. **Chia Seeds**: Chia seeds are rich in omega-3 fatty acids and fiber, which support heart health and digestion. When soaked, they develop a gel-like consistency that adds to the porridge's texture and nutrient profile.

2. **Flaxseeds**: Ground flaxseeds offer fiber and essential fatty acids, which aid in digestion and help maintain regular bowel movements. Adding flaxseeds to slippery elm porridge enhances its benefits for individuals with constipation.

3. **Turmeric**: Known for its anti-inflammatory properties, turmeric can be added to the porridge to further support digestive health and reduce inflammation in the gut. A pinch of black pepper can increase turmeric's bioavailability.

4. **Cinnamon**: Cinnamon not only adds warmth and flavor but also has natural antibacterial properties that support gut health. It may help reduce bloating and improve digestion, making it a valuable addition to slippery elm porridge.

5. **Banana Slices**: Bananas are gentle on the stomach and provide potassium, which supports electrolyte balance. The natural sweetness of bananas can enhance the flavor of the porridge without the need for added sugars.

6. **Honey or Maple Syrup**: For a touch of sweetness, honey or maple syrup can be added. Honey, particularly raw honey, has antimicrobial properties that support immune health and complement the soothing effects of slippery elm.

These additions can be rotated to keep the porridge interesting while providing a range of nutrients. Experimenting with different combinations allows individuals to tailor their porridge to their health needs and taste preferences.

The Role of Slippery Elm in Managing Common Digestive Disorders

Slippery elm porridge can be particularly beneficial for managing specific digestive disorders. Here's how it can support individuals dealing with conditions like acid reflux, IBS, and leaky gut syndrome:

1. **Acid Reflux and Heartburn**: Slippery elm forms a protective barrier along the esophagus, which can shield it from the corrosive effects of stomach acid. Regular consumption of slippery elm porridge may reduce the frequency and severity of acid reflux symptoms by soothing the esophagus and preventing inflammation.

2. **Irritable Bowel Syndrome (IBS)**: IBS often involves symptoms like bloating, gas, and irregular bowel movements. The mucilage in slippery elm helps to regulate bowel function, easing constipation and diarrhea while reducing bloating. Additionally, the prebiotic properties of slippery elm support a healthy gut microbiome, which is often disrupted in individuals with IBS.

3. **Leaky Gut Syndrome**: Leaky gut syndrome occurs when the lining of the intestine becomes permeable, allowing undigested food particles and toxins to enter the bloodstream. Slippery elm's mucilage strengthens the gut lining, reducing permeability and supporting the gut's natural barrier function. This protective effect helps prevent inflammation and supports overall gut health.

4. **Gastritis and Ulcers**: The soothing properties of slippery elm can help alleviate symptoms of gastritis and ulcers by coating the stomach lining and reducing irritation. The protective barrier created by slippery elm also allows inflamed tissues to heal, making it a supportive remedy for these conditions.

Precautions and Considerations When Using Slippery Elm

While slippery elm is generally safe for most individuals, there are a few precautions to keep in mind:

- **Medication Timing**: Slippery elm's mucilage may slow the absorption of certain medications. It's best to take slippery elm at least two hours before or after other medications to avoid interference.

- **Allergies**: Individuals with a known allergy to elm trees should avoid slippery elm. If in doubt, consult with a healthcare provider before using slippery elm as a remedy.

- **Pregnancy and Breastfeeding**: While slippery elm has a long history of use, it's best for pregnant and breastfeeding individuals to consult a healthcare provider before incorporating it into their routine.

Supporting Gut Health Alongside Slippery Elm

Slippery elm porridge is a valuable tool for managing digestive discomfort, but it's even more effective when combined with other gut-friendly practices:

1. **Hydration**: Staying well-hydrated is essential for digestive health, especially when consuming fiber-rich foods like slippery elm. Water supports digestion and helps prevent constipation, making it an important aspect of any gut health regimen.

2. **Fiber-Rich Diet**: A diet rich in fiber from fruits, vegetables, whole grains, and legumes supports regular bowel movements and helps feed beneficial bacteria in the gut. Soluble fiber, in particular, works well with slippery elm to maintain a balanced digestive system.

3. **Probiotics and Prebiotics**: Probiotic-rich foods, such as yogurt, kefir, and sauerkraut, support a healthy gut microbiome. Prebiotic foods, like garlic, onions, and asparagus, feed these beneficial bacteria, creating a balanced environment that reduces the likelihood of digestive discomfort.

4. **Mindful Eating**: Eating slowly and chewing thoroughly can help reduce bloating and gas, making digestion easier on the body. Practicing mindful eating allows the digestive system to function optimally and reduces the risk of indigestion.

5. **Avoiding Common Triggers**: Certain foods, such as highly processed foods, fatty meals, and carbonated drinks, can contribute to bloating and digestive discomfort. Reducing or eliminating these foods can support gut health and enhance the effects of slippery elm.

Slippery Elm as a Natural Healer

For those seeking natural remedies to manage digestive discomfort, slippery elm porridge offers a gentle yet effective solution. Its soothing mucilage provides immediate relief from irritation, while its prebiotic properties promote long-term gut health. Whether used as a daily breakfast or as needed for digestive support, slippery elm porridge is a valuable addition to a holistic approach to health.

By making slippery elm porridge a regular part of a wellness routine, individuals can experience its full range of benefits. This comforting, nutrient-rich meal not only soothes the digestive system but also supports overall vitality, making it an ideal choice for those committed to natural health practices.

Marshmallow root tea, derived from the root of the *Althaea officinalis* plant, has been used for centuries as a natural remedy for various ailments, particularly those related to the digestive and respiratory systems. This herbal tea is well-known for its soothing and anti-inflammatory properties, making it an excellent choice for individuals seeking relief from conditions like indigestion, acid reflux, sore throat, and cough. The root contains mucilage, a gelatinous substance that forms a protective layer over mucous membranes, providing soothing relief to irritated tissues.

In this section, we will delve into the properties of marshmallow root tea, its health benefits, and how it can be incorporated into a wellness routine. Additionally, we'll explore the mechanisms behind its effectiveness, provide usage guidelines, and share practical tips for preparing and consuming this herbal tea.

The Composition and Mechanisms of Marshmallow Root

Marshmallow root contains several bioactive compounds that contribute to its health benefits. Key components include mucilage, flavonoids, tannins, and pectin. Each of these compounds plays a unique role in marshmallow root's therapeutic effects:

- **Mucilage**: The mucilage in marshmallow root is a polysaccharide that swells and forms a gel-like consistency when mixed with water. This property creates a soothing barrier over inflamed tissues, particularly in the digestive and respiratory tracts. The mucilage also helps retain moisture, preventing dryness and further irritation.

- **Flavonoids**: These antioxidants have anti-inflammatory and immune-boosting properties, helping the body fight off infections and reduce inflammation. Flavonoids in marshmallow root contribute to its ability to soothe the gastrointestinal tract and protect against oxidative stress.

- **Tannins**: Known for their astringent qualities, tannins can help tighten tissues, which may reduce inflammation in the throat and digestive tract. Tannins also contribute to the plant's mildly antibacterial properties, making marshmallow root effective for soothing minor infections.

- **Pectin**: This type of soluble fiber supports digestive health by promoting a healthy gut microbiome and helping regulate bowel movements. Pectin is beneficial for both digestive health and immune function, as it encourages the growth of beneficial gut bacteria.

Health Benefits of Marshmallow Root Tea

1. Soothes Digestive Discomfort

One of the most popular uses of marshmallow root tea is for digestive relief. The mucilage forms a protective layer over the stomach and intestinal lining, which can alleviate symptoms of indigestion, acid reflux, and gastritis. This protective coating helps reduce irritation caused by stomach acids, offering relief for people who suffer from frequent heartburn or acid reflux.

Marshmallow root tea may also help manage inflammatory conditions of the digestive tract, such as irritable bowel syndrome (IBS) and Crohn's disease, by reducing inflammation and promoting the healing of the intestinal lining. Although marshmallow root tea is not a cure for these conditions, its soothing effects can provide symptom relief and improve comfort.

2. Relieves Respiratory Issues

Marshmallow root tea is often used as a natural remedy for respiratory conditions such as sore throat, cough, and bronchitis. The mucilage acts as a natural demulcent, coating the throat and reducing irritation, which can alleviate the discomfort of a sore or dry throat.

For individuals with coughs or bronchial inflammation, marshmallow root tea can help soothe the airways and reduce coughing by acting as an expectorant, which helps loosen and expel mucus. This makes it beneficial for colds, respiratory infections, and even asthma. Drinking warm marshmallow root tea can provide instant relief for these symptoms and promote faster recovery from respiratory infections.

3. Supports Skin Health

Marshmallow root is also known for its benefits to skin health, particularly in addressing issues such as dryness, inflammation, and irritation. The mucilage forms a protective barrier on the skin, locking in moisture and providing a soothing effect. Marshmallow root tea, when used both internally and topically, may help treat conditions like eczema, psoriasis, and acne.

By drinking marshmallow root tea regularly, individuals can support their skin from the inside out. The antioxidants in the tea help combat oxidative stress, which can lead to premature aging and skin damage. For topical use, cooled marshmallow root tea can be applied to the skin with a cotton pad to soothe inflamed or irritated areas.

4. Reduces Urinary Tract Irritation

Marshmallow root tea may benefit individuals suffering from urinary tract infections (UTIs) or other forms of urinary tract irritation. The mucilage coats the urinary tract lining, reducing inflammation and providing a soothing effect. Additionally, marshmallow root's mild diuretic properties can increase urine flow, helping to flush out bacteria and reduce the risk of infection.

While marshmallow root tea should not replace antibiotics for treating UTIs, it can be used as a complementary remedy to relieve discomfort and support the healing process.

5. Promotes Wound Healing

Due to its anti-inflammatory and antimicrobial properties, marshmallow root has been traditionally used to promote wound healing. The mucilage forms a protective layer over wounds, preventing infection and promoting moisture retention, which is beneficial for the healing process. Consuming marshmallow root tea can aid in internal recovery from inflammation or infection, while applying the tea externally may support wound healing.

How to Make Marshmallow Root Tea

Making marshmallow root tea is a simple process, but it requires a bit of patience due to the need to extract the mucilage from the root. The following steps will guide you through the preparation:

1. **Ingredients**:
   - 1 tablespoon of dried marshmallow root
   - 1 cup of cold or warm water

2. **Instructions**:
   - **Cold Infusion Method**: The cold infusion method is preferred for maximizing the mucilage content. Place the marshmallow root in a jar or container and add cold water. Cover the jar and let it steep overnight, or for at least 4–6 hours. Strain the tea, discard the root, and enjoy.
   - **Hot Infusion Method**: If you prefer a warm tea, you can use hot water, but avoid boiling water as it can reduce the mucilage content. Place the marshmallow root in a teapot or cup, pour warm water over it, and let it steep for 10–15 minutes. Strain the tea and enjoy.

3. **Flavoring Options**:

o Marshmallow root tea has a mild, slightly sweet flavor. To enhance the taste, you can add a teaspoon of honey or a slice of lemon. Cinnamon or ginger can also be added for additional flavor and potential health benefits.

Practical Tips for Using Marshmallow Root Tea

- **Dosage**: It is generally safe to drink 2–3 cups of marshmallow root tea per day. If you are using it for a specific condition, start with one cup and gradually increase based on your tolerance and response.
- **Storage**: If you prepare a large batch using the cold infusion method, store it in the refrigerator for up to 48 hours. This allows you to have marshmallow root tea readily available.
- **Allergic Reactions**: Although rare, some individuals may experience allergic reactions to marshmallow root. Start with a small dose if you're trying it for the first time, and discontinue use if you notice any signs of an allergic reaction, such as itching or swelling.
- **Interactions**: Marshmallow root may interact with certain medications by affecting absorption. It is advisable to take marshmallow root tea one hour before or after other medications to avoid interference.

When to Use Marshmallow Root Tea

1. **For Digestive Relief**: Drink a cup of marshmallow root tea after meals to help soothe acid reflux, indigestion, or other mild digestive discomforts. The mucilage can protect the stomach lining and reduce irritation.
2. **For Respiratory Support**: Sipping warm marshmallow root tea can relieve sore throat and cough, especially in cases of colds, bronchitis, or seasonal allergies. Drink throughout the day for continuous relief.
3. **For Skin Health**: Consuming marshmallow root tea regularly can help maintain healthy skin. Additionally, for topical use, let the tea cool and apply it with a clean cloth or cotton pad to irritated or dry areas of the skin.
4. **For Urinary Tract Health**: Drink marshmallow root tea at the onset of UTI symptoms to help soothe the urinary tract and promote healing. Pair it with other UTI management practices, such as increased water intake and cranberry juice.

Safety and Considerations

Marshmallow root tea is generally safe for most people, including children and pregnant women, when consumed in moderate amounts. However, there are a few considerations to keep in mind:

- **Pregnancy and Breastfeeding**: While marshmallow root is considered safe during pregnancy and breastfeeding, it is advisable to consult a healthcare provider before use, especially in higher doses.
- **Children**: Marshmallow root tea can be given to children as a gentle remedy for sore throats or mild digestive issues. However, it's best to consult a pediatrician to determine the appropriate dosage based on the child's age and weight.
- **Long-Term Use**: While marshmallow root tea can be consumed daily, prolonged use should be discussed with a healthcare provider to ensure it remains safe and beneficial for your specific health needs.

Marshmallow root tea offers a gentle, natural way to address a variety of health issues, from digestive discomfort to respiratory irritation and beyond. Its soothing properties make it an ideal remedy for calming inflamed tissues and supporting the body's natural healing processes.

Fennel Seed Infusion

Fennel seeds (*Foeniculum vulgare*) have been valued for their therapeutic properties for centuries, particularly in traditional and herbal medicine. Known for their carminative effects, fennel seeds are widely used to relieve digestive discomforts such as bloating, gas, and indigestion. A fennel seed infusion, or tea, is an excellent way to harness these benefits in a simple, natural, and soothing drink that promotes digestive health and offers other holistic advantages.

Beyond its digestive benefits, fennel seed infusion has mild anti-inflammatory, antimicrobial, and antioxidant properties, making it a versatile herbal remedy. It is particularly popular in natural wellness for its gentleness and efficacy, suitable for both adults and children experiencing digestive discomfort.

Health Benefits of Fennel Seed Infusion

The therapeutic value of fennel seed infusion comes from its high content of volatile oils, including anethole, fenchone, and estragole. These compounds are responsible for fennel's distinctive aroma and many of its health benefits. Here's a closer look at how fennel seed infusion supports health:

1. **Relief from Digestive Discomfort**: Fennel seeds are well-known for their ability to reduce gas, bloating, and stomach cramps. The volatile oils in fennel seeds relax the smooth muscles of the digestive tract, allowing trapped gas to pass more easily. This carminative effect is particularly beneficial for individuals suffering from irritable bowel syndrome (IBS) or indigestion.

2. **Anti-Inflammatory Properties**: The anti-inflammatory effects of fennel help reduce inflammation in the digestive tract and beyond. Regular consumption of fennel seed infusion can aid in managing conditions where inflammation plays a role, such as gastritis and inflammatory bowel diseases.

3. **Antimicrobial Activity**: Fennel seeds possess mild antimicrobial properties, which can help prevent the growth of harmful bacteria in the digestive tract. This effect contributes to a balanced gut microbiome and may reduce the risk of infections or imbalances that lead to digestive discomfort.

4. **Hormonal Balance**: Fennel seeds contain phytoestrogens, which are plant compounds that mimic the effects of estrogen in the body. For individuals experiencing hormonal imbalances, particularly women dealing with symptoms of PMS or menopause, fennel seed infusion can offer gentle hormonal support.

5. **Rich in Antioxidants**: Fennel seeds are high in antioxidants, which combat oxidative stress and free radicals in the body. Antioxidants in fennel seeds, such as quercetin and rutin, protect cells from damage and support overall health, including cardiovascular health.

6. **Respiratory Relief**: The expectorant properties of fennel seeds make the infusion beneficial for respiratory health, helping to loosen mucus and relieve coughs. It can be particularly useful during cold and flu season to soothe sore throats and support clear breathing.

How to Make Fennel Seed Infusion

Making fennel seed infusion is simple and requires minimal ingredients. Freshly ground or crushed seeds work best, as they release more of the beneficial oils into the water.

Ingredients:

- 1 teaspoon fennel seeds (crushed or ground)
- 1 cup boiling water
- Optional: honey or lemon for added flavor

Instructions:

1. Crush the fennel seeds slightly to release their oils. You can do this with a mortar and pestle or by placing the seeds in a small plastic bag and crushing them with the back of a spoon.
2. Place the crushed seeds in a teapot or cup.
3. Pour boiling water over the seeds, cover, and let steep for 5-10 minutes.
4. Strain the infusion into a cup, discarding the seeds.
5. Add honey or lemon if desired. Drink warm, preferably after meals for digestive benefits.

This basic infusion can be consumed once or twice daily to support digestion or whenever needed to relieve digestive discomfort.

Practical Tips for Using Fennel Seed Infusion

To get the most out of fennel seed infusion, it's helpful to follow these practical tips:

1. **Enjoy After Meals**: Drinking fennel seed infusion after meals can aid in digestion and reduce the likelihood of bloating or gas. The infusion helps stimulate gastric juices and supports the digestive process.
2. **Combine with Other Herbs**: Fennel pairs well with other digestive herbs like ginger, peppermint, and chamomile. Combining these herbs can enhance the infusion's soothing properties and provide a broader range of digestive benefits.
3. **Use Fresh Seeds**: For the most potent infusion, use fresh fennel seeds. Over time, the oils in fennel seeds can degrade, so it's best to store them in an airtight container and replace them every few months.
4. **Adjust Strength as Needed**: The strength of fennel seed infusion can be adjusted by using more or fewer seeds, depending on individual preference and tolerance. Those who are new to fennel seed infusion may start with a milder strength and gradually increase if desired.

Additional Health Benefits of Fennel Seed Infusion

While fennel seed infusion is best known for its digestive benefits, it also supports various other aspects of health:

1. **Weight Management**: Fennel seed infusion can support weight management by reducing appetite and promoting a feeling of fullness. The fiber content in fennel seeds may help control cravings, making it easier to stick to a balanced diet.

2. **Blood Sugar Control**: Some studies suggest that fennel seeds may help regulate blood sugar levels, which can be beneficial for individuals with diabetes or those at risk. Drinking fennel seed infusion regularly may contribute to more stable blood sugar levels, although it should be part of a broader dietary approach.

3. **Diuretic Properties**: Fennel seeds act as a mild diuretic, promoting the production of urine and helping the body eliminate excess water and toxins. This effect can help reduce bloating caused by water retention and support kidney health.

4. **Stress Relief**: The soothing aroma of fennel seed infusion can promote relaxation and relieve stress. Taking a few moments to enjoy a warm cup of fennel tea can provide a mental break and help reduce feelings of anxiety.

Fennel Seed Infusion for Specific Digestive Conditions

Fennel seed infusion can be particularly beneficial for certain digestive issues. Here's how it can support individuals dealing with common digestive conditions:

1. **Irritable Bowel Syndrome (IBS)**: Fennel seed infusion is a valuable tool for managing IBS symptoms, as it reduces bloating, gas, and cramping. Its muscle-relaxing properties help alleviate spasms in the digestive tract, providing relief from discomfort.

2. **Acid Reflux and Heartburn**: The soothing effect of fennel seed infusion can help reduce the discomfort of acid reflux and heartburn. By promoting smoother digestion, fennel helps prevent the build-up of acid in the stomach, which may alleviate symptoms.

3. **Constipation**: Fennel seed infusion stimulates digestive enzymes and helps regulate bowel movements, making it beneficial for individuals with constipation. When combined with adequate hydration and a fiber-rich diet, fennel seed infusion supports regularity.

4. **Gas and Bloating**: Fennel seeds are known for their ability to reduce gas, making this infusion ideal for those who frequently experience bloating and gas after meals.

The carminative effects encourage the release of gas and reduce the tension in the digestive tract.

Using Fennel Seed Infusion as Part of a Holistic Health Routine

Fennel seed infusion is an accessible and gentle herbal remedy that fits well into a holistic approach to health. To maximize its benefits, individuals can incorporate it into their daily routine in combination with other wellness practices:

1. **Pair with a Balanced Diet**: A diet rich in whole foods, fiber, and low in processed ingredients complements the digestive benefits of fennel seed infusion. Whole grains, fruits, and vegetables provide the nutrients necessary for optimal digestion.

2. **Stay Hydrated**: Adequate hydration is essential for digestive health, and fennel seed infusion can be a soothing addition to daily water intake. Hydration supports regular bowel movements and helps flush out toxins, amplifying the diuretic effects of fennel.

3. **Practice Mindful Eating**: Eating slowly and chewing thoroughly aids in digestion, preventing excessive gas and bloating. Fennel seed infusion after a mindful meal can further support digestion and prevent discomfort.

4. **Include Probiotic Foods**: Consuming probiotic-rich foods like yogurt, sauerkraut, or kombucha can help maintain a healthy gut microbiome. Fennel seed infusion, with its mild antimicrobial properties, complements probiotic foods by preventing the overgrowth of harmful bacteria.

Fennel Seed Infusion for Women's Health

Fennel seed infusion is especially beneficial for women, as it can support menstrual health and alleviate symptoms associated with hormonal changes. Here's how fennel seed infusion can benefit women specifically:

1. **Easing Menstrual Cramps**: The antispasmodic properties of fennel help reduce uterine contractions, making it effective for relieving menstrual cramps. Drinking fennel seed infusion during menstruation can alleviate discomfort and promote relaxation.

2. **Hormonal Balance**: The phytoestrogens in fennel seeds support hormonal balance, particularly during menopause. Women experiencing symptoms of menopause, such

as hot flashes or mood swings, may find relief through regular consumption of fennel seed infusion.

3. **Digestive Support During Pregnancy**: While pregnant individuals should consult a healthcare provider before using herbal remedies, fennel seed infusion can help relieve pregnancy-related digestive issues like gas and bloating. However, caution should be taken with dosage and frequency during pregnancy.

Precautions and Considerations

While fennel seed infusion is generally safe for most people, it's important to keep the following considerations in mind:

1. **Allergies**: Individuals with allergies to fennel or related plants, such as celery or carrots, should avoid fennel seed infusion. Allergic reactions to fennel are rare but possible.

2. **Medication Interactions**: Fennel seeds may interact with certain medications, especially blood thinners. Individuals taking medication should consult a healthcare provider before using fennel seed infusion as a remedy.

3. **Pregnancy and Breastfeeding**: Pregnant and breastfeeding individuals should consult a healthcare provider before consuming fennel seed infusion regularly, as phytoestrogens in fennel could affect hormonal balance.

Fennel Seed Infusion as a Digestive Aid

Fennel seed infusion is a versatile and effective herbal remedy that can be enjoyed as part of a balanced diet and wellness routine. With its ability to relieve digestive discomfort, support hormonal health, and provide antioxidant benefits, fennel seed infusion offers a natural way to promote overall health.

Regular use of fennel seed infusion, especially when combined with other wellness practices, can offer long-lasting support for digestive health and well-being.

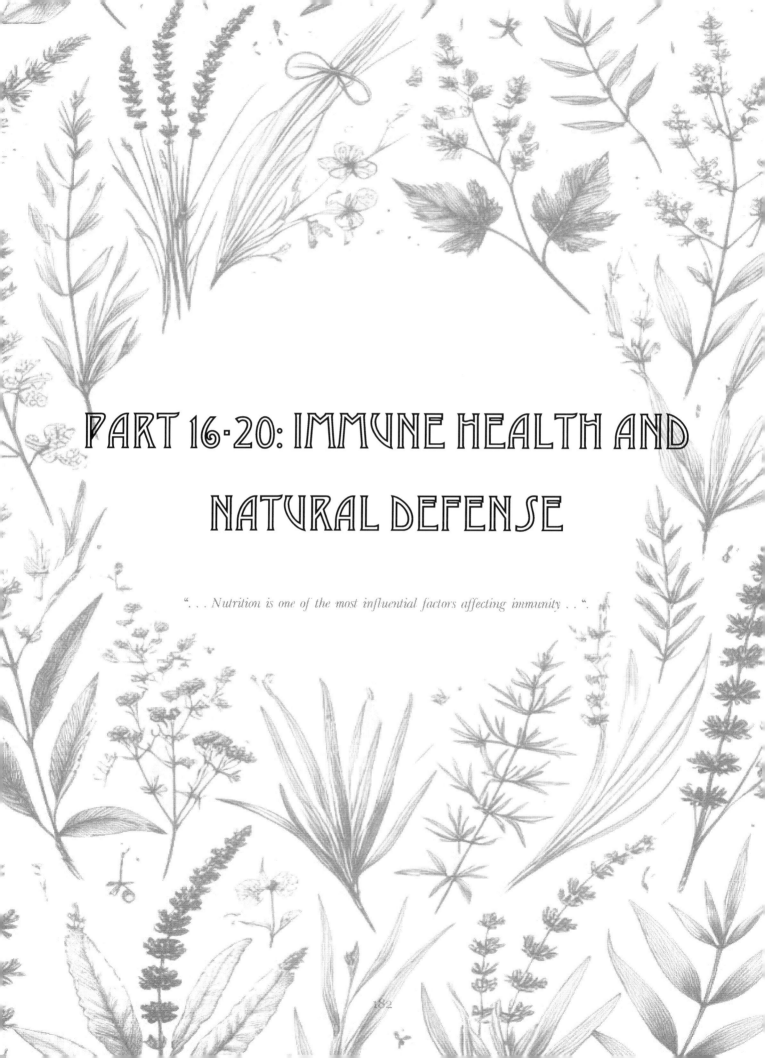

PART 16-20: IMMUNE HEALTH AND NATURAL DEFENSE

". . . Nutrition is one of the most influential factors affecting immunity . . ".

Chapter 1: Building a Strong Immune System

The immune system is a complex network of cells, tissues, and organs that work together to defend the body against harmful pathogens, including viruses, bacteria, and other microorganisms.

Factors that Impact Immunity

This defense mechanism is not static; rather, it is influenced by a wide range of factors, including diet, lifestyle, environmental exposure, and even emotional well-being. Understanding these factors can empower individuals to make informed choices that strengthen their immunity, reduce susceptibility to illness, and promote long-term health.

In this section, we will explore the primary factors that impact immunity, including nutrition, sleep, physical activity, stress, and environmental exposures. By examining each element in depth, this chapter aims to provide a comprehensive overview of how these factors interact to either support or hinder immune function. Additionally, we will explore practical strategies to support immunity naturally, ensuring that each reader feels equipped to make choices that bolster their body's defenses.

Nutrition and Immunity: The Foundation of a Strong Defense

Nutrition is one of the most influential factors affecting immunity. The immune system relies on specific nutrients to perform its functions, including the production of antibodies, activation of immune cells, and signaling between immune cells. A balanced diet rich in vitamins, minerals, antioxidants, and healthy fats provides the necessary fuel for optimal immune function.

1. **Essential Vitamins and Minerals**

Certain vitamins and minerals play a pivotal role in immune health. Deficiencies in these nutrients can lead to weakened immune responses and increased susceptibility to infections.

- **Vitamin C**: Known for its antioxidant properties, vitamin C is essential for the production of white blood cells and supports the skin's natural barriers. Foods rich in vitamin C include citrus fruits, bell peppers, strawberries, and broccoli.
- **Vitamin D**: Often referred to as the "sunshine vitamin," vitamin D is crucial for immune cell function, particularly T-cells. Deficiency in vitamin D has been associated with an increased risk of respiratory infections. While sunlight is the primary source, foods like fatty fish, egg yolks, and fortified dairy products also provide vitamin D.
- **Zinc**: Zinc is necessary for immune cell development and communication. It helps to reduce inflammation and may shorten the duration of illnesses. Zinc-rich foods include shellfish, nuts, seeds, and legumes.
- **Vitamin A**: This fat-soluble vitamin is vital for the maintenance of mucous membranes in the respiratory and digestive tracts, which serve as barriers to infection. Sources include carrots, sweet potatoes, spinach, and fish oils.
- **Vitamin E**: As an antioxidant, vitamin E helps protect immune cells from oxidative damage. It can be found in nuts, seeds, and green leafy vegetables.

2. **Antioxidants and Phytonutrients**

Antioxidants are compounds that protect cells from damage caused by free radicals, which can weaken the immune response. A diet rich in fruits, vegetables, nuts, and seeds provides antioxidants and phytonutrients that support immune health.

Examples of Antioxidant-Rich Foods:
- Berries (blueberries, strawberries, and blackberries) contain anthocyanins, which have anti-inflammatory and immune-boosting properties.
- Leafy greens like spinach and kale are high in beta-carotene, which converts to vitamin A in the body.
- Green tea is rich in catechins, which have been shown to enhance immune response.

Practical Tip: Aim to fill half of your plate with colorful fruits and vegetables at each meal to maximize antioxidant intake. The variety of colors typically represents a range of antioxidants and phytonutrients.

3. **Healthy Fats and Omega-3 Fatty Acids**

Healthy fats, especially omega-3 fatty acids, support immune health by reducing inflammation. Chronic inflammation can suppress the immune system, making it more susceptible to infection. Omega-3s, found in foods like salmon, walnuts, and flaxseeds, help balance the inflammatory response.

Practical Tip: Incorporate sources of omega-3 fatty acids into your diet several times per week. Fatty fish, such as salmon and sardines, provide a direct source of EPA and DHA, two types of omega-3s particularly beneficial for immunity.

Sleep: Restoring and Recharging the Immune System

Sleep is often referred to as the "body's repair mode," as it plays a critical role in restoring and strengthening the immune system. During sleep, the body produces cytokines, proteins that aid in immune response by targeting infection and inflammation. Chronic sleep deprivation can lead to decreased cytokine production, compromising immune function and increasing vulnerability to illness.

1. **The Importance of Sleep Duration and Quality**

Adults typically need 7-9 hours of sleep per night for optimal immune function. Insufficient or poor-quality sleep can weaken immune defenses, making it more challenging for the body to fight off infections. Studies have shown that individuals who sleep fewer than six hours per night are more susceptible to the common cold and other respiratory infections.

Practical Tip: Establish a consistent sleep routine by going to bed and waking up at the same time every day. Avoid screens an hour before bedtime, as the blue light emitted from devices can interfere with melatonin production, a hormone necessary for sleep.

2. **The Role of the Sleep-Wake Cycle**

The sleep-wake cycle, also known as the circadian rhythm, regulates immune function. Immune cells follow a daily rhythm, with certain cells more active at night. Disruptions to this rhythm, such as those caused by shift work or jet lag, can impact immunity. Prioritizing sleep alignment with natural daylight hours can help support the body's immune processes.

Physical Activity: Striking the Balance for Immunity

Regular physical activity can have a positive impact on immune function by promoting circulation, reducing stress, and enhancing immune cell activity. However, there is a balance to be struck, as excessive or intense exercise without adequate recovery can actually suppress immune function.

1. **Moderate Exercise for Immune Support**

Engaging in moderate-intensity exercise, such as walking, cycling, or swimming, for at least 30 minutes most days of the week can enhance immunity by boosting the circulation of immune cells throughout the body. This increase in circulation helps immune cells detect and respond to pathogens more effectively.

Practical Tip: Choose activities that you enjoy and incorporate movement into your daily routine. Exercise should feel energizing, not exhausting, for optimal immune benefits.

2. **Risks of Overtraining**

While regular exercise supports immunity, excessive exercise can have the opposite effect, leading to an "open window" period where the immune system is temporarily weakened. This is particularly common in endurance athletes who engage in prolonged or intense training sessions. Symptoms of overtraining include fatigue, prolonged muscle soreness, and increased susceptibility to infections.

Practical Tip: Ensure adequate rest and recovery if engaging in high-intensity or prolonged exercise. Incorporating rest days and listening to your body's signals can help prevent immune suppression.

Stress Management: Protecting Immunity through Emotional Well-Being

Chronic stress has a profound impact on immunity, as the body's response to stress involves the release of cortisol, a hormone that, in high levels, suppresses immune function. Persistent stress can lead to prolonged inflammation, reduce immune cell production, and increase susceptibility to illness.

1. **The Effects of Chronic Stress on Immune Function**

When the body is under constant stress, it remains in a state of "fight or flight," which diverts resources away from the immune system. Over time, this reduces the body's ability to defend itself against infections and increases the risk of chronic inflammation-related conditions.

2. **Mindfulness and Relaxation Techniques**

Incorporating relaxation techniques, such as meditation, deep breathing exercises, or yoga, can help reduce stress and support immune health. These practices activate the parasympathetic nervous system, encouraging a state of relaxation and reducing cortisol levels.

Practical Tip: Set aside 10–15 minutes each day for stress-reduction practices. Guided meditation apps or simple breathing exercises can be convenient tools to help manage daily stress.

Environmental and Lifestyle Factors

Environmental exposures and lifestyle choices also play a significant role in immunity. These factors can either support or suppress immune function depending on exposure levels and frequency.

1. **Toxin Exposure**

Exposure to environmental toxins, such as pollution, pesticides, and chemicals, can compromise immune health by inducing oxidative stress and damaging immune cells. Over time, chronic exposure can lead to a weakened immune response.

Practical Tip: Reduce toxin exposure by choosing organic foods when possible, using natural cleaning products, and minimizing exposure to air pollution by avoiding outdoor activities during peak pollution times.

2. **Smoking and Alcohol Consumption**

Smoking and excessive alcohol consumption have been shown to impair immune function. Smoking introduces harmful chemicals into the body that damage immune cells and reduce lung capacity, while excessive alcohol disrupts the gut microbiome and weakens the body's ability to fight infections.

Practical Tip: Avoid smoking and limit alcohol intake to moderate levels (up to one drink per day for women and two for men) to minimize immune suppression.

3. **Hand Hygiene and Infection Control**

Simple hygiene practices, such as regular handwashing and avoiding contact with sick individuals, can prevent the spread of infections and reduce the burden on the immune system. Frequent handwashing with soap and water helps remove pathogens that could enter the body and cause illness.

Practical Tip: Practice good hand hygiene by washing hands for at least 20 seconds with soap and water, especially before eating or touching your face.

Hydration and Immune Health

Staying well-hydrated is essential for maintaining immune function. Water is necessary for all cellular functions, including the production and circulation of immune cells. Dehydration can impair the immune system by reducing lymphatic drainage and impeding the removal of toxins from the body.

1. **The Role of Water in Immune Function**

Proper hydration supports the lymphatic system, which is responsible for transporting immune cells throughout the body. Water also helps to thin mucus, making it easier to expel pathogens from the respiratory tract.

Practical Tip: Aim to drink at least 8 cups (64 ounces) of water per day, adjusting intake based on activity level and environmental conditions.

2. Supporting Immunity with Herbal Teas

Herbal teas, such as echinacea, ginger, and elderberry, can provide additional immune-supporting benefits. These herbs contain compounds that support immune health and offer anti-inflammatory and antioxidant properties.

Practical Tip: Incorporate immune-supportive herbal teas into your daily hydration routine for added benefits, especially during cold and flu season.

By considering and addressing these various factors, individuals can take proactive steps to support their immune health naturally. A well-rounded approach that includes proper nutrition, adequate sleep, regular exercise, stress management, and mindful lifestyle choices creates a strong foundation for a resilient immune system capable of protecting the body from illness.

Immunity and Lifestyle Choices

Our immune system is the body's natural defensc mechanism, constantly working to protect us from pathogens like viruses, bacteria, and other harmful invaders. Immunity is not a fixed trait but rather a dynamic system that can be strengthened or weakened depending on various lifestyle choices. Just as herbal remedies can support immunity, so too can lifestyle habits, which form the foundation of our body's defense capabilities. A proactive approach to health can create a resilient immune system that withstands challenges and keeps the body functioning optimally.

Modern life often presents unique challenges to immune health, from stress and poor diet to lack of sleep and sedentary habits. Understanding how daily lifestyle choices impact immunity provides a pathway to building sustainable health. Embracing small, intentional changes can foster long-term resilience, allowing the immune system to perform at its best.

The Impact of Nutrition on Immunity

Nutrition is one of the most critical components of a strong immune system. Nutrient-rich foods provide the building blocks the immune system needs to function efficiently, supporting everything from white blood cell production to the health of mucous membranes that act as barriers against pathogens.

1. **Vitamin C**: Known for its immune-boosting properties, vitamin C supports the production of white blood cells, which are essential in fighting infections. Foods rich in vitamin C include citrus fruits, bell peppers, strawberries, and leafy greens. Consuming these foods regularly can enhance immune response, especially during the cold and flu season.

2. **Vitamin D**: Often called the "sunshine vitamin," vitamin D plays a significant role in modulating the immune response. It helps activate T cells, which are vital in detecting and destroying pathogens. Fatty fish, egg yolks, and fortified foods are good sources, and moderate sun exposure also boosts vitamin D levels.

3. **Zinc**: Zinc is essential for immune cell function and communication. It plays a role in wound healing and may reduce the duration of the common cold. Rich sources of zinc include nuts, seeds, whole grains, and legumes. Maintaining adequate zinc levels supports immune resilience and can help the body recover faster from infections.

4. **Antioxidant-Rich Foods**: Antioxidants protect immune cells from oxidative stress caused by free radicals. Fruits and vegetables, especially those with vibrant colors, are high in antioxidants. Foods like blueberries, spinach, carrots, and tomatoes contribute to a balanced immune response by reducing inflammation and protecting cells from damage.

5. **Probiotics**: A healthy gut microbiome supports immunity by maintaining the integrity of the gut barrier and regulating immune responses. Fermented foods such as yogurt, kefir, sauerkraut, and kombucha contain beneficial bacteria that support gut health. A balanced gut can prevent the overgrowth of harmful bacteria and plays a crucial role in overall immune function.

By incorporating a variety of nutrient-rich foods into the diet, individuals can support their immune systems with the vitamins, minerals, and antioxidants needed to prevent illness and promote healing.

Physical Activity and Its Role in Immune Health

Regular physical activity contributes to immune health by promoting circulation, reducing inflammation, and supporting overall vitality. Exercise mobilizes immune cells, helping them move freely throughout the body, detect potential threats, and respond effectively.

1. **Moderate Exercise**: Moderate-intensity exercise, such as walking, cycling, or swimming, has been shown to enhance immune function. This level of activity increases the circulation of white blood cells and antibodies, making it easier for the immune system to detect and respond to pathogens. Engaging in at least 30 minutes of moderate exercise most days of the week can improve immune surveillance.

2. **High-Intensity Exercise**: While moderate exercise boosts immunity, extreme or prolonged high-intensity exercise can have the opposite effect, temporarily suppressing immune function. Athletes and individuals engaged in intense training should incorporate rest and recovery days to prevent overtaxing the immune system.

3. **Outdoor Activity**: Exercising outdoors combines the benefits of physical activity with exposure to fresh air and sunlight, which boosts vitamin D levels. Activities such as hiking or jogging in nature can reduce stress, enhance mood, and improve immune function, offering a holistic approach to wellness.

Exercise should be tailored to individual fitness levels, with an emphasis on consistency and enjoyment. Regular physical activity is one of the most effective lifestyle choices for supporting long-term immune resilience.

Quality Sleep as the Foundation of Immunity

Sleep is essential for immune health, as it allows the body to recover, repair, and restore. During sleep, the immune system releases cytokines, proteins that help combat infections and inflammation. Chronic sleep deprivation can compromise immune function, making the body more susceptible to illness.

1. **Sleep and Immune Cell Production**: Quality sleep supports the production of immune cells, including T cells and natural killer cells. These cells play a critical role in identifying and neutralizing pathogens. Individuals who consistently get 7-9 hours

of sleep per night are less likely to catch common infections and have stronger immune responses.

2. **Improving Sleep Hygiene**: Creating a restful sleep environment can enhance sleep quality. Avoiding screens before bedtime, establishing a relaxing pre-sleep routine, and maintaining a cool, dark, and quiet bedroom contribute to better rest. Consistency is key, as a regular sleep schedule helps regulate the body's internal clock.

3. **Reducing Sleep Disruptors**: Limiting caffeine intake in the afternoon, managing stress, and avoiding heavy meals before bed can prevent sleep disruptions. Alcohol, while initially sedating, disrupts sleep cycles, leading to poor sleep quality and diminished immune function.

Prioritizing sleep is an act of self-care that directly impacts immune health. By maintaining a regular sleep schedule and creating an environment conducive to rest, individuals can support their immune system's ability to protect against illness.

Managing Stress for a Stronger Immune Response

Chronic stress is one of the most significant lifestyle factors that negatively impact immunity. When the body is under stress, it produces cortisol, a hormone that suppresses immune function. Long-term exposure to high cortisol levels can lead to chronic inflammation, leaving the body vulnerable to infections.

1. **Stress and Immune Suppression**: Elevated cortisol levels decrease the body's ability to produce antibodies and impair immune cell function. This suppression leaves the body more susceptible to infections and may delay recovery times.

2. **Mindfulness Practices**: Mindfulness techniques, such as meditation, deep breathing exercises, and yoga, are effective for reducing stress and promoting relaxation. These practices help lower cortisol levels and reduce inflammation, supporting a balanced immune response. Just a few minutes of mindfulness each day can have lasting effects on overall well-being.

3. **Social Connections**: Maintaining strong social connections also reduces stress. Positive relationships provide emotional support, which can buffer against the effects of stress. Studies show that individuals with strong social ties have more robust immune responses and are better equipped to cope with life's challenges.

4. **Hobbies and Leisure**: Engaging in activities that bring joy, such as reading, gardening, or crafting, allows the mind and body to relax, releasing tension and

lowering stress levels. These activities provide a healthy distraction and encourage a positive mindset, indirectly supporting immune function.

Managing stress is essential for immune resilience. By cultivating a balanced approach to stress through mindfulness, meaningful relationships, and enjoyable activities, individuals can protect their immune system from the harmful effects of chronic stress.

Avoiding Immune-Suppressing Habits

Certain lifestyle choices can undermine immune health, particularly when practiced regularly. Recognizing and minimizing these habits supports a stronger immune system.

1. **Smoking**: Smoking damages the respiratory system and weakens immune defenses, making the body more susceptible to respiratory infections. Quitting smoking not only improves lung health but also enhances the immune system's ability to fight infections.

2. **Excessive Alcohol Consumption**: High alcohol intake suppresses immune function and reduces the ability of white blood cells to fight infections. Moderation is key, as small amounts of alcohol may not have significant effects, but excessive consumption weakens immunity.

3. **High Sugar Intake**: Diets high in refined sugars can suppress immune function and increase inflammation. Excessive sugar intake reduces the ability of white blood cells to combat pathogens, making it more challenging for the immune system to function effectively.

4. **Sedentary Lifestyle**: Lack of physical activity is linked to poor immune function. Incorporating movement into daily routines, even if it's a short walk, can counteract the effects of a sedentary lifestyle and enhance immune health.

Avoiding these habits or incorporating healthier alternatives can make a meaningful difference in supporting immunity and overall health.

Natural Remedies and Immune-Boosting Herbs

Herbal remedies can further enhance immune health by providing additional nutrients and bioactive compounds. Herbs like echinacea, elderberry, and astragalus have been used for centuries to support immune function and ward off infections.

1. **Echinacea**: Known for its immune-stimulating effects, echinacea may reduce the severity and duration of colds. It supports the body's natural defenses, especially when taken at the first sign of illness.

2. **Elderberry**: Elderberries are rich in antioxidants and have antiviral properties. Elderberry extract or syrup is often used to support respiratory health and reduce flu symptoms.

3. **Astragalus**: Astragalus root is an adaptogen that strengthens the immune system and increases resistance to stress. Regular consumption can provide ongoing support for immune resilience.

4. **Ginger and Turmeric**: Both ginger and turmeric have anti-inflammatory properties that support immune health. Turmeric's active compound, curcumin, is particularly effective in reducing inflammation and boosting the body's natural defenses.

Herbs should complement, not replace, a balanced diet and healthy lifestyle choices. Incorporating these remedies as part of a holistic approach provides additional immune support, especially during cold and flu season.

Building an Immune-Resilient Lifestyle

Creating a lifestyle that supports immunity involves a balance of nutrition, exercise, sleep, and stress management. Small, consistent efforts in each area contribute to long-term health and wellness, empowering the body's natural defenses. By adopting positive lifestyle habits and avoiding those that weaken immunity, individuals can create a foundation of resilience. The immune system is intricately linked to lifestyle, responding to the choices we make each day. Embracing a proactive approach to immunity allows the body to function at its best, providing lasting protection and resilience in the face of life's challenges.

Importance of Sleep

Sleep is an essential component of human health and well-being, impacting nearly every system in the body, from the brain and immune system to metabolism and mental health. Despite its vital role, sleep is often one of the first aspects of self-care to be sacrificed in favor of productivity, social activities, or even late-night screen time. However, quality sleep is a cornerstone of maintaining a strong immune system, optimal brain function, emotional balance, and physical health. Without adequate sleep, the body becomes more susceptible to disease, mental health issues, and chronic conditions.

In this section, we'll explore the importance of sleep, the mechanisms by which it supports the body, the consequences of sleep deprivation, and practical strategies to improve sleep quality. Understanding the profound impact of sleep on various aspects of health can encourage individuals to prioritize rest as an integral part of their wellness routines.

The Science of Sleep: Stages and Cycles

Sleep is a complex process that occurs in stages, each playing a unique role in physical and mental restoration. The sleep cycle consists of two main types: non-rapid eye movement (NREM) and rapid eye movement (REM) sleep, which cycle several times throughout the night.

1. NREM Sleep

NREM sleep comprises three stages, each progressively deeper than the last. The first stage is a light sleep, during which the body begins to relax, and brain activity slows. This stage transitions into the second stage, where heart rate and breathing slow down further. The final NREM stage is deep sleep, often referred to as "slow-wave sleep," which is essential for physical restoration, muscle repair, immune function, and the release of growth hormones. Deep sleep is crucial for the body to recover and restore itself, particularly after physical activity or stress.

2. REM Sleep

REM sleep, which follows each cycle of NREM sleep, is when most dreaming occurs. This stage is essential for brain health, emotional processing, and memory consolidation. During REM sleep, brain activity resembles that of wakefulness, but the body remains mostly paralyzed, preventing physical reactions to dreams. REM sleep is believed to be particularly important for cognitive function, emotional health, and the ability to process experiences.

3. Sleep Cycles

Each complete sleep cycle lasts approximately 90 minutes, and adults typically go through 4-6 cycles per night. The first half of the night usually contains more NREM sleep, particularly deep sleep, while REM sleep dominates the latter half of the night. This distribution is why getting adequate sleep time is critical; cutting the night short or waking frequently can disrupt these cycles, leading to inadequate restoration and mental function.

How Sleep Impacts Immune Function

One of the most significant roles of sleep is its impact on immune health. During sleep, the immune system is in a heightened state of alertness, producing cytokines, proteins that play a role in fighting off infection and inflammation. Sleep deprivation can weaken the immune system, making the body more susceptible to infections, from the common cold to more severe illnesses.

1. **Cytokine Production**

Cytokines are crucial in the immune response, particularly for inflammation and defense against infections. During sleep, the body increases the production of certain cytokines, especially those that help fight infection and inflammation. When sleep is inadequate, cytokine production is reduced, weakening the immune response. This reduction explains why people who are sleep-deprived are more likely to get sick after exposure to viruses.

2. **Antibody Formation**

Antibodies are proteins that help the immune system recognize and neutralize pathogens. Adequate sleep supports the production of antibodies, enhancing the body's ability to fight off infections. Studies show that sleep-deprived individuals respond less effectively to vaccines, as they produce fewer antibodies in response. This finding highlights how sleep is essential for immune memory and resilience.

3. **Sleep and Inflammation**

Chronic sleep deprivation is associated with increased levels of inflammation in the body, a condition that contributes to many chronic diseases, including heart disease, diabetes, and autoimmune disorders. By allowing the body time to rest and recover, sleep helps keep inflammation in check, reducing the risk of these conditions. Prioritizing sleep can thus be viewed as a preventive measure for long-term health.

The Impact of Sleep on Mental Health and Cognitive Function

Sleep is critical for cognitive processes, including memory, learning, problem-solving, and emotional regulation. During sleep, the brain processes and organizes information from the day, strengthens neural connections, and prepares itself for new learning. A lack of sleep can impair these cognitive functions, leading to difficulties in focus, decision-making, and emotional stability.

1. **Memory Consolidation**

During sleep, particularly during REM sleep, the brain consolidates memories, organizing information and transferring it from short-term to long-term storage. This process is crucial for learning and retaining new information. Sleep deprivation can disrupt this process, making it harder to remember information and reducing cognitive performance.

2. Emotional Regulation

Sleep also plays a vital role in regulating emotions. Sleep-deprived individuals are more prone to mood swings, irritability, and stress. Sleep helps the brain process and recover from emotional experiences, which is why a good night's sleep can make challenges feel more manageable. Chronic sleep deprivation is linked to a higher risk of mental health conditions such as anxiety and depression, underscoring the need for adequate sleep for emotional well-being.

3. Focus and Decision-Making

Inadequate sleep impairs executive function, affecting one's ability to focus, plan, and make decisions. This can lead to increased errors, decreased productivity, and difficulty in managing complex tasks. Over time, this cognitive decline can affect both personal and professional life, creating a cycle of stress and reduced sleep quality.

Physical Health and Sleep: The Body's Nightly Repair Mode

Sleep is essential for physical recovery and energy restoration, as the body undergoes various repair processes during rest. For instance, muscles recover and grow during deep sleep, and tissues repair themselves, which is particularly important for those who engage in regular physical activity or lead active lives.

1. Muscle Recovery and Growth

Growth hormone, essential for tissue growth and muscle repair, is released during deep sleep. This hormone promotes cell regeneration and helps the body heal from physical exertion. Athletes and those who exercise regularly need sufficient sleep to recover properly, as inadequate sleep can lead to fatigue, muscle soreness, and a higher risk of injury.

2. Metabolic Health

Sleep also plays a role in regulating metabolism. During sleep, the body balances hormones that control hunger and satiety, such as leptin and ghrelin. When sleep is disrupted, these hormones become imbalanced, leading to increased appetite, particularly for high-calorie foods. This disruption contributes to weight gain and increases the risk of metabolic disorders such as obesity and type 2 diabetes.

3. Cardiovascular Health

Cardiovascular health is closely linked to sleep quality. Poor sleep can lead to an increase in blood pressure and stress hormone levels, putting strain on the heart and blood vessels. Chronic sleep deprivation is associated with a higher risk of heart disease, stroke, and hypertension. By supporting cardiovascular function, sleep acts as a protective factor against these serious health conditions.

Practical Strategies for Improving Sleep Quality

Improving sleep quality involves both creating a conducive sleep environment and establishing healthy sleep habits. Simple changes to one's bedtime routine, sleep environment, and lifestyle can significantly enhance sleep quality and overall well-being.

1. **Establish a Consistent Sleep Schedule**

Going to bed and waking up at the same time each day helps regulate the body's internal clock, known as the circadian rhythm. Consistency reinforces the sleep-wake cycle, making it easier to fall asleep and wake up at the desired times. Even on weekends, maintaining a consistent schedule can help improve sleep quality.

2. **Create a Relaxing Bedtime Routine**

A calming pre-sleep routine can signal to the body that it's time to wind down. This routine might include activities such as reading, gentle stretching, or practicing mindfulness. Avoid stimulating activities like watching TV or scrolling through social media, as these can delay the onset of sleep.

3. **Optimize the Sleep Environment**

Creating a sleep-friendly environment is essential for quality rest. Consider these factors:

   o **Darkness**: Use blackout curtains or an eye mask to eliminate light, which can disrupt sleep.

   o **Noise Control**: Reduce noise with earplugs or a white noise machine if necessary.

   o **Temperature**: Keep the room cool, as lower temperatures are conducive to better sleep.

4. **Limit Caffeine and Alcohol Intake**

Both caffeine and alcohol can interfere with sleep. Caffeine is a stimulant that can stay in the body for several hours, so it's best to avoid it in the afternoon and evening. Alcohol, although it may initially make you feel drowsy, can disrupt sleep cycles and lead to poorer quality rest. Limiting or eliminating these substances can improve sleep duration and quality.

5. Physical Activity

Regular exercise can promote better sleep, especially when done earlier in the day. Physical activity increases the amount of time spent in deep sleep, which is restorative. However, intense exercise close to bedtime may have the opposite effect, as it raises adrenaline and cortisol levels.

The Role of Natural Remedies in Supporting Sleep

In addition to lifestyle changes, certain natural remedies may help support sleep by promoting relaxation and reducing anxiety. These remedies can complement healthy sleep habits and offer additional support for those struggling with sleep issues.

1. **Herbal Teas**: Chamomile, valerian root, and lavender teas are popular choices for promoting relaxation before bed. Chamomile contains apigenin, an antioxidant that binds to receptors in the brain, potentially inducing a mild sedative effect. Valerian root may reduce the time it takes to fall asleep and improve sleep quality.

2. **Melatonin Supplements**: Melatonin, the hormone that regulates sleep-wake cycles, can be taken as a supplement for short-term sleep support. It may be helpful for individuals with circadian rhythm disruptions, such as shift workers or those experiencing jet lag. It's best used under the guidance of a healthcare professional.

3. **Magnesium**: Magnesium is a mineral that supports muscle relaxation and may improve sleep quality. Foods rich in magnesium, such as leafy greens, nuts, and seeds, can be incorporated into the diet, or magnesium supplements can be taken before bed to support restful sleep.

Reducing Stress for Immunity

The connection between stress and immunity is powerful and immediate, as chronic stress can significantly weaken the body's natural defenses. When the body experiences stress, it releases cortisol and other hormones that, while beneficial in short bursts, can be detrimental when elevated for prolonged periods. Chronic stress impairs immune function, making individuals more susceptible to illness, inflammation, and slower recovery from infections. Therefore, effectively managing and reducing stress is not only beneficial for mental well-being but also essential for a strong, resilient immune system.

Understanding the relationship between stress and immunity empowers individuals to make lifestyle changes that support both physical and mental health. By cultivating practices that reduce stress, one can help fortify the immune system, leading to enhanced overall wellness and a greater ability to resist illness.

The Physiological Impact of Stress on Immunity

Stress triggers the body's "fight-or-flight" response, a mechanism designed to prepare for potential danger. This response involves the release of cortisol and adrenaline, hormones that temporarily suppress non-essential functions, including immune response, to prioritize survival. In the short term, this response is adaptive and beneficial; however, when stress becomes chronic, the ongoing release of these hormones can disrupt immune balance.

1. **Suppression of Immune Cells**: Chronic stress reduces the number of lymphocytes, which are white blood cells crucial for fighting off infections. Lower lymphocyte levels mean the body is less capable of combating foreign invaders like viruses and bacteria, making it easier for infections to take hold.

2. **Increased Inflammation**: While inflammation is a natural part of the immune response, chronic stress causes persistent, low-level inflammation that can damage tissues and organs. This inflammation is linked to various health issues, including heart disease, diabetes, and autoimmune disorders.

3. **Impaired Antibody Production**: Stress also hinders the production of antibodies, which are proteins that recognize and neutralize pathogens. A reduction in antibodies can delay the body's response to infections, allowing them to spread more easily and potentially become more severe.

Recognizing the profound impact that stress has on immune function is the first step toward actively reducing stress levels. Through intentional lifestyle changes, individuals can help restore balance to the immune system, ensuring it operates at full capacity.

Mindfulness and Meditation as Tools for Stress Reduction

Mindfulness and meditation have gained widespread recognition for their effectiveness in managing stress and supporting mental clarity. These practices encourage individuals to focus on the present moment, reducing worry about the past or future, which often exacerbates stress.

1. **Mindfulness Techniques**: Mindfulness involves observing thoughts, feelings, and bodily sensations without judgment. This process helps create a sense of calm and acceptance, reducing stress levels and supporting a healthy immune response. Practicing mindfulness daily, even for just 10-15 minutes, can lower cortisol levels, decrease inflammation, and improve immune function over time.

2. **Meditation Practices**: Meditation, particularly focused breathing exercises, deepens relaxation and reduces stress hormones. Techniques like deep diaphragmatic breathing activate the body's parasympathetic nervous system, which counters the stress response and promotes relaxation. Guided meditation, visualization, and progressive muscle relaxation are also helpful for reducing tension and anxiety.

3. **Incorporating Mindfulness into Daily Life**: Mindfulness does not require special settings or long periods. Simple practices, such as mindful eating or mindful walking, encourage people to focus fully on their current activity, allowing for a brief mental reset. These practices make it easier to manage stress in daily life and contribute to long-term immune health.

Mindfulness and meditation are powerful tools for transforming one's response to stress, and over time, they lead to a calmer, more resilient mindset. Regular practice can enhance immune resilience, creating a foundation for lasting well-being.

Physical Activity as a Natural Stress Reliever

Exercise is a proven method for reducing stress and supporting immune health. Physical activity promotes the release of endorphins, chemicals that elevate mood and reduce perceptions of pain, which helps counteract the effects of stress.

1. **Moderate Exercise for Immunity**: Moderate-intensity exercise, such as walking, cycling, or swimming, effectively reduces cortisol levels and improves immune function. Regular activity strengthens the cardiovascular system, improves circulation, and aids in the removal of waste products, supporting overall health and immunity.

2. **The Role of Outdoor Activities**: Exercising outdoors combines the physical benefits of activity with the mental health benefits of exposure to nature. Studies suggest that spending time in green spaces reduces stress, anxiety, and depression. Activities like hiking, jogging, or even yoga in nature provide a natural way to manage stress and boost immune function.

3. **Consistency Over Intensity**: While intense exercise has its benefits, excessive or high-intensity workouts can actually weaken immunity due to increased cortisol production. A balanced approach, focusing on moderate but consistent exercise, yields the best results for immunity and stress reduction.

Incorporating exercise into daily routines provides a natural and enjoyable way to reduce stress. Not only does regular activity improve mood and mental clarity, but it also contributes to a more resilient immune system, enhancing the body's ability to fight illness.

The Power of Social Connections

Positive social interactions are essential for reducing stress and supporting immunity. Human connection fosters feelings of belonging, safety, and comfort, which can offset the negative effects of stress.

1. **Building a Support System**: A strong support system of friends, family, or community members provides a buffer against stress. Talking to loved ones about concerns or simply spending time with them can reduce anxiety, lower cortisol levels, and foster emotional well-being.

2. **Participating in Group Activities**: Group activities, such as volunteering, joining clubs, or participating in hobby-based groups, create a sense of community and purpose. These activities also distract from stressors and provide enjoyable, shared experiences that boost mood and reduce anxiety.

3. **Maintaining Connections in Times of Stress**: During difficult times, people may withdraw from social interaction, but staying connected is crucial for managing stress. Reaching out to friends or family, even through a brief phone call or message, can provide a valuable emotional lift and mitigate the effects of stress on the immune system.

Social support plays an irreplaceable role in mental and physical health. By cultivating relationships and nurturing connections, individuals can build a network of support that aids in stress management and enhances immune resilience.

Sleep: The Ultimate Stress Management Tool

Quality sleep is one of the most critical factors in managing stress and supporting immune function. Sleep allows the body to recover, regenerate, and prepare for the day ahead. Chronic sleep deprivation leads to elevated stress hormones, impaired immune responses, and reduced overall resilience.

1. **Establishing a Bedtime Routine**: A consistent sleep routine improves sleep quality and reduces stress. Activities such as reading, taking a warm bath, or practicing relaxation techniques before bed signal the body that it's time to wind down. Consistency in bedtime and wake-up time also helps regulate the body's internal clock.

2. **Creating a Sleep-Friendly Environment**: A dark, quiet, and cool room creates an optimal sleep environment. Limiting screen exposure, especially blue light from devices, in the evening prevents disruptions in melatonin production, which is essential for quality sleep.

3. **Limiting Stimulants**: Reducing caffeine intake, particularly in the afternoon, prevents sleep disturbances. Alcohol, while initially sedating, can also disrupt sleep cycles, leading to poor sleep quality and increased stress levels.

Quality sleep is essential for stress resilience. By prioritizing sleep and creating a restful environment, individuals can improve their ability to manage stress and support their immune system.

Nutritional Support for Stress Reduction

Diet plays a critical role in managing stress and supporting immune health. Certain foods can help regulate stress hormones, reduce inflammation, and stabilize blood sugar levels, all of which contribute to a calmer, more resilient state of mind.

1. **Complex Carbohydrates**: Foods like whole grains, legumes, and sweet potatoes provide a steady release of energy, which helps stabilize blood sugar and prevent mood swings. Complex carbohydrates also support serotonin production, which is known to enhance mood.

2. **Healthy Fats**: Omega-3 fatty acids, found in fatty fish, walnuts, and flaxseeds, have anti-inflammatory properties that support brain function and reduce stress levels.

Regular consumption of these fats may help regulate cortisol and improve resilience to stress.

3. **Magnesium-Rich Foods**: Magnesium plays a role in relaxing muscles and reducing anxiety. Leafy greens, nuts, seeds, and whole grains are excellent sources of magnesium, which supports a calm nervous system and reduces stress-related tension.

4. **Hydration**: Dehydration can exacerbate stress and increase cortisol levels. Staying hydrated with water, herbal teas, and low-sugar beverages supports optimal cognitive function and mood stability.

Choosing a balanced, nutrient-rich diet provides the body with the resources needed to manage stress effectively and maintain immune resilience.

Herbs and Natural Remedies for Stress Management

In addition to lifestyle changes, certain herbs can support stress management by promoting relaxation and balance. Herbal remedies have been used for centuries to soothe the nervous system, improve mood, and reduce anxiety.

1. **Ashwagandha**: Known as an adaptogen, ashwagandha helps the body adapt to stress by regulating cortisol levels. Regular use of ashwagandha can improve mood, reduce fatigue, and enhance overall resilience to stress.

2. **Chamomile**: Chamomile is a gentle herb with calming properties. Drinking chamomile tea in the evening promotes relaxation, aids sleep, and can help reduce feelings of anxiety, making it beneficial for stress relief.

3. **Lavender**: Lavender's calming scent has been shown to reduce anxiety and improve mood. Using lavender essential oil in a diffuser or applying it topically can create a sense of calm, supporting both sleep and stress management.

4. **Lemon Balm**: Lemon balm is a member of the mint family and has mild sedative properties. It helps reduce anxiety, ease nervous tension, and promote restful sleep, making it an excellent choice for managing stress.

Incorporating herbs into daily routines provides natural support for stress management. These herbs can be used in teas, tinctures, or essential oils to enhance relaxation and balance, complementing other stress-reducing lifestyle practices.

Mindful Breathing and Relaxation Techniques

Breathing exercises and relaxation techniques are simple yet effective methods for managing stress. By focusing on the breath and practicing deep, intentional breathing, individuals can activate the body's relaxation response, countering the effects of stress.

1. **Deep Breathing**: Deep breathing involves taking slow, full breaths from the diaphragm. This technique slows the heart rate, lowers blood pressure, and reduces cortisol levels. Practicing deep breathing for a few minutes each day can help maintain a calm state.

2. **Progressive Muscle Relaxation**: This technique involves tensing and relaxing each muscle group in the body, moving from head to toe. Progressive muscle relaxation helps release physical tension associated with stress, promoting a sense of calm.

3. **Guided Imagery**: Guided imagery involves visualizing a peaceful scene or place, which can help shift the mind away from stressors. This technique encourages relaxation and can be practiced anytime, especially before sleep or during stressful moments.

Mindful breathing and relaxation techniques are accessible to everyone and can be practiced anytime. These techniques are powerful tools for managing stress, supporting mental clarity, and enhancing immune function.

Creating a Personalized Stress-Reduction Plan

Reducing stress is not a one-size-fits-all approach. Each person has unique needs, preferences, and stressors. Creating a personalized stress-reduction plan, incorporating nutrition, exercise, sleep, social support, and relaxation techniques, enables individuals to develop a resilient response to life's challenges.

Building a plan that incorporates a variety of stress-reducing practices ensures a balanced approach to mental and physical well-being. By prioritizing stress reduction, individuals can support their immune systems, fostering a healthier, more fulfilling life.

Chapter 2: Nutrition for Immune Support

Antioxidants play a crucial role in protecting the body from oxidative stress, a process that occurs when free radicals—unstable molecules that damage cells—accumulate. This oxidative stress can lead to chronic inflammation and contribute to various health issues, including aging, heart disease, cancer, and neurodegenerative conditions. Antioxidants neutralize free radicals, reducing or preventing cell damage.

Antioxidant-Rich Foods

One of the most effective ways to increase antioxidant levels is through diet, focusing on foods that are naturally high in these protective compounds.

In this section, we'll examine the importance of antioxidants, explore the different types found in foods, and discuss the best antioxidant-rich foods to include in a balanced diet. By understanding and incorporating these foods, individuals can support overall health, enhance their body's natural defenses, and prevent disease.

Why Antioxidants Matter: The Role in Health and Disease Prevention

Free radicals are produced in the body as a natural part of processes like metabolism. However, external factors such as pollution, UV radiation, smoking, and poor diet can increase their production. When the body is overwhelmed by free radicals, it enters a state of oxidative stress, leading to cellular damage. Over time, oxidative stress contributes to inflammation, weakens the immune system, and plays a role in various chronic diseases.

Antioxidants counteract this effect by donating an electron to free radicals, stabilizing them and preventing them from damaging cells. Different antioxidants work in various parts of the body, some protecting the eyes and skin, while others support the heart and immune system. A diet rich in antioxidants can help prevent chronic conditions, boost immune function, and even slow the aging process by protecting cellular health.

Types of Antioxidants in Foods

There are many types of antioxidants, each with specific benefits. The most well-known categories include vitamins, flavonoids, polyphenols, and carotenoids. Each type has a unique role in the body and can be found in various foods:

1. **Vitamin C**

Vitamin C is a powerful water-soluble antioxidant that plays a vital role in immune health, skin protection, and iron absorption. It also regenerates other antioxidants, such as vitamin E, enhancing their effects. Found in high concentrations in citrus fruits, strawberries, and bell peppers, vitamin C is essential for maintaining cellular health and preventing oxidative damage.

2. **Vitamin E**

Vitamin E is a fat-soluble antioxidant that protects cell membranes from damage. It is particularly beneficial for skin health, preventing damage from UV exposure, and has anti-inflammatory properties. Nuts, seeds, and leafy greens are excellent sources of vitamin E.

3. **Carotenoids**

Carotenoids are pigments that give fruits and vegetables their vibrant colors. They include beta-carotene, lycopene, and lutein. Beta-carotene, found in carrots and sweet potatoes, is converted to vitamin A in the body and supports vision and immune health. Lycopene, found in tomatoes, supports heart health, while lutein, found in spinach and kale, promotes eye health.

4. **Flavonoids**

Flavonoids are a group of antioxidants found in many fruits, vegetables, and herbs. They are known for their anti-inflammatory and immune-boosting properties. Flavonoids are abundant in berries, citrus fruits, tea, and dark chocolate. Quercetin, a flavonoid found in apples and onions, has shown potential benefits in reducing allergy symptoms and inflammation.

5. **Polyphenols**

Polyphenols are potent antioxidants found in foods like red wine, berries, green tea, and dark chocolate. They have been linked to improved heart health, better cognitive function, and reduced inflammation. Resveratrol, a polyphenol found in red wine, grapes, and peanuts, has gained attention for its anti-aging properties.

Top Antioxidant-Rich Foods to Include in Your Diet

1. **Berries**

Berries are one of the richest sources of antioxidants, particularly flavonoids and vitamin C. Blueberries, strawberries, raspberries, and blackberries contain anthocyanins, which give them their deep colors and provide powerful anti-inflammatory effects.

- **Blueberries**: Known for their high levels of anthocyanins, blueberries help reduce oxidative stress, improve cognitive function, and support heart health.
- **Strawberries**: High in vitamin C, strawberries enhance immune health and protect the skin from environmental damage.
- **Raspberries**: Raspberries are rich in quercetin and vitamin C, supporting heart health and reducing inflammation.

2. **Dark Leafy Greens**

Leafy greens, such as spinach, kale, and Swiss chard, contain a range of antioxidants, including vitamins C and E, beta-carotene, and lutein. These antioxidants support eye health, immune function, and cellular repair.

- **Spinach**: Rich in beta-carotene and lutein, spinach helps protect the eyes from oxidative damage and supports skin health.
- **Kale**: A potent source of vitamins C and E, kale helps neutralize free radicals and supports immune health.
- **Swiss Chard**: Swiss chard contains betalains, antioxidants that provide anti-inflammatory and detoxifying benefits.

3. **Nuts and Seeds**

Nuts and seeds, particularly almonds, walnuts, sunflower seeds, and flaxseeds, are packed with vitamin E, selenium, and omega-3 fatty acids, all of which have strong antioxidant properties.

- **Almonds**: High in vitamin E, almonds help protect skin and cell membranes from oxidative stress.
- **Walnuts**: Walnuts contain polyphenols, which reduce inflammation and support brain health.
- **Sunflower Seeds**: A rich source of vitamin E, sunflower seeds support immune function and skin health.

4. **Cruciferous Vegetables**

Vegetables such as broccoli, cauliflower, and Brussels sprouts are rich in antioxidants, particularly vitamin C and sulforaphane, a compound with potent anti-cancer properties.

- **Broccoli**: High in vitamin C and sulforaphane, broccoli supports immune health and detoxification.
- **Cauliflower**: Contains vitamin C and glucosinolates, which support liver function and reduce inflammation.
- **Brussels Sprouts**: Rich in vitamin K and antioxidants, Brussels sprouts support heart health and have anti-inflammatory benefits.

5. Tomatoes

Tomatoes are high in lycopene, an antioxidant known for its heart-protective and anti-cancer properties. Cooking tomatoes increases the bioavailability of lycopene, making it easier for the body to absorb.

- **Cherry Tomatoes**: These smaller tomatoes have a concentrated level of lycopene and vitamin C, supporting skin health and reducing the risk of chronic diseases.
- **Sun-Dried Tomatoes**: Sun-dried tomatoes contain higher levels of antioxidants due to their concentrated form, supporting immune and cardiovascular health.

6. Tea and Coffee

Both green tea and coffee contain antioxidants that support brain function, reduce inflammation, and protect against certain diseases.

- **Green Tea**: Contains catechins, particularly epigallocatechin gallate (EGCG), which has been shown to support heart health, brain function, and weight management.
- **Black Tea**: Contains theaflavins and catechins, which have anti-inflammatory and immune-boosting effects.
- **Coffee**: A rich source of polyphenols, coffee has been linked to a reduced risk of neurodegenerative diseases and improved liver health.

7. Dark Chocolate

Dark chocolate, particularly varieties with a high cocoa content, is rich in polyphenols and flavonoids. These antioxidants support heart health, improve blood flow, and reduce inflammation.

- **Cocoa Powder**: Pure cocoa powder is a concentrated source of antioxidants, making it beneficial for heart health and reducing oxidative stress.

- o **Dark Chocolate (70% or Higher Cocoa Content)**: The higher the cocoa content, the more antioxidants are present. Dark chocolate can support brain health and improve mood.

8. **Citrus Fruits**

Citrus fruits, including oranges, lemons, and grapefruits, are high in vitamin C and flavonoids, which support immune function, skin health, and collagen production.

- o **Oranges**: Rich in vitamin C, oranges help boost immune health and protect the skin from environmental damage.
- o **Grapefruit**: Contains lycopene and vitamin C, supporting heart health and reducing oxidative stress.
- o **Lemons**: High in vitamin C, lemons enhance iron absorption and support immune function.

Incorporating Antioxidant-Rich Foods into Your Daily Diet

Incorporating a variety of antioxidant-rich foods into your diet can provide a comprehensive range of benefits, from immune support to heart health. Here are some practical strategies for adding more of these foods to your meals:

1. **Start with a Berry-Loaded Breakfast**

Begin your day with a bowl of oatmeal or yogurt topped with mixed berries. This breakfast provides a rich dose of antioxidants from blueberries, strawberries, and raspberries, as well as fiber and protein.

2. **Add Leafy Greens to Lunch**

Incorporate spinach, kale, or Swiss chard into your lunch as a salad, wrap, or smoothie ingredient. Adding a handful of leafy greens to your daily diet is an easy way to increase your antioxidant intake.

3. **Snack on Nuts and Seeds**

Keep a mix of almonds, walnuts, and sunflower seeds as a snack. They're high in antioxidants, healthy fats, and protein, making them a perfect choice for a midday energy boost.

4. **Include Cruciferous Vegetables at Dinner**

Add broccoli, cauliflower, or Brussels sprouts as a side dish for dinner. These vegetables are packed with antioxidants that support detoxification and immune health.

5. **Enjoy a Square of Dark Chocolate**

For dessert, have a piece of dark chocolate with at least 70% cocoa content. This treat provides polyphenols and flavonoids, supporting heart health and reducing oxidative stress.

Antioxidant-Rich Food Choices for Special Diets

If you follow a specific diet, such as vegan, gluten-free, or ketogenic, you can still enjoy a wide range of antioxidant-rich foods. Here are some ideas:

- **Vegan**: Focus on berries, leafy greens, nuts, and seeds to meet your antioxidant needs. Avoid processed vegan snacks that may lack nutritional value.
- **Gluten-Free**: Choose gluten-free grains like quinoa or amaranth and add antioxidant-rich fruits and vegetables to each meal.
- **Ketogenic**: Stick to low-carb, antioxidant-rich foods such as dark leafy greens, nuts, seeds, and low-sugar berries like raspberries and blackberries.

A diet rich in antioxidants supports long-term health, prevents disease, and improves vitality. By incorporating a diverse array of these foods, individuals can protect their bodies from oxidative stress and promote overall wellness, building a strong foundation for a healthy life.

Barbara's Anti-Inflammatory Tips

Inflammation is the body's natural response to injury or infection, but when it becomes chronic, it can lead to various health issues, including arthritis, cardiovascular disease, and autoimmune disorders. Reducing inflammation is crucial for long-term health, and through a natural approach, you can mitigate the effects of chronic inflammation. Barbara's holistic anti-inflammatory tips focus on incorporating specific dietary and lifestyle adjustments, herbal remedies, and mindfulness practices that empower the body to heal itself. By embracing these practical strategies, you can experience reduced inflammation and a renewed sense of well-being.

The Role of Diet in Reducing Inflammation

Barbara emphasizes that what we eat can either fuel inflammation or fight it. Choosing anti-inflammatory foods, limiting inflammatory triggers, and practicing mindful eating are essential elements in her approach.

1. **Incorporate Anti-Inflammatory Superfoods**: Certain foods are renowned for their anti-inflammatory properties, thanks to their high levels of antioxidants, polyphenols, and omega-3 fatty acids. Barbara's recommended anti-inflammatory superfoods include:
   - **Leafy Greens**: Vegetables like spinach, kale, and Swiss chard are rich in vitamins and minerals and contain antioxidants that help reduce oxidative stress in the body.
   - **Berries**: Blueberries, strawberries, and blackberries are rich in antioxidants, particularly anthocyanins, which help reduce inflammation and support cellular health.
   - **Fatty Fish**: Salmon, mackerel, and sardines provide omega-3 fatty acids, which reduce the production of inflammatory compounds and are linked to improved heart and brain health.
   - **Nuts and Seeds**: Almonds, walnuts, chia seeds, and flaxseeds are rich in healthy fats, fiber, and vitamin E, all of which support the body's natural defenses against inflammation.

Barbara recommends incorporating these foods into daily meals as a foundation for reducing inflammation. A simple way to start is by adding berries to your breakfast, leafy greens to your lunch, and fatty fish or nuts to your dinner. Over time, these additions help balance inflammation levels naturally.

2. **Avoid Common Inflammatory Foods**: Certain foods and ingredients exacerbate inflammation, particularly those high in trans fats, refined sugars, and processed additives. Foods that Barbara encourages limiting include:
   - **Refined Carbohydrates**: White bread, pastries, and sugary cereals can cause blood sugar spikes, which contribute to inflammation.
   - **Processed Meats**: Sausages, hot dogs, and bacon contain preservatives and other additives that may lead to chronic inflammation.
   - **Sugary Drinks**: Sodas and sweetened beverages are loaded with sugar and may trigger inflammatory responses in the body.
   - **Fried Foods**: Foods cooked in trans fats, such as French fries and doughnuts, promote inflammation and are linked to increased risk of disease.

Reducing the intake of these foods and replacing them with healthier alternatives like whole grains, lean proteins, and water or herbal teas can make a significant difference in managing inflammation.

3. **Mindful Eating and Digestion**: Barbara believes that eating mindfully not only helps with digestion but also reduces stress, a known contributor to inflammation. Taking time to chew thoroughly, appreciating the flavors and textures, and avoiding distractions while eating allow the body to fully engage in the digestive process. This practice reduces bloating, improves nutrient absorption, and contributes to an overall reduction in inflammation.

Herbal Remedies for Inflammation

Herbs play a significant role in Barbara's anti-inflammatory toolkit, as many have natural compounds that support immune balance and reduce pain and swelling associated with chronic inflammation.

1. **Turmeric and Curcumin**: Turmeric is widely recognized for its anti-inflammatory properties, primarily due to curcumin, a powerful compound that can inhibit inflammatory pathways. Consuming turmeric regularly, whether in meals, as a supplement, or as a golden milk latte, can help lower inflammation. Barbara recommends combining turmeric with black pepper to enhance absorption, as piperine (found in black pepper) increases curcumin's bioavailability.

2. **Ginger**: Known for its warming and soothing properties, ginger contains gingerol, a compound with potent anti-inflammatory and antioxidant effects. Barbara advises drinking ginger tea or adding freshly grated ginger to meals. Not only does ginger aid digestion, but it also reduces inflammation in the body, especially for those suffering from joint pain or arthritis.

3. **Boswellia**: Often referred to as Indian frankincense, boswellia has been used in traditional medicine to treat inflammatory conditions. The active compounds in boswellia inhibit the production of inflammatory molecules, making it beneficial for managing arthritis and similar conditions. Barbara recommends taking boswellia as a supplement after consulting with a healthcare provider.

4. **Green Tea**: Rich in catechins, particularly epigallocatechin gallate (EGCG), green tea is known for its antioxidant properties. Drinking green tea regularly can reduce

inflammation and improve metabolic health. Barbara suggests incorporating one to two cups of green tea daily for optimal anti-inflammatory benefits.

Using these herbs either individually or in combination provides natural support for managing inflammation. Many of these can be easily added to meals, teas, or taken as supplements, providing versatile options for reducing inflammation naturally.

The Importance of Hydration in Managing Inflammation

Staying hydrated is often overlooked in discussions of inflammation, but it is a crucial component in Barbara's anti-inflammatory strategy. Proper hydration helps flush out toxins and supports cellular health, both of which are essential for reducing inflammation.

1. **Water as a Primary Anti-Inflammatory Tool**: Drinking sufficient water daily aids in the removal of waste and helps maintain optimal cellular function. Barbara recommends drinking filtered water and aiming for at least eight glasses a day, more if active or in hot climates.

2. **Herbal Teas for Added Benefits**: In addition to water, herbal teas offer a way to stay hydrated while delivering anti-inflammatory compounds. Teas made from chamomile, ginger, turmeric, or peppermint have calming effects on the body and can soothe inflammation. Barbara suggests rotating between these herbal teas throughout the day to enjoy their unique benefits.

3. **Avoid Dehydrating Beverages**: Beverages high in caffeine, alcohol, or sugar can contribute to dehydration and increase inflammation in the body. While moderate coffee or alcohol intake is acceptable for some, it's essential to balance these with ample water and to limit sugary drinks entirely.

Hydration plays a foundational role in Barbara's approach, supporting the body's ability to process nutrients and expel toxins, which is crucial for reducing inflammation.

Lifestyle Practices to Support Anti-Inflammatory Goals

Barbara emphasizes the need for lifestyle changes alongside dietary adjustments to address inflammation holistically. Regular movement, adequate sleep, and stress reduction are all essential components of her anti-inflammatory plan.

1. **Regular Movement**: Physical activity promotes circulation, aids in the removal of toxins, and reduces inflammation. Barbara encourages incorporating low-impact exercises, such as walking, swimming, and yoga, into daily routines. These forms of

movement reduce joint stiffness, improve flexibility, and support cardiovascular health, which collectively combat inflammation.

2. **Quality Sleep**: Sleep is a natural anti-inflammatory agent, as the body undergoes repair and regeneration during rest. Lack of sleep disrupts immune function and increases inflammation. Barbara suggests maintaining a consistent sleep schedule, creating a calming bedtime routine, and ensuring the sleep environment is comfortable and dark to promote restful sleep.

3. **Stress Management Techniques**: Chronic stress triggers inflammatory responses in the body, making stress management crucial for reducing inflammation. Barbara advocates for mindfulness practices, such as meditation, deep breathing, and gratitude exercises, to help manage stress levels. Spending time in nature, engaging in hobbies, and cultivating supportive relationships also contribute to a balanced, lower-stress lifestyle.

Anti-Inflammatory Supplements and Oils

For those seeking additional support, Barbara recommends specific supplements and oils that can further aid in managing inflammation. These should be used in conjunction with a healthy diet and lifestyle for optimal effectiveness.

1. **Omega-3 Fatty Acids**: Omega-3 supplements, particularly those derived from fish oil or algae, provide EPA and DHA, which are known to reduce inflammation. Barbara suggests choosing high-quality omega-3 supplements to support cardiovascular health and reduce joint pain.

2. **Vitamin D**: Low levels of vitamin D are linked to increased inflammation, making it an essential nutrient in Barbara's anti-inflammatory protocol. Spending time in sunlight, consuming vitamin D-rich foods, and taking a supplement as needed can help maintain adequate levels.

3. **Magnesium**: Magnesium plays a role in muscle relaxation and supports numerous biochemical reactions that reduce inflammation. Foods rich in magnesium include

leafy greens, nuts, and seeds, but supplementation can be beneficial for those who are deficient.

4. **Essential Oils**: Essential oils, such as lavender, frankincense, and eucalyptus, have anti-inflammatory properties that can be used topically or in aromatherapy. Barbara advises diluting essential oils with a carrier oil and applying them to areas of discomfort or using them in a diffuser to support relaxation and reduce inflammation.

Creating a Personalized Anti-Inflammatory Plan

Barbara advocates for a personalized approach to inflammation management, as each person's needs, lifestyle, and sensitivities are unique. Creating a tailored anti-inflammatory plan involves identifying individual triggers, testing various foods and remedies, and observing their effects on the body.

1. **Identify Inflammatory Triggers**: Everyone's body reacts differently to specific foods, stressors, or environmental factors. Keeping a journal to track symptoms, foods consumed, and lifestyle habits can help identify patterns and triggers that lead to inflammation.

2. **Test and Adjust**: Implementing changes gradually allows individuals to observe the effects of each adjustment. For example, introducing anti-inflammatory foods one at a time helps determine how each impacts well-being.

3. **Listen to Your Body**: Paying close attention to how the body responds to different foods, herbs, and lifestyle practices helps refine the anti-inflammatory approach. By tuning into physical and emotional responses, individuals can make adjustments that support their unique needs.

Chapter 3: Immune-Boosting Practices

Supporting immunity is not just about responding to illness; it's about building a lifestyle that promotes resilience, strength, and long-term health. While the immune system is complex and influenced by numerous factors, certain daily habits can significantly contribute to its optimal functioning.

Daily Habits to Support Immunity

These habits help maintain a strong defense against infections, reduce inflammation, and support the body's natural ability to heal.

In this section, we'll explore specific daily practices that can foster a robust immune system. These habits focus on nutrition, sleep, stress management, physical activity, and mindfulness, creating a holistic approach that addresses both the body and mind.

Prioritizing Balanced Nutrition

Nutrition forms the foundation of immune health. The body needs a consistent supply of vitamins, minerals, and other nutrients to maintain and repair tissues, create antibodies, and sustain energy. A balanced diet that includes a variety of whole foods supports immune function and reduces the risk of nutrient deficiencies that could weaken the body's defenses.

1. **Focus on a Rainbow of Fruits and Vegetables**

Each color in fruits and vegetables represents different antioxidants and phytochemicals, which support immunity by neutralizing free radicals, reducing inflammation, and protecting cells. A diet rich in colorful produce supplies essential nutrients like vitamin C, beta-carotene, and flavonoids, which are known for their immune-boosting properties.

   o **Examples**: Include a variety of berries, leafy greens, sweet potatoes, carrots, and bell peppers in daily meals. Each of these provides antioxidants that enhance cellular health and protect against illness.

2. **Incorporate Probiotic-Rich Foods for Gut Health**

A significant portion of the immune system resides in the gut, making gut health crucial for immunity. Probiotics, found in foods like yogurt, kefir, sauerkraut, and kombucha, help maintain a healthy balance of gut bacteria, which in turn supports immune responses.

- o **Practical Tip**: Include at least one probiotic-rich food in your daily diet. If probiotics are new to you, start with small portions to allow your digestive system to adjust, gradually increasing as tolerated.

3. **Stay Hydrated**

Hydration is vital for immune function, as it helps flush toxins from the body, keeps mucosal tissues moist, and facilitates the circulation of immune cells. Water also supports lymph production, which is essential for transporting immune cells throughout the body.

- o **Daily Goal**: Aim for at least eight cups of water per day, adjusting based on activity levels, climate, and individual needs. Herbal teas, particularly those with immune-supportive herbs like ginger or echinacea, can also be beneficial additions.

Prioritize Quality Sleep

Sleep is a natural immune booster. During sleep, the body releases cytokines, proteins that help the immune system fight off infections and reduce inflammation. Chronic sleep deprivation can disrupt the production of these protective cytokines, leaving the body more vulnerable to illness.

1. **Establish a Consistent Sleep Routine**

Going to bed and waking up at the same time each day helps regulate the body's internal clock, or circadian rhythm, which supports sleep quality. A consistent schedule reinforces the sleep-wake cycle, making it easier to fall asleep and wake up refreshed.

- o **Practical Strategy**: Create a pre-sleep routine that signals the body it's time to wind down. This routine might include reading, gentle stretching, or a warm bath to help relax the muscles.

2. **Optimize the Sleep Environment**

A comfortable sleep environment enhances rest. Keep the bedroom dark, cool, and quiet, and reserve it for sleep to strengthen the association between the space and relaxation. Limit screen time before bed, as blue light from devices can disrupt melatonin production, the hormone that regulates sleep.

- o **Simple Adjustments**: Invest in blackout curtains, wear an eye mask, and use earplugs or a white noise machine if necessary. These adjustments can reduce disturbances and promote deeper, restorative sleep.

Manage Stress Through Mindfulness and Relaxation Techniques

Chronic stress suppresses immune function by increasing the production of cortisol, a hormone that, when elevated for extended periods, can impair immune response and increase inflammation. Regularly engaging in stress-reducing activities helps modulate cortisol levels and supports immune resilience.

1. **Practice Mindfulness Meditation**

Mindfulness meditation can reduce stress by promoting relaxation and enhancing mental clarity. Regular meditation has been shown to lower cortisol levels, reduce anxiety, and improve mood, all of which contribute to stronger immunity.

- o **Starting Point**: Begin with a simple five to ten-minute meditation each day. Focus on your breath, and let go of any thoughts that arise without judgment. Gradually increase your meditation time as you become more comfortable with the practice.

2. **Engage in Deep Breathing Exercises**

Deep breathing exercises can help activate the body's relaxation response, counteracting the effects of stress. Techniques like diaphragmatic breathing stimulate the vagus nerve, which plays a role in calming the nervous system.

- o **Practical Tip**: Practice deep breathing by inhaling deeply through your nose, allowing your belly to rise, and exhaling slowly through your mouth. Repeat for five to ten breaths, especially during moments of stress or before sleep.

3. **Make Time for Hobbies and Social Connections**

Engaging in enjoyable activities and maintaining social connections can provide a mental break from daily stressors, lifting mood and promoting relaxation. Positive social interactions, even brief ones, can increase levels of oxytocin, a hormone that reduces stress and promotes a sense of well-being.

- o **Suggestion**: Schedule regular phone calls or meetups with friends and family, or pursue hobbies like painting, cooking, or gardening. These activities offer a mental reset and support emotional health, indirectly benefiting immunity.

Maintain Regular Physical Activity

Exercise supports immune function by promoting circulation, reducing inflammation, and supporting cardiovascular health. Regular physical activity enhances the movement of immune cells, allowing them to patrol the body more effectively.

1. **Engage in Moderate Exercise**

Moderate exercise, such as brisk walking, swimming, or cycling, has been shown to support immune health without overstressing the body. High-intensity exercise, while beneficial in moderation, can sometimes lead to temporary immune suppression, so finding a balance is key.

   o **Practical Approach**: Aim for at least 150 minutes of moderate exercise per week, as recommended by the CDC. Break this time into manageable segments throughout the week, incorporating activities that are enjoyable and sustainable.

2. **Include Muscle-Strengthening Exercises**

In addition to cardiovascular exercise, muscle-strengthening activities contribute to overall health by supporting bone density, metabolic function, and balance. Resistance training, using weights or body weight, can help maintain muscle mass, which is particularly beneficial as we age.

   o **Tip**: Incorporate strength exercises two to three times per week, focusing on all major muscle groups. Simple exercises like squats, lunges, and push-ups can be done at home with minimal equipment.

Practice Good Hygiene

Good hygiene is essential for preventing the spread of infections and maintaining immune health. Simple daily hygiene practices reduce the body's exposure to harmful pathogens, supporting overall immunity.

1. **Regular Handwashing**

Washing hands frequently, especially before meals and after using the bathroom, is one of the most effective ways to prevent the spread of infections. Use soap and water, scrubbing for at least 20 seconds to remove germs effectively.

   o **Tip**: Carry hand sanitizer when soap and water are not available, and avoid touching the face, as this can introduce pathogens through the eyes, nose, and mouth.

2. **Practice Oral Hygiene**

Oral health is closely linked to immune health. Poor oral hygiene can lead to gum infections, which can contribute to systemic inflammation. Brushing, flossing, and regular dental check-ups can help maintain a healthy mouth, reducing the risk of inflammation that could compromise immunity.

- o **Daily Routine**: Brush twice daily and floss once a day to remove plaque and prevent gum disease. Rinsing with a mouthwash can provide additional antibacterial benefits.

Get Sunlight Exposure and Consider Supplementing with Vitamin D

Vitamin D plays a critical role in immune function, helping to modulate the body's response to infections. While the body produces vitamin D when exposed to sunlight, modern lifestyles and winter months can make it challenging to get enough. Low levels of vitamin D are associated with a weakened immune response and a higher risk of infections.

1. **Spend Time Outdoors Daily**

Aim to get at least 10-30 minutes of sunlight exposure several times a week, depending on skin tone, location, and season. Sunlight exposure supports natural vitamin D synthesis, which enhances immune health and contributes to bone strength.

- o **Tip**: Enjoy outdoor activities like walking, gardening, or picnicking during midday hours when UVB rays are most available. However, be mindful of skin protection if you're outdoors for prolonged periods.

2. **Consider Vitamin D Supplements if Needed**

For those with limited sun exposure or during winter months, a vitamin D supplement can help maintain adequate levels. It's advisable to consult with a healthcare professional to determine the appropriate dosage based on individual needs.

- o **Note**: A blood test can assess vitamin D levels, ensuring you take the correct amount. Excessive supplementation should be avoided, as very high levels of vitamin D can lead to adverse effects.

Limit Alcohol and Avoid Smoking

Both excessive alcohol consumption and smoking can suppress immune function, making it easier for pathogens to infect the body. Limiting or eliminating these substances can have a significant impact on immune health.

1. **Moderate Alcohol Consumption**

Alcohol can impair immune responses, especially when consumed in excess. It disrupts the balance of gut bacteria and affects the function of immune cells. Limiting alcohol to moderate levels—up to one drink per day for women and two for men—can reduce the risk of immune suppression.

   o **Alternative Choices**: Opt for herbal teas, flavored water, or sparkling water with a splash of fruit juice as healthier beverage alternatives.

2. **Avoid Smoking and Exposure to Secondhand Smoke**

Smoking harms the respiratory system and weakens immune function, making the body more susceptible to infections. If quitting smoking is challenging, seeking support from a healthcare provider or support groups can make the process more manageable.

   o **First Step**: Gradually reduce smoking or seek alternative strategies to manage cravings. Nicotine replacement therapies or behavioral counseling can be helpful tools in the journey to quit.

Developing daily habits to support immunity takes time and consistency, but the benefits are substantial. By prioritizing nutrition, sleep, stress management, physical activity, and good hygiene, individuals can fortify their immune systems and enhance overall well-being.

Seasonal Immunity Routines

Maintaining a robust immune system year-round requires adjustments that align with seasonal changes. Each season presents unique challenges and environmental factors that impact immunity, from harsh winter conditions to the allergens of spring. By tailoring daily routines and incorporating season-specific practices, individuals can naturally strengthen their immune defenses throughout the year. Barbara's approach to seasonal immunity focuses on lifestyle adjustments, dietary choices, and herbal remedies that adapt to each season's demands, ensuring that immunity remains strong and balanced.

Winter Immunity: Boosting Defense During Cold Months

Winter often brings cold and flu season, with shorter daylight hours and colder temperatures that challenge the immune system. Barbara emphasizes the importance of warming foods, protective herbs, and habits that compensate for reduced sunlight and lower temperatures.

1. **Embrace Warming Foods and Herbs**: In winter, incorporating warming foods and spices into the diet helps stimulate circulation, supports digestion, and keeps the body's core temperature stable. Foods like soups, stews, and broths made with root vegetables and spices such as cinnamon, ginger, and turmeric are excellent choices.
   - **Ginger and Turmeric**: Both spices have powerful anti-inflammatory and immune-boosting properties. Ginger can help prevent respiratory infections and soothe sore throats, while turmeric, when combined with black pepper, enhances immune function and fights inflammation.
   - **Garlic and Onions**: These foods have natural antibacterial and antiviral properties, making them ideal for winter immunity support. Adding garlic and onions to meals can help ward off colds and flu.
2. **Support with Vitamin D**: During winter, sunlight exposure is often limited, leading to reduced vitamin D levels, which are crucial for immune function. Barbara recommends supplementing vitamin D or spending time outdoors on sunny days. Vitamin D is known for its role in strengthening the immune system and reducing susceptibility to infections.
3. **Herbal Teas for Warmth and Immunity**: Hot herbal teas provide warmth and offer immune-boosting benefits. Barbara suggests teas made from elderberry, echinacea, and chamomile to support immunity. Elderberry, in particular, is rich in antioxidants and has been shown to reduce the severity and duration of colds.
4. **Moisturizing the Air**: Winter's dry air can dry out mucous membranes, making it easier for pathogens to enter the respiratory tract. Barbara advises using a humidifier to maintain optimal humidity levels in indoor environments. Adding a few drops of eucalyptus or tea tree essential oil to the humidifier can provide additional respiratory support.
5. **Daily Gentle Exercise**: Regular movement, even in winter, helps keep the immune system active. Barbara recommends gentle exercises like yoga or brisk walking indoors or outdoors (if weather permits) to stimulate circulation and maintain immune function without the risk of exposure to harsh outdoor conditions.

Spring Immunity: Managing Allergies and Detoxifying

Spring is a time of renewal but also a season that triggers allergies for many. Barbara's spring immunity practices focus on supporting respiratory health, reducing allergens, and cleansing the body after winter.

1. **Introduce Seasonal Greens**: Fresh greens, such as dandelion, arugula, and spinach, help detoxify the liver and prepare the body for the change in season. Dandelion greens, in particular, support liver function and help flush toxins accumulated over winter, reducing the burden on the immune system.

2. **Herbs for Respiratory Health**: Spring's blooming plants release pollen that can trigger allergies. Herbs like nettle, butterbur, and quercetin-rich foods help manage allergy symptoms and support respiratory health.

   o **Nettle**: Known for its antihistamine properties, nettle can help alleviate symptoms like sneezing and itchy eyes caused by seasonal allergies. Barbara suggests drinking nettle tea daily to support immune and respiratory health.

   o **Butterbur**: This herb is often used to relieve sinus congestion and headaches, which are common during spring allergy season. Butterbur can be taken as a supplement to ease respiratory symptoms.

3. **Hydrate to Flush Allergens**: Staying hydrated is essential in spring to help the body flush out allergens and keep mucous membranes moist. Barbara recommends drinking water with a splash of lemon, which provides vitamin C and supports liver detoxification.

4. **Spring Cleansing Routine**: Spring is an ideal time for a gentle detox. Barbara's approach to cleansing includes incorporating fiber-rich foods, increasing water intake, and using herbs like milk thistle to support liver health. A spring cleanse can help eliminate toxins and prepare the immune system for the year ahead.

5. **Outdoor Exercise with Precautions**: Enjoying the outdoors is part of embracing spring, but taking precautions against allergens is essential. Barbara advises exercising in the early morning when pollen levels are lower, and wearing sunglasses to reduce eye exposure to pollen.

Summer Immunity: Staying Cool and Protecting Skin

Summer's heat, sun exposure, and increased outdoor activity can impact immune health. Barbara's summer immunity routine emphasizes hydration, skin protection, and cooling foods.

1. **Stay Hydrated**: The body loses more water through sweating in summer, making hydration critical for immune health. Dehydration can weaken immunity, so Barbara suggests drinking plenty of water and adding electrolyte-rich drinks like coconut water for optimal hydration.

2. **Consume Cooling Foods**: Fresh fruits and vegetables with high water content, such as cucumbers, melons, and berries, help cool the body and support hydration. These foods also provide antioxidants that combat sun-induced oxidative stress.

3. **Herbal Sun Protection**: Sun exposure increases the risk of skin damage and immune suppression. Barbara recommends using aloe vera topically to soothe skin after sun exposure and drinking green tea, which contains polyphenols that support skin health.

4. **Avoid Sugary and Processed Foods**: In summer, it's easy to indulge in sugary treats and processed snacks, but these foods can contribute to inflammation. Instead, Barbara encourages whole foods, like salads, smoothies, and grilled vegetables, to keep the body nourished and immune function strong.

5. **Moderate Sun Exposure for Vitamin D**: While prolonged sun exposure can harm the skin, moderate sun exposure helps maintain vitamin D levels, which supports immunity. Barbara suggests short, regular sun exposure during non-peak hours (morning or late afternoon) to balance vitamin D intake.

6. **Natural Insect Repellents**: Spending time outdoors increases exposure to insects, which can carry pathogens. Barbara recommends natural insect repellents made from essential oils like citronella, eucalyptus, and lavender to protect against bites without harsh chemicals.

Fall Immunity: Preparing for Colder Months

Fall is a time to strengthen the immune system in preparation for winter. Barbara's fall immunity routine emphasizes grounding foods, immune-boosting herbs, and practices that reinforce resilience before winter.

1. **Nourish with Root Vegetables**: Root vegetables like sweet potatoes, carrots, and beets provide grounding energy and essential nutrients that prepare the body for colder weather. These vegetables are rich in vitamins A and C, which support immune health.

2. **Increase Intake of Vitamin C**: Fall is an excellent time to boost vitamin C intake to enhance immunity for winter. Foods like oranges, bell peppers, and kale are packed with vitamin C, which supports white blood cell function and helps the body fight off infections.

3. **Immune-Boosting Herbs**: Barbara recommends incorporating herbs like astragalus, echinacea, and reishi mushroom in fall to build immunity. These herbs help strengthen immune defenses and can be taken as teas, tinctures, or supplements.

   o **Astragalus**: Known for its immune-stimulating properties, astragalus supports the body's resilience to infections. Barbara advises using astragalus regularly in fall to prepare the immune system for winter.

   o **Echinacea**: Echinacea is effective for stimulating immune function and is often used at the first sign of illness. Barbara recommends having echinacea on hand in fall to use as needed.

4. **Practice Grounding Exercises**: Fall is a time for grounding, which involves connecting with the earth and slowing down. Barbara encourages grounding exercises, such as walking barefoot outdoors or practicing yoga, to calm the mind and strengthen the body's natural defenses.

5. **Regular Sleep Schedule**: As daylight hours shorten, Barbara emphasizes the importance of establishing a regular sleep schedule to align with natural circadian rhythms. Consistent sleep patterns support immune function and prepare the body for the winter season.

6. **Moderate Use of Immune Supplements**: Barbara advises adjusting immune-support supplements like vitamin C and zinc as winter approaches, using them in moderation to avoid overloading the system. By building immunity gradually, the body becomes more resilient to seasonal changes.

Year-Round Immunity Essentials

In addition to seasonal routines, certain immunity-boosting practices are valuable year-round. Barbara highlights essential habits that keep the immune system in balance regardless of the season.

1. **Maintain Gut Health**: A healthy gut is foundational to a strong immune system. Barbara recommends consuming probiotic-rich foods like yogurt, kefir, and

fermented vegetables regularly. These foods support the gut microbiome, which plays a critical role in immunity.

2. **Reduce Chronic Stress**: Chronic stress weakens the immune system and makes the body more susceptible to infections. Barbara advocates for regular stress-reducing practices, such as meditation, deep breathing, and spending time in nature, to maintain immune resilience.

3. **Exercise Consistently**: Regular exercise enhances circulation, helps flush out toxins, and promotes overall immune health. Barbara suggests varying exercise routines based on the season to keep the body active and adaptive.

4. **Eat a Balanced Diet**: Regardless of the season, a diet rich in whole foods, lean proteins, healthy fats, and plenty of fruits and vegetables supports immune health. Avoiding excessive sugar and processed foods helps maintain balance and reduces inflammation.

5. **Mindful Supplementation**: Supplements can be beneficial when used mindfully. Barbara recommends using supplements to fill dietary gaps and support seasonal needs, but not as a replacement for nutrient-rich foods.

Spring Detox Tips

Spring is an ideal season to rejuvenate the body, clear away winter sluggishness, and prepare for a season of renewed energy. A detox regimen can support this natural transition by gently helping the body eliminate accumulated toxins, reset digestive health, and boost energy levels. Detoxing in the spring can be both invigorating and refreshing, fostering a sense of lightness and clarity. In this section, we'll explore various safe and effective strategies for a gentle yet thorough spring detox that aligns with the rhythms of the body.

Understanding Detoxification and Its Benefits

Detoxification, or detox, is the body's natural process of eliminating toxins through organs like the liver, kidneys, lungs, and skin. These organs work continuously to filter and expel waste products, environmental pollutants, and metabolic by-products. A spring detox doesn't "replace" these functions but rather supports them, promoting optimal function.

Detoxing can offer benefits beyond simple toxin elimination. Many people experience enhanced mental clarity, improved digestion, reduced inflammation, and boosted immune function. A well-structured detox can also help reset cravings, especially for sugar and processed foods, leading to healthier choices that last long after the detox is over.

Starting with Hydration: The Foundation of Detox

Water is essential to any detox regimen. Proper hydration supports all the body's detoxifying organs by helping flush out toxins more efficiently. Without adequate water intake, these organs can become sluggish, leading to fatigue, dull skin, and bloating.

1. **Begin Each Morning with Lemon Water**

Starting your day with a warm glass of water with fresh lemon juice can help stimulate the liver and promote digestion. Lemon juice contains vitamin C and antioxidants that support liver health and metabolism.

- **Tip**: Squeeze half a lemon into a glass of warm water and drink it on an empty stomach. This practice can also improve hydration levels after a night's sleep.

2. **Drink Herbal Detox Teas**

Herbal teas can be a gentle and effective way to support the body's natural detox pathways. Teas like dandelion root, ginger, peppermint, and nettle have specific properties that aid digestion, improve liver function, and reduce bloating.

- **Suggested Routine**: Replace one or two cups of coffee with detoxifying herbal teas throughout the day. Dandelion root tea, for instance, is known for its liver-supportive properties and can help reduce water retention.

3. **Increase Overall Water Intake**

Aim to drink at least 8 to 10 glasses of water daily during a detox to help flush out toxins. For additional benefits, try infused water with fresh cucumber slices, mint, or berries. These add flavor and antioxidants without added sugars.

- **Hydration Reminder**: Carry a refillable water bottle and take sips regularly throughout the day. This habit not only improves hydration but can also help prevent overeating, as thirst is often mistaken for hunger.

Incorporate Nutrient-Dense Foods

A detox is an opportunity to nourish the body with clean, whole foods that provide essential vitamins, minerals, and antioxidants. Instead of focusing on deprivation, think of a detox as a way to enrich your diet with foods that are particularly supportive of the liver, kidneys, and digestive system.

1. **Focus on Fiber-Rich Vegetables**

Vegetables like broccoli, Brussels sprouts, cauliflower, and spinach are high in fiber, which supports digestion and regularity, essential components of detoxification. Fiber binds to toxins in the digestive tract, aiding in their elimination.

   o **Meal Idea**: Create colorful salads with a variety of raw and cooked vegetables, adding a handful of fresh herbs like parsley or cilantro, which have mild detoxifying effects.

2. **Add Cruciferous Vegetables for Liver Support**

Cruciferous vegetables, such as kale, cabbage, and arugula, contain sulfur compounds that enhance liver enzyme activity, helping the liver break down and remove toxins more effectively.

   o **Daily Addition**: Incorporate at least one serving of cruciferous vegetables into your meals, whether in a morning smoothie, salad, or stir-fry.

3. **Incorporate Probiotic-Rich Foods for Gut Health**

A healthy gut is essential for an effective detox. Probiotics, found in foods like sauerkraut, kimchi, kefir, and yogurt, help maintain a balanced gut flora, which plays a crucial role in digestion and immunity.

   o **Probiotic Tip**: Start with small servings if probiotics are new to you, as introducing too many at once can sometimes lead to bloating. Gradually increase your intake as your body adjusts.

Include Gentle Detox Practices

A detox can go beyond diet alone. Incorporating practices that promote relaxation, circulation, and gentle cleansing can enhance the body's natural detox processes, improving energy levels and overall well-being.

1. **Dry Brushing to Stimulate the Lymphatic System**

Dry brushing is a technique that uses a natural bristle brush to stimulate the skin and lymphatic system, which plays a key role in detoxification. By brushing the skin in upward strokes towards the heart, dry brushing encourages lymphatic flow, removing toxins and dead skin cells.

- o **How-To**: Before showering, gently brush your skin, starting from your feet and moving upwards. Use circular motions on your stomach and chest, and gentle strokes on sensitive areas.

2. **Epsom Salt Baths for Detoxification and Relaxation**

Epsom salt, or magnesium sulfate, can help draw out toxins through the skin while relaxing the muscles. An Epsom salt bath is an excellent way to unwind after a long day, relieve tension, and support detoxification.

- o **Bath Ritual**: Add 1-2 cups of Epsom salt to a warm bath and soak for 15-20 minutes. Avoid using very hot water, as this can dehydrate the body. Follow with a glass of water to rehydrate.

3. **Incorporate Deep Breathing or Meditation**

Detoxing is not just physical; it's also an opportunity to clear mental clutter. Deep breathing and meditation can help reduce stress and support immune health. Chronic stress impairs detoxification, as it disrupts digestion and increases inflammation.

- o **Practice**: Dedicate 5-10 minutes each day to deep breathing exercises or guided meditation. Find a quiet place, close your eyes, and focus on slow, deep breaths. This practice promotes relaxation and mindfulness, complementing your physical detox efforts.

Engage in Gentle Movement

Physical activity supports detoxification by promoting blood circulation, which delivers oxygen to tissues and removes waste products from cells. Gentle exercises can also aid in digestion, reduce bloating, and improve mood, enhancing the overall detox experience.

1. **Walking for Circulation and Mental Clarity**

Walking is a low-impact way to increase circulation, release stress, and stimulate the lymphatic system. A brisk walk in nature can also be incredibly grounding and uplifting, aligning with the spirit of spring renewal.

- o **Suggestion**: Aim for a 20-30 minute walk daily. If possible, walk outdoors to enjoy fresh air and sunlight, which can further enhance mood and support vitamin D production.

2. **Try Yoga or Stretching**

Yoga combines movement with breath, making it an ideal exercise during detox. Certain poses, like twists, support digestion by gently massaging the abdominal organs, while stretches release muscle tension and improve circulation.

- o **Routine**: Begin with a short stretching or yoga routine each morning. Simple poses like the seated twist, child's pose, and downward-facing dog can help stretch muscles, improve posture, and promote relaxation.

Experiment with Seasonal Herbs and Natural Remedies

Certain herbs and natural remedies align with spring's energy and can enhance detoxification by supporting the liver, digestion, and overall energy levels.

1. **Dandelion Root for Liver Support**

Dandelion root is a traditional herbal remedy that aids digestion and liver health. It acts as a natural diuretic, helping the body eliminate excess fluids and toxins.

- o **How to Use**: Enjoy dandelion root tea as part of your morning or evening routine. Brew one tea bag or 1-2 teaspoons of dried dandelion root in hot water, letting it steep for 5-10 minutes.

2. **Nettle Leaf for Allergy Relief and Detox**

Nettle leaf is known for its detoxifying properties and can be helpful in managing seasonal allergies. It contains minerals and antioxidants that reduce inflammation and support kidney health.

- o **Practical Tip**: Nettle tea can be consumed daily during your detox. Drink one to two cups for a gentle way to support kidney function and reduce seasonal allergy symptoms.

3. **Add Fresh Ginger for Digestion and Warmth**

Ginger is warming and stimulating, making it perfect for spring detoxes. It enhances digestion, reduces bloating, and has anti-inflammatory properties, which support overall detoxification.

- o **Usage**: Add fresh ginger to smoothies, salads, or herbal teas. A simple ginger tea can be made by slicing a piece of fresh ginger and steeping it in hot water for 10 minutes.

Spring Detox Dos and Don'ts

- **Do Listen to Your Body**: Detoxing should feel gentle and supportive. Pay attention to how you feel and adjust your detox practices as needed. If you feel fatigued or overwhelmed, consider reducing the intensity of your detox.

- **Do Focus on Whole Foods**: A detox is an opportunity to consume more whole, unprocessed foods that nourish your body without adding unnecessary toxins.

- **Don't Attempt Extreme Fasting or Restriction**: Extreme detox methods, like prolonged fasting or very restrictive diets, can stress the body and weaken the immune system. Focus on nourishment rather than deprivation.

- **Don't Skip Meals**: Regular meals stabilize blood sugar and prevent cravings, keeping energy levels balanced throughout the day.

- **Avoid Overdoing Caffeine or Sugar**: While caffeine and sugar can offer temporary energy, they can contribute to dehydration and blood sugar crashes, which undermine detox efforts.

A spring detox should be about refreshment, not stress. By focusing on natural, supportive practices, you can harness the energy of spring to cleanse, rejuvenate, and empower your body and mind.

Winter Immune Boosting

Winter brings cold temperatures, reduced sunlight, and an increase in respiratory illnesses, all of which challenge the immune system. During this season, it's essential to adopt habits and dietary practices that fortify the body's natural defenses. Barbara's approach to winter immunity combines warming foods, strategic use of vitamins and herbs, and lifestyle adjustments to help individuals stay healthy and resilient.

The Role of Warming Foods in Winter Immunity

In winter, the body expends more energy to maintain its core temperature, and it's common to crave foods that provide warmth and nourishment. According to Barbara, warming foods play a crucial role in supporting digestion and circulation, both of which are key for a well-functioning immune system.

1. **Root Vegetables and Winter Squash**: Vegetables like sweet potatoes, carrots, beets, and winter squash are nutrient-dense and rich in beta-carotene, an antioxidant

that supports immunity. When consumed regularly, these vegetables help the body stay energized and resilient.

2. **Spices with Warming Properties**: Spices like cinnamon, ginger, cayenne, and turmeric not only add warmth but also offer powerful anti-inflammatory and antioxidant benefits. Barbara recommends incorporating these spices into meals or warm beverages to keep the body's defenses strong.

   o **Ginger**: Known for its antiviral and antibacterial properties, ginger helps to relieve sore throats and prevent respiratory infections. A daily ginger tea can be beneficial for maintaining respiratory health during winter.

   o **Turmeric**: When combined with black pepper, turmeric's bioavailability increases, enhancing its anti-inflammatory effects. Turmeric can be added to soups, stews, or warm milk as an immunity-boosting elixir.

3. **Bone Broth and Herbal Soups**: Bone broth is a warming, nutrient-rich liquid that Barbara often recommends in winter. Packed with collagen, amino acids, and minerals, bone broth supports gut health, which is vital for a robust immune system. Adding garlic, onions, and herbs like thyme to the broth further enhances its immunity-boosting qualities.

Essential Vitamins for Winter Immunity

Winter's limited sunlight can lead to a decrease in vitamin D levels, impacting immune function. Barbara advises monitoring and supplementing essential vitamins to support the immune system.

1. **Vitamin D**: Vitamin D is essential for immune health, and its deficiency is common in winter due to reduced sunlight exposure. Barbara recommends getting at least 10-20 minutes of sunlight exposure whenever possible, as well as considering a high-quality vitamin D supplement if natural sunlight is scarce.

2. **Vitamin C**: Known for its immune-boosting properties, vitamin C helps stimulate the production of white blood cells and strengthens the body's defense against pathogens. Foods high in vitamin C, such as citrus fruits, bell peppers, and broccoli, should be included daily. For added convenience, a vitamin C supplement may be beneficial during winter's peak cold and flu season.

3. **Zinc**: Zinc plays a critical role in immune function and helps shorten the duration of colds. Barbara suggests incorporating zinc-rich foods, such as pumpkin seeds,

chickpeas, and lentils, into the diet. Zinc lozenges can also be helpful at the onset of cold symptoms to provide additional support.

Immune-Boosting Herbs for Winter

Herbs have been used for centuries to support the immune system, and several are particularly effective during winter. Barbara emphasizes the use of adaptogenic and antiviral herbs to keep the body resilient.

1. **Elderberry**: Rich in antioxidants, elderberry helps strengthen the immune system and reduces the severity and duration of colds and flu. Barbara suggests making elderberry syrup at home or purchasing it as a supplement to take regularly throughout winter.

2. **Echinacea**: Known for its immune-stimulating properties, echinacea can be used at the first sign of a cold. This herb activates white blood cells and helps the body fight infections more effectively. Echinacea tea or tincture is an easy way to incorporate this herb into daily winter routines.

3. **Astragalus**: An adaptogen with immune-modulating effects, astragalus supports the body in resisting infections. Barbara recommends taking astragalus as a tea or supplement to help the immune system adapt to winter's physical and environmental stresses.

4. **Garlic**: Garlic is a natural antibacterial and antiviral agent. Consuming garlic regularly can help prevent colds and flu. For maximum potency, Barbara suggests eating raw or lightly cooked garlic, as high heat may reduce some of its beneficial compounds.

5. **Thyme and Oregano**: These herbs have powerful antimicrobial and respiratory-supportive properties. Adding fresh or dried thyme and oregano to meals or drinking them as tea can be particularly helpful in keeping the respiratory system clear and strong.

Hydration and Humidity

Winter's dry air can dry out mucous membranes, which are the body's first line of defense against pathogens. Staying hydrated and maintaining indoor humidity levels help protect these membranes.

1. **Drink Plenty of Water**: Although people may feel less thirsty in winter, staying hydrated is crucial. Water supports cellular function and flushes out toxins. Barbara suggests warm water with a splash of lemon for hydration and an added vitamin C boost.

2. **Use a Humidifier**: Indoor heating often leads to dry air, which can irritate the respiratory tract. Barbara recommends using a humidifier in bedrooms and common areas to maintain optimal humidity levels. Adding a few drops of eucalyptus or tea tree oil to the humidifier can provide additional respiratory support.

Daily Winter Habits for Immune Health

Beyond diet and herbs, lifestyle habits play a vital role in keeping the immune system strong during winter. Barbara's winter routine includes practices that reduce stress, support the body's natural rhythms, and enhance well-being.

1. **Prioritize Sleep**: Quality sleep is essential for a strong immune system. Barbara advises maintaining a regular sleep schedule, aiming for 7-9 hours per night. Winter's longer nights align well with natural circadian rhythms, making it an ideal time to reinforce healthy sleep patterns.

2. **Moderate Physical Activity**: While outdoor exercise may be limited in winter, Barbara encourages daily movement to keep circulation strong and maintain immune health. Activities such as indoor yoga, stretching, or brisk walking (even indoors) support both physical and mental well-being.

3. **Limit Stress**: Chronic stress can weaken the immune system, making the body more susceptible to illness. Barbara suggests incorporating stress-relief practices, such as meditation, journaling, or listening to calming music, as part of a daily winter routine.

4. **Warmth and Layering**: Keeping the body warm, especially around the core and extremities, helps maintain immune function. Barbara emphasizes the importance of dressing in layers, using scarves and hats, and keeping the indoor environment comfortably warm to avoid taxing the body's energy reserves.

Immune-Supportive Winter Recipes

1. **Ginger-Turmeric Immunity Tea**: This tea is a powerful blend of ginger, turmeric, lemon, and honey. Ginger and turmeric provide anti-inflammatory benefits, while

lemon and honey add immune-boosting vitamin C and antibacterial properties. Barbara's recipe:

- o Slice fresh ginger and turmeric (or use a pinch of turmeric powder).
- o Simmer in water for 10-15 minutes.
- o Add lemon juice and a teaspoon of honey.
- o Drink this tea daily to support immune health.

2. **Elderberry Syrup**: Making elderberry syrup at home is a simple way to ensure a daily dose of immunity support. Barbara's recipe includes:

   - o 1 cup dried elderberries, 3 cups water, 1 cinnamon stick, and 1 tablespoon fresh ginger.
   - o Simmer ingredients for 30-45 minutes, then strain and add honey to taste.
   - o Take 1-2 teaspoons daily as an immune booster or up to 1 tablespoon if symptoms arise.

3. **Garlic and Onion Soup**: This soup combines the immunity-enhancing properties of garlic and onions with other winter vegetables.

   - o Sauté garlic, onions, and leeks in olive oil.
   - o Add root vegetables like carrots, parsnips, and sweet potatoes, and simmer in bone broth until tender.
   - o This nourishing soup provides warmth, vitamins, and minerals to bolster the immune system.

Consistent Self-Care Practices

Winter immune boosting is as much about consistency as it is about any single practice. Barbara encourages building daily routines that provide small but steady support for the immune system.

1. **Mindful Eating**: Winter meals should be enjoyed slowly and mindfully, allowing the body to digest and absorb nutrients fully. Barbara recommends focusing on whole, nutrient-dense foods and avoiding processed sugars and refined carbs that can suppress immune function.

2. **Breathing Exercises**: Indoor air quality can become stagnant in winter. Practicing deep breathing or opening windows for a few minutes each day helps refresh the air and encourages respiratory health.

3. **Outdoor Time, When Possible**: Getting outside during daylight hours provides a mental boost and some exposure to natural light, which can help with vitamin D synthesis. Even a short walk on sunny winter days can support mood and immune function.

Tailoring to Individual Needs

Barbara understands that everyone has unique needs, and winter immunity practices should be adaptable. She encourages individuals to listen to their bodies and adjust these routines as needed. For instance, those with respiratory conditions may benefit more from steam inhalation with eucalyptus oil, while others may find extra vitamin D supplementation essential.

Winter immune boosting is not about overloading the system with supplements and practices; rather, it's a balanced approach that aligns with nature and respects the body's rhythms.

Chapter 4: Immune-Enhancing Recipes

Echinacea tea has long been revered as a powerful natural remedy, especially renowned for its immune-boosting properties. Derived from the Echinacea plant, native to North America, this herb has been used for centuries by Native American tribes to treat a variety of ailments, from infections to wounds.

Echinacea Tea

Today, Echinacea tea is a staple in natural wellness routines, particularly for individuals looking to bolster their immunity, prevent seasonal illnesses, and support overall health. In this section, we will explore the origins, benefits, preparation, and practical applications of Echinacea tea, making it a versatile tool for those interested in natural remedies.

The Origins and Varieties of Echinacea

Echinacea, also known as the coneflower, is a flowering plant that belongs to the daisy family. There are several species of Echinacea, but the three most commonly used for medicinal purposes are *Echinacea purpurea*, *Echinacea angustifolia*, and *Echinacea pallida*. These species are rich in compounds like alkamides, polysaccharides, glycoproteins, and flavonoids, which are thought to be responsible for their health benefits.

The plant's vibrant purple flowers and distinctive shape have made it a popular garden plant, but it's the roots, leaves, and flowers that hold its medicinal qualities. Native American tribes, including the Lakota, Pawnee, and Cheyenne, were among the first to recognize the healing powers of Echinacea, using it as a remedy for snakebites, wounds, and respiratory infections. Today, Echinacea remains one of the most widely studied herbal remedies, with research highlighting its immune-modulating, anti-inflammatory, and antioxidant properties.

Key Health Benefits of Echinacea Tea

The benefits of Echinacea tea extend beyond immune support, making it a valuable addition to a holistic wellness routine. Here are some of the primary health benefits associated with this herbal tea:

1. **Immune System Support**

Echinacea is best known for its immune-boosting capabilities. Compounds within the plant stimulate the activity of white blood cells, which play a critical role in defending the body against infections. Drinking Echinacea tea regularly, especially during the colder months, may help reduce the frequency and severity of colds and other respiratory infections.

- **How it Works**: Echinacea promotes the production of interferons, proteins that signal the immune system to respond to infections. Additionally, alkamides in Echinacea have been shown to enhance the activity of macrophages, immune cells responsible for engulfing and destroying pathogens.

2. **Anti-Inflammatory Properties**

Echinacea tea may benefit those suffering from inflammation-related conditions, including arthritis, respiratory infections, and skin disorders. The plant's anti-inflammatory properties stem from compounds like cichoric acid and rosmarinic acid, which have been shown to reduce inflammation markers in the body.

- **Practical Use**: For individuals with chronic inflammatory conditions, Echinacea tea can be a gentle way to manage symptoms. Unlike pharmaceutical anti-inflammatories, Echinacea does not carry a risk of gastrointestinal side effects when consumed in moderate amounts.

3. **Antioxidant Protection**

Echinacea contains antioxidants, including flavonoids, cichoric acid, and rosmarinic acid, which help combat oxidative stress in the body. Oxidative stress occurs when there's an imbalance between free radicals and antioxidants, leading to cell damage and contributing to aging and chronic diseases.

- **Why It's Important**: By drinking Echinacea tea, individuals may support their body's natural defenses against oxidative damage, reducing the risk of age-related diseases and promoting youthful skin and overall vitality.

4. **Skin Health and Wound Healing**

Traditionally, Echinacea was used topically to treat wounds, infections, and insect bites due to its antibacterial and anti-inflammatory properties. Drinking Echinacea tea may benefit the skin from within, promoting a clear complexion and accelerating the healing process for minor cuts and abrasions.

- o **Application**: While Echinacea tea supports skin health when consumed, it can also be applied topically. Brew a strong batch of Echinacea tea, allow it to cool, and use it as a natural rinse or compress for minor skin irritations.

5. **Respiratory Health**

Echinacea tea is frequently used as a natural remedy for respiratory infections, including the common cold, bronchitis, and sinusitis. It may help alleviate symptoms such as a sore throat, congestion, and coughing.

- o **Benefit in Daily Life**: For individuals prone to seasonal allergies or frequent colds, incorporating Echinacea tea into their daily routine can provide preventative support. Its natural anti-inflammatory properties also help soothe the respiratory tract, making it an effective remedy for sore throats and sinus congestion.

How to Prepare Echinacea Tea

To experience the full benefits of Echinacea tea, it's essential to prepare it correctly. Echinacea tea can be made from dried roots, leaves, or flowers, each of which has unique properties. The following method provides a straightforward approach to making a potent Echinacea tea.

1. **Ingredients**:
   - o 1 teaspoon of dried Echinacea roots, leaves, or flowers, or a combination of all three
   - o 1 cup of water
2. **Instructions**:
   - o Bring water to a boil in a small pot or kettle.
   - o Add the dried Echinacea to a teapot or infuser.
   - o Pour boiling water over the Echinacea and let it steep for 10-15 minutes.
   - o Strain and enjoy the tea warm. For added benefits, consider adding a slice of lemon or a teaspoon of honey.

- Frequency: For immune support, consider drinking one to two cups of Echinacea tea daily. However, Echinacea should not be consumed continuously for extended periods. Taking a break after two weeks of daily use is generally recommended to maintain the herb's effectiveness.

Echinacea Tea Recipes and Variations

While Echinacea tea is beneficial on its own, combining it with other herbs can enhance its properties and provide additional health benefits. Here are a few popular combinations:

1. **Echinacea and Ginger for Immune Support**

Adding ginger to Echinacea tea provides an extra boost of immune support and anti-inflammatory benefits. Ginger also adds a warming, spicy flavor that complements the earthy taste of Echinacea.

- **Recipe**: Brew Echinacea tea as usual and add a few slices of fresh ginger root. Let steep for an additional 5 minutes before straining.

2. **Echinacea and Peppermint for Respiratory Health**

Peppermint adds a cooling effect that can be soothing for sore throats and nasal congestion. This combination is particularly beneficial for respiratory health during cold and flu season.

- **Recipe**: Combine 1 teaspoon of dried Echinacea with 1 teaspoon of dried peppermint leaves. Steep in hot water for 10-15 minutes.

3. **Echinacea and Lemon Balm for Relaxation**

Lemon balm has calming properties, making this combination ideal for individuals experiencing stress or tension. This blend also has a refreshing flavor and is perfect for evening relaxation.

- **Recipe**: Brew Echinacea tea as directed, then add 1 teaspoon of dried lemon balm. Steep for an additional 5 minutes and enjoy.

Potential Side Effects and Precautions

While Echinacea tea is generally safe for most people, it's essential to be aware of potential side effects and contraindications.

1. **Allergic Reactions**: Individuals with allergies to plants in the daisy family (such as ragweed) may experience allergic reactions to Echinacea. Symptoms may include itching, rash, or swelling.

2. **Autoimmune Disorders**: People with autoimmune conditions should consult a healthcare provider before using Echinacea, as it may stimulate the immune system and worsen symptoms.

3. **Pregnancy and Breastfeeding**: Pregnant and breastfeeding women should consult a healthcare provider before incorporating Echinacea tea into their routine.

4. **Medication Interactions**: Echinacea may interact with certain medications, including immunosuppressants. If you are on prescription medication, discuss Echinacea use with your doctor.

When to Drink Echinacea Tea

For optimal benefits, drink Echinacea tea during times when you feel your immune system needs a boost, such as at the onset of cold or flu symptoms. Many people also enjoy drinking it during the winter months as a preventive measure. However, Echinacea tea can be enjoyed year-round in moderate amounts, especially when combined with other herbs.

- **Timing**: Drinking Echinacea tea in the evening can be particularly soothing, as it promotes relaxation and supports the immune system overnight. However, it can also be consumed in the morning or afternoon, depending on personal preference.

The Benefits of Incorporating Echinacea Tea into a Wellness Routine

Echinacea tea's versatility makes it easy to incorporate into daily life. Whether used as a preventive measure, a remedy for colds, or simply a way to support overall health, Echinacea tea offers a range of benefits for those seeking natural health solutions. Its immune-boosting properties make it especially valuable during colder months, while its gentle support for inflammation, respiratory health, and skin healing adds to its appeal as a comprehensive wellness aid.

By understanding its origins, benefits, and best practices for use, you can make the most of Echinacea tea as part of a holistic, natural approach to health.

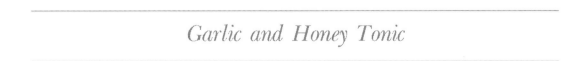

Garlic and Honey Tonic

Garlic and honey may seem like an unusual combination, but together, they form a powerful natural remedy that's been trusted for generations. This tonic harnesses the health-boosting properties of both garlic and honey to support immune health, improve cardiovascular function, and combat infections. Known for their complementary medicinal qualities, garlic and honey make an ideal pairing in holistic health practices. In this section, we'll delve into the benefits, preparation, and uses of a garlic and honey tonic, as well as discuss why it's a must-have in a natural health regimen, especially during times when immunity is paramount.

The Powerful Benefits of Garlic

Garlic, scientifically known as *Allium sativum*, is a bulbous plant related to onions, leeks, and shallots. Used since ancient times, garlic has been revered for its medicinal and culinary uses. Its potent health benefits stem primarily from a compound called allicin, which is released when garlic is crushed or chopped. Allicin gives garlic its signature odor and is responsible for its immune-boosting and antimicrobial effects.

1. **Antibacterial and Antiviral Properties**: Allicin in garlic is known to fight a range of bacteria, viruses, and even fungi. Studies have shown that garlic can inhibit the growth of common illness-causing bacteria like *E. coli* and *Salmonella*. This property makes garlic an invaluable tool during cold and flu season or any time the body needs additional immune support.

2. **Anti-Inflammatory Effects**: Garlic's anti-inflammatory effects can benefit those with chronic inflammation or autoimmune issues. The compounds in garlic inhibit pro-inflammatory enzymes, making it a valuable food for reducing inflammation throughout the body, which is beneficial not only for immune health but also for joint and cardiovascular health.

3. **Supports Cardiovascular Health**: Garlic is well-known for its ability to improve heart health by reducing blood pressure, lowering cholesterol levels, and promoting circulation. Consuming garlic regularly has been linked to a reduction in the risk of cardiovascular disease, partly due to its anti-inflammatory and antioxidant properties, which help protect blood vessels from damage.

4. **Rich in Antioxidants**: Garlic contains antioxidants that combat oxidative stress, which is known to accelerate aging and damage cells. By reducing oxidative stress, garlic helps the body maintain a balanced immune response, preventing damage to healthy cells while protecting against potential threats.

5. **Detoxification Support**: Garlic supports liver health and detoxification by enhancing the body's natural detox processes. Sulfur compounds in garlic stimulate

the liver to produce enzymes that filter out toxins, which is essential for maintaining overall health and immune function.

The Healing Properties of Honey

Honey has been valued for its medicinal qualities for thousands of years, and it's a staple in many traditional healing practices around the world. Raw honey, in particular, is rich in nutrients, antioxidants, and enzymes, making it a valuable addition to natural remedies. Unlike pasteurized honey, raw honey retains all of its natural compounds and is highly effective in supporting immune health.

1. **Natural Antibacterial Agent**: Raw honey contains hydrogen peroxide, which gives it antibacterial properties. This is why honey has been used to treat wounds and prevent infections for centuries. When ingested, honey can also soothe sore throats and prevent bacterial growth in the digestive system, providing a protective effect.

2. **High in Antioxidants**: Honey is a rich source of antioxidants, including phenolic compounds, which protect cells from damage. These antioxidants help strengthen the immune system and reduce the body's susceptibility to illness. Darker varieties of honey, like buckwheat honey, are especially high in antioxidants.

3. **Anti-Inflammatory Effects**: Chronic inflammation is at the root of many diseases, including heart disease and autoimmune conditions. Honey's anti-inflammatory properties make it an ideal addition to any anti-inflammatory regimen. When consumed regularly, honey helps to lower inflammation, benefiting joint health, cardiovascular health, and immune function.

4. **Soothes the Digestive System**: Honey's natural enzymes can aid in digestion and support gut health. A healthy gut is essential for a robust immune system, as it helps the body efficiently absorb nutrients and combat pathogens. Honey's prebiotic properties also promote the growth of healthy bacteria in the gut, further supporting immune health.

5. **Energy Boosting**: Unlike refined sugars, honey provides a steady source of energy without causing a sharp spike in blood glucose. Its natural sugars and trace minerals make it an ideal sweetener for those looking for a healthier energy boost, especially when they're fighting off an illness.

How Garlic and Honey Work Together

When combined, garlic and honey create a potent synergy that enhances each of their individual properties. The honey not only improves the taste of raw garlic but also helps preserve it, creating a mixture that can be stored and used regularly. Together, garlic and honey provide a range of benefits that support immune health, improve digestion, and enhance overall well-being.

- **Enhanced Immune Defense**: The antibacterial, antiviral, and antifungal properties of garlic are amplified when paired with honey, creating a tonic that can help prevent and treat infections. This combination is especially effective against respiratory infections, colds, and flu.
- **Digestive Health and Detoxification**: Honey soothes the digestive tract, while garlic stimulates digestion and helps remove toxins. Together, they provide comprehensive support for digestive health, which is crucial for immunity, as a healthy gut is central to a well-functioning immune system.
- **Sustained Energy for Recovery**: Honey's natural sugars provide sustained energy, which is especially beneficial for those recovering from illness or dealing with chronic fatigue. The steady release of glucose helps the body heal and recover without causing energy crashes.

Making a Garlic and Honey Tonic

Creating a garlic and honey tonic is simple, and it requires only two ingredients: raw garlic and raw honey. Here's how to make it:

1. **Ingredients**:
   - 10-12 cloves of fresh garlic, peeled
   - 1 cup of raw honey (preferably organic and unprocessed)
2. **Preparation**:
   - Begin by lightly crushing each garlic clove. Crushing activates the allicin in the garlic, enhancing its medicinal properties.
   - Place the crushed garlic cloves in a glass jar and pour the honey over them, ensuring the garlic is fully submerged.
   - Seal the jar with a lid and store it in a cool, dark place for a week. During this time, the garlic will infuse into the honey, creating a potent tonic.
3. **Storage**:

- After a week, the tonic is ready to use. Store it in the refrigerator to keep it fresh. The honey may thicken over time, but it will remain effective.

4. **Dosage**:
   - Take one clove and a spoonful of honey daily as a preventive measure. For acute symptoms like a sore throat or the onset of a cold, take a clove and honey mixture two to three times per day.

Practical Uses and Scenarios

1. **Preventive Daily Tonic**: Many people use garlic and honey as a preventive measure against colds and flu, especially during peak seasons. Consuming a small spoonful each day provides a regular dose of immune-boosting compounds, helping the body stay resilient.

2. **Cold and Flu Relief**: When symptoms of cold or flu appear, taking extra doses of garlic and honey can help reduce the severity and duration of the illness. Garlic's antiviral properties help the body fight off the infection, while honey soothes sore throats and provides comfort.

3. **Digestive Health**: The garlic and honey tonic can also be taken to support digestive health, especially when experiencing symptoms like bloating or indigestion. The tonic's antibacterial properties help maintain a healthy balance of gut bacteria, while honey's prebiotics support digestive function.

4. **Skin Health**: Due to its antibacterial and anti-inflammatory properties, the garlic and honey mixture can also be applied topically to treat minor cuts or acne. Apply a small amount directly to the affected area, leave it on for a few minutes, and then rinse with warm water. Be cautious when using garlic topically, as it can be potent and may cause skin irritation in some individuals.

Tips for Maximizing the Benefits of Garlic and Honey

1. **Use Raw Ingredients**: To preserve the potency of the tonic, always use raw garlic and raw honey. Processing can strip these ingredients of their beneficial compounds, reducing their effectiveness.

2. **Allow Garlic to Rest After Crushing**: After crushing or chopping garlic, let it rest for about 10 minutes before combining it with honey. This waiting period maximizes allicin production, enhancing the health benefits of the tonic.

3. **Incorporate into Meals**: While taking the tonic directly is beneficial, you can also add it to warm (not hot) dishes like salads or toast. However, avoid heating the mixture, as high temperatures can degrade allicin and the enzymes in honey.

4. **Monitor for Sensitivity**: Garlic can be potent, and some people may experience digestive discomfort if they consume it in large amounts. Start with a small dose and gradually increase it to ensure your body tolerates it well.

Frequently Asked Questions

1. **Can I use powdered garlic and processed honey?**
   - Fresh, raw garlic and raw honey are essential for maximum benefits. Powdered garlic lacks allicin, and processed honey may contain added sugars and lack the natural enzymes that make raw honey beneficial.

2. **How long does the tonic last?**
   - When stored in the refrigerator, the garlic and honey tonic can last for several months. The honey acts as a natural preservative, preventing spoilage.

3. **Can I give this tonic to children?**
   - For children over one year, a small dose of honey alone can be beneficial. However, garlic's potency may be too strong for young children, so consult a healthcare professional before administering it.

Enhancing the Tonic with Additional Ingredients

For those looking to enhance their garlic and honey tonic, consider adding lemon, ginger, or turmeric for extra immune support. Lemon adds vitamin C, ginger provides additional anti-inflammatory benefits, and turmeric's curcumin works synergistically with garlic and honey to reduce inflammation.

1. **Lemon**: Add a slice of lemon or a few drops of lemon juice to each dose of tonic for a vitamin C boost.

2. **Ginger**: Grate fresh ginger into the mixture to enhance its warming properties and improve circulation.

3. **Turmeric**: A pinch of turmeric powder can be added to provide additional anti-inflammatory benefits, especially beneficial during cold and flu season.

The garlic and honey tonic is an ancient remedy that combines the healing power of two potent natural ingredients. When taken consistently, this simple tonic can be a valuable tool in supporting overall health and resilience, especially during times when the immune system needs extra support. By incorporating this tonic into your daily routine, you're embracing a timeless approach to wellness that's both effective and rooted in natural medicine.

Oregano Oil Capsules

Oregano oil capsules have garnered significant attention in the realm of natural health due to their powerful antimicrobial, anti-inflammatory, and antioxidant properties. Made from the concentrated essential oil of the oregano plant (*Origanum vulgare*), these capsules offer a convenient and effective way to harness the therapeutic benefits of oregano without the strong taste often associated with the oil itself. Known for centuries in Mediterranean regions, oregano oil has been traditionally used for its ability to treat infections, support immune health, and aid digestion. In this section, we will delve into the history, benefits, uses, and considerations of incorporating oregano oil capsules into a daily wellness routine.

Origins and Composition of Oregano Oil

Oregano, native to the Mediterranean, has been used as a culinary and medicinal herb for thousands of years. Ancient Greeks and Romans recognized its healing properties, using it to treat wounds, respiratory ailments, and digestive issues. The word "oregano" derives from the Greek phrase "joy of the mountains," reflecting the plant's significance in ancient Mediterranean culture.

The therapeutic benefits of oregano oil come from its rich concentration of active compounds, particularly carvacrol and thymol. These compounds are potent phenols known for their antibacterial, antifungal, and anti-inflammatory effects. Other notable constituents include terpenes, which give oregano its distinct aroma and contribute to its antimicrobial action, and rosmarinic acid, a powerful antioxidant that supports the body in neutralizing free radicals.

- **Carvacrol**: Carvacrol is the primary component in oregano oil, responsible for most of its antimicrobial properties. Studies suggest that carvacrol can inhibit the growth of several bacterial strains, including *E. coli*, *Staphylococcus aureus*, and *Salmonella*.
- **Thymol**: Another significant compound in oregano oil, thymol, exhibits antiseptic properties and aids in protecting against toxins and infections. Thymol is commonly

used in mouthwashes and antiseptic solutions due to its effectiveness against pathogens.

Health Benefits of Oregano Oil Capsules

Oregano oil capsules offer a range of health benefits, primarily due to their ability to support the immune system, combat infections, and reduce inflammation. Below are some of the key benefits associated with this potent herbal supplement.

1. Immune System Support

One of the primary uses of oregano oil capsules is to bolster immune health, especially during cold and flu season. The antimicrobial properties of carvacrol and thymol make oregano oil highly effective against a wide spectrum of pathogens, including bacteria, viruses, and fungi. By incorporating oregano oil capsules into a daily routine, individuals may experience increased resilience against infections and a reduction in the duration of illnesses.

- **Use in Daily Life**: Taking oregano oil capsules during seasonal transitions, when immunity may be lower, can offer a preventive shield against common infections. People who frequently experience colds or sinus issues may find oregano oil capsules particularly beneficial.

2. Antibacterial and Antiviral Properties

Oregano oil's most notable attribute is its powerful antibacterial and antiviral properties. Research has shown that carvacrol can disrupt bacterial cell membranes, effectively neutralizing harmful bacteria without harming beneficial gut bacteria when taken in moderation. Additionally, carvacrol has demonstrated antiviral activity, making it a potential natural remedy for viral infections, such as the flu.

- **Practical Applications**: For individuals exposed to environments with high pathogen levels, such as schools, offices, or public transportation, oregano oil capsules can serve as a proactive defense. They can also be helpful for individuals traveling to regions with high rates of infectious diseases.

3. Anti-Inflammatory Effects

Oregano oil contains compounds that help reduce inflammation, making it a valuable supplement for individuals with inflammatory conditions such as arthritis, asthma, or digestive disorders. Chronic inflammation is linked to numerous health issues, including autoimmune diseases, cardiovascular disease, and metabolic syndrome. By reducing inflammation, oregano oil capsules may aid in managing symptoms and improving overall health.

- **Use for Chronic Conditions**: Regular use of oregano oil capsules can be beneficial for those managing inflammatory conditions. For instance, individuals with arthritis may find relief from joint pain and swelling by incorporating oregano oil capsules as part of their regimen.

4. Digestive Health Support

Oregano oil has been traditionally used to support digestive health, particularly by combatting harmful bacteria in the gut and promoting a healthy balance of gut flora. Its antimicrobial properties help inhibit the growth of pathogens that can lead to digestive issues, such as bloating, gas, and cramps. Additionally, oregano oil is known to stimulate bile production, aiding in the digestion of fats and enhancing nutrient absorption.

- **Benefit in Daily Life**: For individuals with frequent digestive issues, such as irritable bowel syndrome (IBS) or small intestinal bacterial overgrowth (SIBO), oregano oil capsules may provide relief by restoring balance to gut bacteria and reducing symptoms. However, as with any potent herb, moderation and professional guidance are key.

5. Antioxidant Protection

Oregano oil is rich in antioxidants, particularly rosmarinic acid and thymol. Antioxidants play a crucial role in neutralizing free radicals, unstable molecules that can damage cells and contribute to aging and disease. By providing antioxidant support, oregano oil capsules may protect cells from oxidative stress, supporting healthy skin, immune function, and cardiovascular health.

- **Practical Use**: For individuals exposed to high levels of environmental toxins or oxidative stress, such as smokers or those living in polluted areas, oregano oil capsules offer a convenient way to incorporate antioxidant protection into their routine.

How to Take Oregano Oil Capsules

Oregano oil is highly concentrated and potent, so taking it in capsule form offers an effective, controlled method for consumption. Here's how to use oregano oil capsules safely and effectively:

1. **Dosage**: Most oregano oil capsules contain 150-200 mg of oregano oil per serving, with a standardized concentration of carvacrol. The recommended dosage typically ranges from 1-2 capsules per day, but it's essential to follow the specific instructions on the product label.

2. **Timing**: Oregano oil capsules are best taken with food to prevent gastrointestinal discomfort. Taking the capsules with a meal also aids in nutrient absorption and reduces the risk of an upset stomach.

3. **Duration**: For immune support, oregano oil capsules can be taken daily for short periods (up to two weeks). For ongoing use, such as for chronic conditions, it's recommended to take breaks periodically to maintain effectiveness and prevent potential tolerance.

4. **Precautions**: Because oregano oil is a natural antibiotic, prolonged use may impact gut health by disturbing beneficial bacteria. For extended use, consider incorporating a probiotic supplement to maintain gut flora balance.

Safety and Potential Side Effects

While oregano oil capsules are generally safe for most people, there are some potential side effects and contraindications to be aware of:

- **Allergic Reactions**: Individuals with allergies to plants in the mint family, such as basil, mint, or lavender, may also be allergic to oregano. Symptoms may include skin rashes, itching, or gastrointestinal discomfort.

- **Pregnancy and Breastfeeding**: Pregnant and breastfeeding women should avoid oregano oil capsules unless recommended by a healthcare provider, as the herb may stimulate the uterus and affect pregnancy.

- **Blood Clotting**: Oregano oil may have a mild blood-thinning effect, so individuals on anticoagulant medications should use it with caution.

- **Digestive Upset**: In some cases, high doses of oregano oil may lead to digestive discomfort, such as heartburn or upset stomach. Taking the capsules with food usually alleviates this issue.

Practical Applications and Daily Use

Oregano oil capsules are versatile and can be used in various ways to support overall health:

- **Seasonal Use for Immune Support**: Many people take oregano oil capsules as part of a seasonal immune-boosting routine during the fall and winter months when colds and flu are more prevalent.
- **For Digestive Health**: Individuals with IBS, bloating, or digestive infections may benefit from a short course of oregano oil capsules to address underlying bacterial imbalances. Taking the capsules for two weeks, followed by a break, is often effective for digestive support.
- **Support for Travel**: Traveling can expose individuals to various pathogens, especially in regions with different hygiene standards. Taking oregano oil capsules before and during travel can help bolster immunity and reduce the risk of gastrointestinal issues.
- **For Skin Health**: The antioxidant properties of oregano oil make it beneficial for skin health. Some people find that regular use of oregano oil capsules supports a clearer complexion and protects against oxidative stress, which contributes to aging.

The Benefits of Choosing Capsules Over Liquid Oregano Oil

Oregano oil is available in both liquid and capsule form, each with distinct advantages. However, capsules are often preferred for several reasons:

1. **Convenience**: Capsules are easier to take and eliminate the strong, often overwhelming taste of oregano oil, which can be quite intense.
2. **Controlled Dosage**: Capsules provide a pre-measured dosage, reducing the risk of taking too much or too little. This is especially important given the potency of oregano oil.
3. **Travel-Friendly**: Capsules are portable and less likely to spill, making them ideal for travel and on-the-go use.
4. **Reduced Irritation**: Direct ingestion of oregano oil can sometimes cause mouth or throat irritation. Capsules provide a buffered delivery method, reducing the risk of irritation and ensuring that the oil reaches the stomach and intestines.

By incorporating oregano oil capsules into a daily wellness routine, individuals can experience a variety of health benefits, from immune support to improved digestion and antioxidant protection. The convenience, potency, and versatility of these capsules make them a valuable addition to natural health practices, providing a safe and effective way to harness the therapeutic power of oregano oil.

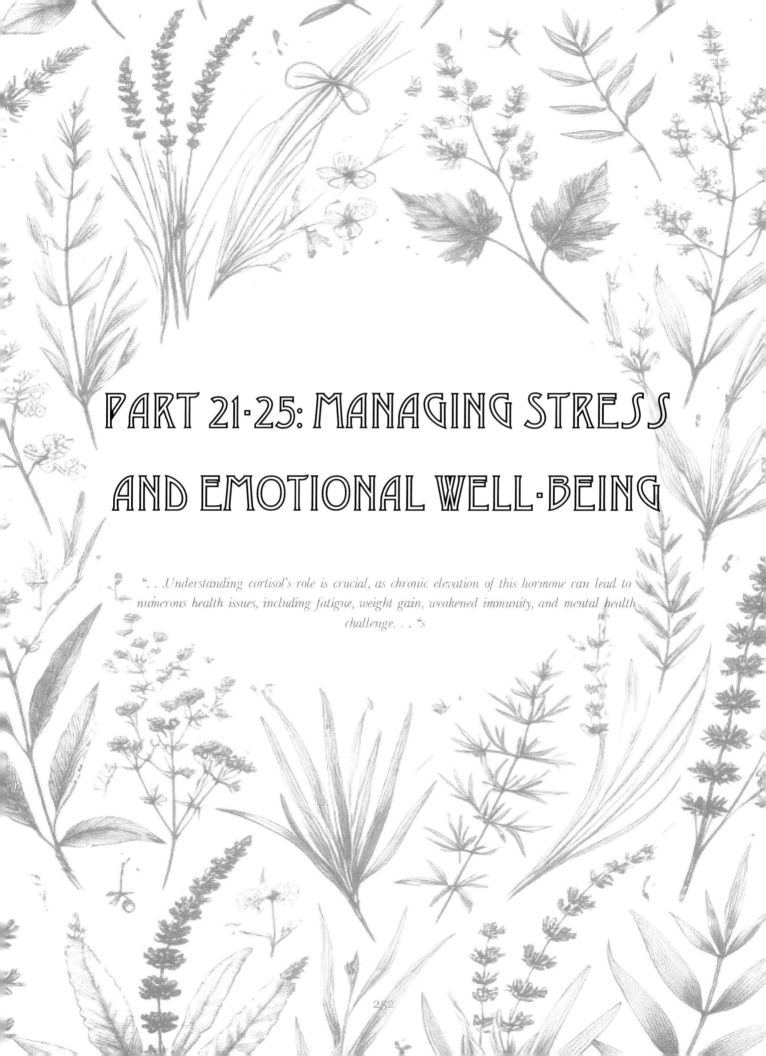

PART 21-25: MANAGING STRESS AND EMOTIONAL WELL-BEING

"...Understanding cortisol's role is crucial, as chronic elevation of this hormone can lead to numerous health issues, including fatigue, weight gain, weakened immunity, and mental health challenge..."

Chapter 1: Impact of Stress on Health

Cortisol, often called the "stress hormone," plays a pivotal role in how our bodies respond to stress and various physical demands. Produced by the adrenal glands, cortisol affects nearly every organ system, influencing everything from metabolism to immune function and even cognitive performance.

Cortisol and Body Response

Understanding cortisol's role is crucial, as chronic elevation of this hormone can lead to numerous health issues, including fatigue, weight gain, weakened immunity, and mental health challenges. In this section, we'll explore the mechanisms of cortisol, its impact on the body, and effective strategies for managing cortisol levels to promote holistic well-being.

What is Cortisol?

Cortisol is a steroid hormone produced by the adrenal glands, small organs located on top of each kidney. It is released in response to signals from the hypothalamus and pituitary gland in the brain. This communication pathway, known as the hypothalamic-pituitary-adrenal (HPA) axis, is activated whenever the body perceives stress—whether physical, emotional, or environmental. When the HPA axis signals the adrenal glands, they release cortisol into the bloodstream, preparing the body for a "fight or flight" response.

Functions of Cortisol in the Body

Cortisol's role in the body is multifaceted. It influences various physiological processes, adapting the body to stress and regulating functions that are critical for survival.

1. **Energy Mobilization**: When cortisol is released, it increases blood sugar levels by converting stored glycogen into glucose. This provides the body with quick energy, allowing muscles and the brain to respond effectively to stressors. This energy mobilization is essential for handling acute stress but can become problematic when cortisol remains elevated over long periods.

2. **Immune System Regulation**: Cortisol has a suppressive effect on the immune system, which can be beneficial in short bursts, as it prevents the body from

overreacting to minor injuries or infections. However, chronic elevation of cortisol weakens the immune system, making the body more susceptible to infections, colds, and other illnesses.

3. **Anti-Inflammatory Effects**: One of cortisol's primary functions is to reduce inflammation. In short-term stress, this is beneficial, helping to prevent swelling and pain. However, if cortisol levels remain high, this anti-inflammatory effect can dampen the body's ability to heal, as the immune response is suppressed. Long-term suppression of inflammation can also increase the risk of autoimmune diseases.

4. **Blood Pressure Regulation**: Cortisol increases blood pressure to ensure that the body's organs and muscles receive adequate blood flow during times of stress. While this is useful during an emergency, chronic high blood pressure resulting from elevated cortisol can lead to cardiovascular issues over time.

5. **Cognitive Function**: Cortisol has a direct effect on the brain, particularly the hippocampus, which is involved in memory formation and learning. Moderate levels of cortisol can enhance memory and focus, but chronic stress and elevated cortisol can impair cognitive function, leading to memory problems and difficulties with concentration.

6. **Mood and Mental Health**: Cortisol influences neurotransmitters in the brain, such as serotonin and dopamine, which are associated with mood regulation. Chronic stress can alter cortisol levels, contributing to mood disorders like anxiety and depression. High cortisol levels can make it difficult to feel calm or happy, as the body remains in a prolonged state of alertness.

The Impact of Chronic Elevated Cortisol

While cortisol serves many vital functions, chronic stress keeps cortisol levels elevated, which can have detrimental effects on both physical and mental health. Let's examine some of the ways prolonged cortisol elevation impacts well-being.

1. **Fatigue and Burnout**: Chronic stress places a significant demand on the adrenal glands, which can lead to adrenal fatigue. When the body constantly produces cortisol, it eventually exhausts itself, leading to fatigue, low energy, and difficulty recovering from stress. This state of burnout can affect all aspects of life, from physical health to mental clarity.

2. **Weight Gain and Metabolic Issues**: Cortisol encourages the storage of fat, particularly in the abdominal area, which is linked to metabolic issues and an increased risk of cardiovascular disease. Additionally, high cortisol levels can lead to insulin resistance, making it difficult for the body to regulate blood sugar and potentially leading to type 2 diabetes.

3. **Weakened Immune System**: Chronic cortisol elevation suppresses immune function, making the body more vulnerable to infections, viruses, and other pathogens. People with prolonged high cortisol levels often experience frequent illnesses, such as colds and respiratory infections, and may take longer to recover from these conditions.

4. **Mental Health Challenges**: Prolonged high cortisol levels can lead to mental health issues, such as anxiety, depression, and irritability. The constant state of alertness can make it difficult to relax or experience joy, and over time, it can lead to more severe mental health challenges.

5. **Disrupted Sleep Patterns**: Cortisol follows a natural daily rhythm, with levels peaking in the morning and gradually decreasing throughout the day. However, chronic stress can disrupt this rhythm, leading to elevated cortisol at night. This disruption interferes with sleep quality, making it hard to fall asleep or stay asleep, which further impacts mental and physical health.

Managing Cortisol Levels Naturally

Fortunately, there are natural ways to manage and balance cortisol levels. Implementing these strategies can help reduce chronic stress, allowing the body to return to a balanced state.

1. **Adaptogens**: Adaptogens are herbs that help the body adapt to stress, supporting adrenal health and helping balance cortisol levels. Examples include ashwagandha, rhodiola, and holy basil. These herbs work by modulating the HPA axis, helping the body cope with stress more effectively without overproducing cortisol.

2. **Mindfulness and Meditation**: Practicing mindfulness and meditation has been shown to reduce cortisol levels significantly. These practices help the mind relax, reducing the body's stress response. Just 10-20 minutes of meditation per day can lower cortisol levels, improve mood, and enhance mental clarity.

3. **Physical Activity**: Exercise, especially moderate aerobic activities like walking or swimming, can help manage cortisol levels. Physical activity releases endorphins, which improve mood and reduce stress. However, it's essential to avoid excessive, high-intensity exercise, as this can increase cortisol levels further.

4. **Sleep Hygiene**: Quality sleep is essential for balancing cortisol. Establishing a regular sleep schedule, avoiding caffeine and electronic screens before bed, and creating a calming pre-sleep routine can help maintain healthy cortisol levels. Ensuring seven to eight hours of restful sleep each night is crucial for overall hormonal balance.

5. **Diet and Nutrition**: Eating a balanced diet rich in antioxidants, vitamins, and minerals supports adrenal health and helps regulate cortisol. Foods high in vitamin C, magnesium, and B vitamins are particularly beneficial. Avoiding refined sugars and caffeine can also prevent unnecessary spikes in cortisol levels.

6. **Social Support and Connection**: Maintaining healthy relationships and having a supportive social network can reduce stress and improve resilience. Engaging in positive social interactions releases oxytocin, which counteracts cortisol and promotes relaxation and well-being.

Herbal Remedies for Cortisol Balance

1. **Ashwagandha**: Known as a powerful adaptogen, ashwagandha helps the body adapt to stress and lowers cortisol levels. Studies have shown that ashwagandha can reduce cortisol by up to 30%, making it an effective remedy for chronic stress.

2. **Rhodiola Rosea**: This herb is known for its ability to enhance physical and mental resilience. It supports the adrenal glands, helping them manage stress without becoming overactive. Rhodiola is particularly helpful for those experiencing burnout and fatigue due to prolonged stress.

3. **Holy Basil**: Also called tulsi, holy basil is revered in Ayurvedic medicine for its stress-relieving properties. It reduces cortisol levels and promotes a sense of calm, making it beneficial for managing anxiety and mental fatigue.

4. **Licorice Root**: Licorice root supports adrenal function by modulating cortisol levels. However, it should be used with caution, as it can raise blood pressure in some individuals. Working with a healthcare provider can help determine the correct dosage.

5. **Lemon Balm**: Known for its calming effects, lemon balm helps reduce anxiety and stress. This herb also improves sleep quality, which is essential for maintaining balanced cortisol levels.

The Mind-Body Connection in Cortisol Management

Cortisol is more than just a chemical response; it's influenced by our perceptions, thoughts, and emotions. Learning to manage stress mindfully is crucial for controlling cortisol levels and improving overall health. Practicing gratitude, positive self-talk, and self-compassion can help shift the mind's perspective on stress, reducing the intensity of the body's cortisol response.

1. **Gratitude Practice**: Focusing on what you're grateful for has been shown to reduce stress hormones and improve mental resilience. A daily gratitude practice helps the mind view stressors with more balance, reducing the impact of cortisol on the body.

2. **Breathing Techniques**: Deep, diaphragmatic breathing activates the parasympathetic nervous system, which reduces cortisol and promotes relaxation. Techniques like 4-7-8 breathing or box breathing are effective in managing immediate stress responses.

3. **Mindful Movement**: Yoga and tai chi combine physical activity with mindfulness, offering a dual approach to managing cortisol. These practices promote relaxation while also improving physical fitness, providing a holistic approach to cortisol management.

Supporting Adrenal Health for Balanced Cortisol

The adrenal glands play a central role in cortisol production, and supporting their health can help regulate cortisol levels. In addition to stress management practices, dietary and lifestyle choices can support adrenal health.

- **Balanced Diet**: Ensuring a diet rich in whole foods, healthy fats, and lean proteins supports adrenal health and hormone production. Foods like avocados, nuts, and

Chronic stress is a pervasive issue affecting millions, with consequences that extend far beyond temporary discomfort. While short-term stress responses can be beneficial—enabling focus, energy, and even survival—prolonged exposure to stress can lead to detrimental effects on both physical and mental health. This section examines the long-term effects of chronic stress on various body systems, providing insights into the mechanisms at play and practical approaches to mitigate these impacts.

Understanding Chronic Stress and Its Mechanisms

Stress is the body's natural reaction to perceived threats or demands, activating the "fight or flight" response through the release of hormones such as cortisol and adrenaline. In acute situations, this response prepares the body to respond effectively. However, in cases of chronic stress, these physiological reactions become continuously activated, keeping the body in a prolonged state of alert. Over time, this constant state of stress can lead to wear and tear on the body, affecting vital functions and increasing susceptibility to illnesses.

Chronic stress involves complex interactions between the brain, endocrine system, and immune system. The primary stress hormone, cortisol, is produced by the adrenal glands and regulated by the hypothalamic-pituitary-adrenal (HPA) axis. When stress becomes chronic, this axis can become dysregulated, leading to elevated cortisol levels and imbalances in other hormones, which in turn affect multiple body systems.

Impact on the Cardiovascular System

Chronic stress has a profound effect on cardiovascular health. The continuous release of stress hormones increases heart rate and blood pressure, placing strain on the heart and blood vessels. Over time, this can lead to high blood pressure (hypertension), increasing the risk of serious cardiovascular events such as heart attacks and strokes.

Research indicates that individuals under chronic stress are more prone to developing atherosclerosis, a condition characterized by the buildup of plaque in the arteries. This buildup restricts blood flow, further elevating the risk of heart disease. Additionally, stress-related behaviors, such as overeating, smoking, or a sedentary lifestyle, can compound these cardiovascular risks, creating a vicious cycle that is difficult to break without intervention.

- **Example Scenario**: Consider a corporate executive working in a high-stakes environment with constant deadlines. The sustained stress not only raises their blood pressure but also leads them to cope through unhealthy eating habits. These combined factors place the individual at significant risk for cardiovascular complications over time.

Digestive System Disturbances

The digestive system is highly sensitive to stress. Chronic stress can alter the gut's natural motility, leading to symptoms like bloating, cramping, constipation, or diarrhea. Stress has also been shown to disrupt the delicate balance of gut microbiota, which plays a critical role in digestion, immune function, and mental health.

Increased cortisol levels can reduce blood flow to the digestive system, impairing nutrient absorption and leading to inflammation in the gut lining. This inflammation is linked to conditions such as irritable bowel syndrome (IBS) and inflammatory bowel disease (IBD). Furthermore, individuals experiencing chronic stress often turn to comfort foods high in fat and sugar, which can exacerbate digestive issues and contribute to obesity.

- **Practical Application**: For individuals experiencing digestive issues tied to stress, incorporating practices like mindful eating, stress management techniques, and dietary adjustments can provide relief and support gut health.

Immune System Suppression

Chronic stress weakens the immune system, making the body more susceptible to infections and illnesses. Under stress, the body prioritizes immediate survival over long-term immune function, suppressing white blood cell production and reducing the body's ability to fight off pathogens.

High cortisol levels also interfere with cytokine production, proteins that regulate immune responses, which can lead to chronic inflammation. In the long term, this suppression and dysregulation of the immune system increase vulnerability to both acute infections, like colds and the flu, and more severe autoimmune conditions.

- **Impact on Daily Life**: Individuals under prolonged stress may notice they are more likely to catch colds or experience frequent infections. For those with autoimmune conditions, chronic stress can lead to more frequent flare-ups and a worsening of symptoms.

Endocrine and Hormonal Imbalances

The endocrine system, which regulates hormones, is profoundly affected by chronic stress. Elevated cortisol disrupts the balance of other hormones, such as insulin, thyroid hormones, and sex hormones like estrogen and testosterone.

- **Insulin Resistance**: Chronic stress can lead to insulin resistance, a condition where the body's cells become less responsive to insulin, increasing blood sugar levels. Insulin resistance is a precursor to type 2 diabetes, and stress is a significant contributing factor.
- **Thyroid Dysfunction**: Stress can impair thyroid function, leading to symptoms like fatigue, weight gain, and mood disturbances. Hypothyroidism, a condition where the thyroid gland underproduces hormones, is often exacerbated by chronic stress.
- **Reproductive Health**: In both men and women, chronic stress can disrupt reproductive health. For women, stress can lead to irregular menstrual cycles, exacerbating conditions like polycystic ovary syndrome (PCOS). For men, prolonged stress may reduce testosterone levels, impacting fertility and libido.

Scenario Application

Imagine an individual with a demanding job, chronic sleep deprivation, and frequent family responsibilities. This combination of stressors not only raises their cortisol levels but also contributes to insulin resistance and fatigue, leading to weight gain and increasing their risk for metabolic syndrome.

Mental Health Effects

The mental health implications of chronic stress are significant. Long-term exposure to stress is associated with anxiety, depression, and even cognitive decline. Chronic stress reduces serotonin production and alters brain structure, particularly in areas involved in memory, decision-making, and emotional regulation.

Studies have shown that stress can shrink the hippocampus, a region of the brain crucial for learning and memory, while enlarging the amygdala, which is involved in fear and anxiety responses. This imbalance can lead to heightened anxiety, making it more challenging to cope with future stressors and perpetuating a cycle of stress and mental health challenges.

- **Daily Coping Strategies**: Engaging in regular exercise, practicing mindfulness, and building a support network can alleviate some of these mental health effects. Therapy or counseling can also provide tools for managing chronic stress more effectively.

Effects on Sleep Quality

One of the earliest signs of chronic stress is often a disruption in sleep. High cortisol levels make it difficult to fall asleep and stay asleep, leading to a cycle of poor sleep quality that further exacerbates stress. Sleep is essential for the body's recovery, memory consolidation, and immune function. When stress interferes with sleep, it diminishes the body's ability to repair itself, perpetuating the adverse effects of stress on overall health.

- **Example**: For individuals struggling with sleep due to chronic stress, practices like setting a regular bedtime, avoiding caffeine late in the day, and practicing relaxation techniques can be beneficial. Supplements like magnesium or herbal teas, such as chamomile, may also support restful sleep.

Muscular and Skeletal Health

Chronic stress often leads to muscle tension, particularly in the neck, shoulders, and back. Over time, this muscle tension can contribute to musculoskeletal pain and discomfort. Additionally, chronic stress may increase inflammation in the body, exacerbating joint pain and contributing to conditions like arthritis.

Stress also affects bone health by reducing calcium absorption and bone density, which can increase the risk of osteoporosis. Individuals who experience high levels of stress throughout life may have a higher risk of developing brittle bones and fractures as they age.

- **Physical Relief**: Regular exercise, stretching, and massage can relieve muscle tension, while practices like yoga and Tai Chi can help improve flexibility, support joint health, and lower stress levels.

Skin Health and Appearance

The skin is highly responsive to hormonal changes, and chronic stress can significantly impact skin health. Elevated cortisol levels increase oil production, leading to acne and other skin issues. Chronic stress may also impair skin barrier function, making the skin more susceptible to irritation, redness, and sensitivity.

Additionally, stress accelerates aging by reducing collagen production, leading to fine lines, wrinkles, and dullness. For individuals with conditions like eczema or psoriasis, chronic stress can exacerbate symptoms, leading to more frequent flare-ups.

- **Daily Skin Care Tips**: For those experiencing stress-related skin issues, adopting a skincare routine that includes gentle cleansing, moisturizing, and SPF protection can be beneficial. Antioxidant-rich serums, along with practices like facial massages, can also support skin health.

Strategies to Combat Chronic Stress

While it's impossible to eliminate all sources of stress, developing effective strategies to manage stress can prevent or mitigate many of its long-term effects. Here are some evidence-based practices for managing chronic stress:

1. **Mindfulness and Meditation**: Practicing mindfulness or meditation can help reduce stress by promoting relaxation and enhancing awareness of present-moment experiences. These practices have been shown to lower cortisol levels and improve emotional resilience.

2. **Exercise**: Regular physical activity is a proven method for reducing stress. Exercise increases endorphins, which improve mood and reduce anxiety. Activities like walking, swimming, and yoga are particularly beneficial for stress management.

3. **Social Support**: Building a support network of friends, family, or a therapist can provide emotional relief during stressful times. Talking to someone who listens and offers support can alleviate feelings of isolation and anxiety.

4. **Dietary Adjustments**: Nutritional choices impact stress levels. A diet rich in whole foods, particularly those high in antioxidants, can reduce oxidative stress in the body. Omega-3 fatty acids, found in foods like salmon and walnuts, are known to have anti-inflammatory effects, benefiting both mental and physical health.

5. **Adequate Sleep**: Ensuring consistent, restful sleep is essential for managing chronic stress. Developing a bedtime routine, minimizing screen time, and creating a calming sleep environment can support better sleep quality.

6. **Herbal Supplements**: Natural remedies, including adaptogenic herbs like ashwagandha, rhodiola, and holy basil, may help reduce the body's stress response. These herbs support adrenal function and help the body adapt to stress over time.

Impacts on Mental Health

In the modern world, mental health has become an area of critical concern. As daily stress levels continue to rise, so too does the toll on our mental well-being. While physical health often garners attention, mental health is equally essential to leading a balanced, fulfilling life. Interestingly, mental health is not isolated from physical health; the two are deeply interconnected. This section explores how mental health impacts every facet of life, with a particular focus on how natural remedies, lifestyle choices, and nutrition can influence mental well-being.

The Mind-Body Connection

The connection between mind and body is a concept as old as medicine itself, rooted in holistic practices. Many natural remedies used to treat mental health recognize that the state of the mind affects the body and vice versa. In this view, mental health is inseparable from physical health, with each exerting influence over the other. For example, stress and anxiety can manifest physically through headaches, digestive issues, or fatigue. Conversely, chronic pain or physical ailments often contribute to depression or mood instability.

The hypothalamic-pituitary-adrenal (HPA) axis is a key player in this connection. When a person experiences stress, the hypothalamus (a small region in the brain) sends signals to the pituitary and adrenal glands, which release hormones like cortisol and adrenaline. These hormones impact both mental and physical states, preparing the body for "fight or flight" responses. This mechanism is beneficial in short-term stress but becomes harmful when activated over extended periods.

Effects of Chronic Stress on Mental Health

Stress, especially when experienced chronically, is one of the most influential factors affecting mental health. Chronic stress can alter brain chemistry, creating a state of hypervigilance that is difficult to shut off. Some of the ways chronic stress influences mental health include:

1. **Anxiety and Overthinking**: When stress is chronic, it fosters a loop of anxious thoughts that can be hard to break. This hyperactive state makes it difficult to relax and creates an ongoing sense of unease or dread, even when the original stressor has passed.

2. **Depression**: Extended periods of stress exhaust mental and emotional reserves, contributing to symptoms of depression. The body's natural response to protect itself from stress, in this case, can manifest as withdrawal, lethargy, or sadness.

3. **Sleep Disturbances**: Stress impacts sleep cycles by keeping the body in a state of alertness. People with high-stress levels often report difficulty falling asleep, staying asleep, or waking up rested. Poor sleep exacerbates other mental health issues, creating a cycle that's challenging to break.

4. **Emotional Dysregulation**: Chronic stress can disrupt neurotransmitters like serotonin and dopamine, leading to emotional instability. People may experience intense mood swings, irritability, or even aggression, which affects personal relationships and overall well-being.

The Role of Nutrition in Mental Health

Nutrition plays an unexpectedly powerful role in mental health. What we eat can influence mood, energy levels, and mental clarity. Nutrients from food help create neurotransmitters, hormones, and other chemicals essential for brain health. Certain vitamins, minerals, and amino acids are particularly important for mental well-being:

- **Omega-3 Fatty Acids**: Found in fatty fish, walnuts, and flaxseeds, omega-3 fatty acids are essential for brain health. These fats are anti-inflammatory and have been shown to reduce symptoms of depression and anxiety.

- **Vitamin D**: Often called the "sunshine vitamin," vitamin D is crucial for mood regulation. Low levels of vitamin D are associated with increased risk of depression and seasonal affective disorder (SAD).

- **B Vitamins**: B vitamins, especially B6, B9 (folate), and B12, support cognitive function and mood regulation. These vitamins are found in leafy greens, legumes, eggs, and fortified grains.

- **Magnesium**: Known as nature's tranquilizer, magnesium helps calm the nervous system. It can reduce anxiety and improve sleep quality, supporting overall mental health.

- **Amino Acids**: Amino acids like tryptophan and tyrosine are building blocks for neurotransmitters such as serotonin and dopamine. Serotonin, in particular, is a key player in mood regulation, and many anti-depressants aim to increase its levels.

Herbal Remedies for Mental Health

Natural remedies have long been used to support mental health. Many herbs possess calming, anti-inflammatory, and mood-boosting properties. Here are some well-regarded herbs for mental health support:

1. **Ashwagandha**: This adaptogenic herb helps the body handle stress by modulating the release of cortisol. Ashwagandha is often used to reduce anxiety, improve mood, and support mental clarity. As an adaptogen, it supports overall resilience to stress.

2. **St. John's Wort**: Known as an herbal antidepressant, St. John's Wort has been used to treat mild to moderate depression. It works by increasing levels of serotonin, a neurotransmitter linked to mood regulation. However, it should be used with caution as it can interact with other medications.

3. **Chamomile**: Chamomile has a gentle sedative effect and is commonly used to reduce anxiety and promote sleep. Chamomile tea, in particular, is a soothing bedtime ritual that supports relaxation.

4. **Rhodiola Rosea**: This herb helps alleviate fatigue and improves the body's response to stress. Rhodiola is commonly used to improve energy levels and mental focus, which can suffer during periods of high stress.

5. **Passionflower**: Known for its calming effects, passionflower is often used to relieve anxiety and improve sleep quality. It can be particularly helpful for those experiencing insomnia or restlessness due to stress.

Lifestyle Choices to Support Mental Health

Lifestyle choices have a profound impact on mental well-being. Creating a supportive routine, engaging in physical activity, and building a social support network are essential components of a healthy lifestyle that supports mental health.

1. **Physical Exercise**: Physical activity is a natural mood booster, releasing endorphins that counteract stress. Activities such as walking, jogging, yoga, or swimming are particularly beneficial. Exercise has also been shown to improve sleep quality, reduce anxiety, and increase mental resilience.

2. **Mindfulness and Meditation**: Practicing mindfulness helps calm the mind and reduces the body's stress response. Mindfulness techniques, such as meditation and deep breathing, activate the parasympathetic nervous system, which promotes relaxation.

3. **Social Connections**: Humans are inherently social creatures, and a strong support system is crucial for mental health. Positive relationships provide a sense of belonging and security, reducing feelings of loneliness and anxiety. Engaging in social activities and reaching out to loved ones during stressful times can mitigate mental strain.

4. **Sleep Hygiene**: Good sleep hygiene is essential for mental well-being. Going to bed and waking up at consistent times, avoiding screens before bed, and creating a restful environment can improve sleep quality. Quality sleep helps regulate mood, reduce stress, and restore mental clarity.

The Role of Gut Health in Mental Health

Recent studies have shown a significant link between gut health and mental health, often referred to as the gut-brain axis. The gut houses a large portion of the body's serotonin, a neurotransmitter closely linked to mood. An imbalance in gut bacteria, caused by poor diet or stress, can impact mental health, contributing to depression, anxiety, and mood swings.

1. **Probiotics**: Probiotics are beneficial bacteria that support gut health. Foods rich in probiotics, such as yogurt, kefir, sauerkraut, and kimchi, can promote a healthy gut microbiome, which in turn supports mental well-being.

2. **Prebiotics**: Prebiotics are fibers that feed beneficial gut bacteria. Foods like garlic, onions, bananas, and oats serve as prebiotics, encouraging the growth of healthy bacteria that support mental health.

3. **Avoiding Processed Foods**: Processed foods high in sugar and unhealthy fats can disrupt gut health, leading to inflammation that affects both body and mind. Eating whole foods, rich in nutrients, supports a balanced microbiome that positively impacts mental health.

The Influence of Cortisol and Adrenal Health on Mental Health

Cortisol, the stress hormone, affects both physical and mental health. Elevated cortisol levels are associated with anxiety, irritability, and mood swings. When cortisol is chronically high, it taxes the adrenal glands, leading to a state called adrenal fatigue. Adrenal fatigue exacerbates symptoms of mental health challenges, including feelings of exhaustion, anxiety, and depression.

1. **Adaptogens for Adrenal Support**: Adaptogens like ashwagandha, holy basil, and rhodiola support adrenal health, helping regulate cortisol levels. Lower cortisol levels promote a sense of calm and resilience, improving mental well-being.

2. **Cortisol-Balancing Activities**: Activities that reduce cortisol, such as gentle exercise, meditation, and creative hobbies, can improve mood and reduce symptoms of anxiety. These activities promote parasympathetic nervous system activity, counteracting the effects of chronic stress.

The Impact of Seasonal Changes on Mental Health

Seasonal changes, particularly during the winter months, can impact mental health. Seasonal Affective Disorder (SAD) is a form of depression that occurs in response to changes in light exposure. Lack of sunlight affects serotonin production, contributing to mood fluctuations and low energy levels.

1. **Light Therapy**: Exposure to light, especially in the morning, can help mitigate symptoms of SAD. Light therapy lamps that mimic sunlight can improve mood and energy, helping the body regulate its circadian rhythms.

2. **Vitamin D Supplementation**: Low vitamin D levels are common in winter, contributing to mood disorders. Supplementing with vitamin D during colder months supports mood regulation and can prevent winter-related depression.

3. **Physical Activity Outdoors**: Spending time outdoors, even in cold weather, can improve mood. Outdoor activities expose the body to natural light, which supports mental well-being.

Practicing Gratitude and Positivity

Focusing on positivity can improve mental health by changing neural pathways. Practicing gratitude, for example, encourages the mind to focus on what is going well rather than what is going wrong. Techniques to cultivate a positive mindset include:

- **Gratitude Journaling**: Writing down three things you are grateful for each day helps the mind focus on positive experiences.

- **Mindful Reflection**: Taking a few minutes each day to reflect on small achievements or acts of kindness can foster positivity.

Mental health is integral to overall well-being, and nurturing it requires a comprehensive approach that includes nutrition, lifestyle, and mindful practices. By embracing a balanced approach that supports both mind and body, individuals can cultivate resilience and improve their quality of life.

Physical Health Risks

Understanding the physical health risks associated with modern lifestyle choices, environmental factors, and chronic stress is essential for maintaining long-term well-being. This section delves into the various physical health risks prevalent today, exploring how they arise, how they impact the body, and strategies to mitigate their effects. From cardiovascular diseases to immune suppression, each aspect of physical health risk underscores the need for proactive lifestyle choices and, where applicable, natural remedies to support overall health.

Cardiovascular Health Risks

Cardiovascular diseases (CVDs) remain one of the most significant health risks worldwide. These include heart attacks, strokes, and conditions such as high blood pressure and atherosclerosis. A sedentary lifestyle, high-stress levels, poor dietary choices, and exposure to environmental pollutants increase the risk of developing cardiovascular issues. The body's response to chronic stress also plays a role; prolonged stress leads to elevated cortisol levels, which can raise blood pressure and increase heart rate over time.

- **Example**: Imagine an individual with a demanding job, often skipping exercise and relying on fast food for convenience. Over time, these habits increase their blood pressure, leading to hypertension. Combined with the stress of a high-paced job, this individual is at greater risk for a heart attack.

Maintaining cardiovascular health requires a comprehensive approach that combines regular exercise, a balanced diet rich in omega-3 fatty acids, and stress management techniques. Omega-3s, found in fatty fish and flaxseeds, have been shown to support heart health by reducing inflammation and improving blood vessel function.

Metabolic Syndrome and Obesity

Metabolic syndrome is a cluster of conditions that includes obesity, high blood pressure, high blood sugar, and abnormal cholesterol levels. These factors increase the risk of heart disease, stroke, and type 2 diabetes. Obesity, in particular, is a physical health risk that exacerbates almost every other condition, from joint problems to respiratory issues.

The causes of metabolic syndrome are often lifestyle-related, including a diet high in sugars and processed foods, physical inactivity, and stress. Chronic stress, as mentioned, leads to elevated cortisol levels, which can contribute to weight gain, particularly in the abdominal area, increasing the risk for metabolic disorders.

- **Practical Scenario**: For those dealing with metabolic syndrome, incorporating natural remedies such as ginger or green tea can help support metabolism. These substances are known to aid in digestion and can potentially increase calorie burning. However, the foundation of prevention lies in balanced eating, regular physical activity, and stress reduction techniques.

Diabetes and Blood Sugar Dysregulation

Type 2 diabetes is another serious health risk with profound long-term effects. It occurs when the body becomes resistant to insulin or when the pancreas cannot produce enough insulin to maintain normal blood glucose levels. Risk factors include obesity, poor diet, and a sedentary lifestyle, with genetic predispositions also playing a role.

Chronic stress and hormonal imbalances can contribute to blood sugar dysregulation by causing insulin resistance. Elevated cortisol levels trigger glucose release for immediate energy, but if the body is not utilizing that energy—due to inactivity, for example—blood sugar levels remain elevated, contributing to insulin resistance.

Incorporating a balanced diet with low-glycemic foods, regular physical activity, and stress management can help regulate blood sugar levels. Natural supplements like cinnamon and berberine may help to improve insulin sensitivity, though they should be used as part of a comprehensive approach under professional guidance.

Digestive Health Risks

Digestive health issues, such as irritable bowel syndrome (IBS), acid reflux, and inflammatory bowel disease (IBD), are common in today's fast-paced world. These conditions are often exacerbated by poor dietary habits, chronic stress, and lack of physical activity. The gut-brain axis, a bidirectional communication pathway between the gut and brain, means that stress and anxiety can directly impact digestive health, leading to symptoms such as bloating, cramps, and irregular bowel movements.

Prolonged digestive issues can lead to nutrient deficiencies, as the body's ability to absorb vitamins and minerals is compromised. Inflammation in the digestive tract can also increase the risk of autoimmune diseases, as the immune system becomes dysregulated.

- **Scenario**: An individual with a high-stress job may frequently experience acid reflux and bloating due to poor eating habits and high-stress levels. Incorporating digestive-friendly foods such as ginger, peppermint, and fiber-rich foods can provide some relief. Additionally, probiotics can help restore the gut's balance of beneficial bacteria, improving digestive health and potentially alleviating symptoms over time.

Immune System Suppression

A weakened immune system is one of the more serious long-term effects of chronic stress, poor diet, and lack of exercise. The immune system is responsible for defending the body against infections and diseases, and when it's compromised, the risk of illness increases. Chronic stress, in particular, has been shown to suppress the immune response by reducing the production of lymphocytes, white blood cells that are critical to fighting infections.

The immune system also relies on a healthy gut microbiome, as a significant portion of the immune system resides in the digestive tract. An imbalance in gut bacteria due to poor diet, stress, or lack of sleep can weaken the immune response and increase the risk of infections and chronic illnesses.

- **Supporting Immune Health**: Consuming antioxidant-rich foods, engaging in regular physical activity, and managing stress are all essential for a healthy immune system. Herbs such as echinacea, elderberry, and astragalus are known for their immune-boosting properties and can be incorporated as natural remedies.

Respiratory Health and Environmental Toxins

Exposure to environmental toxins, such as air pollution, chemicals, and allergens, poses significant respiratory health risks. Chronic exposure to these toxins can lead to conditions like asthma, bronchitis, and even lung cancer. Respiratory issues can also be exacerbated by smoking, lack of exercise, and a weakened immune system.

Indoor pollutants, including mold, dust, and chemicals from cleaning products, can further impact respiratory health. Additionally, the stress of urban living, with high levels of pollutants, places individuals at greater risk of respiratory conditions.

- **Detoxification and Protection**: Supporting respiratory health involves reducing exposure to environmental toxins, maintaining a clean indoor environment, and engaging in practices like deep breathing exercises. Herbs like eucalyptus and peppermint can be used in teas or essential oils to open airways and improve respiratory function. Regular outdoor activities in natural settings, away from urban pollution, can also help to clear the lungs and reduce the impact of toxins.

Bone and Joint Health Risks

Sedentary lifestyles, lack of physical activity, and poor dietary habits can contribute to bone and joint health risks. Osteoporosis, characterized by weakened bones, and arthritis, marked by inflammation of the joints, are prevalent among older adults but are increasingly affecting younger individuals due to lifestyle factors.

Chronic inflammation is a key contributor to joint problems, as it can wear down cartilage and cause pain and stiffness. Calcium and vitamin D deficiencies, often seen in those with poor dietary habits or limited sun exposure, further increase the risk of weakened bones and fractures.

- **Maintaining Bone Health**: Engaging in weight-bearing exercises, such as walking, running, or resistance training, helps to strengthen bones. A diet rich in calcium, vitamin D, and magnesium supports bone health, while anti-inflammatory foods like turmeric and ginger can help reduce joint pain and inflammation.

Mental Health Risks and the Physical Body

Mental health conditions, such as depression and anxiety, have physical manifestations that can affect various aspects of health. Chronic stress and untreated mental health conditions can lead to physical symptoms such as headaches, muscle tension, and insomnia. In some cases, mental health conditions contribute to unhealthy coping mechanisms like substance abuse, poor diet, and lack of exercise, which further exacerbate physical health risks.

The physical toll of untreated mental health conditions can lead to burnout, adrenal fatigue, and, in severe cases, suicidal ideation. Addressing mental health with a holistic approach that includes physical activity, balanced nutrition, and natural remedies can help alleviate physical symptoms and support mental well-being.

- **Herbal Support**: Adaptogenic herbs like ashwagandha and rhodiola may help regulate the body's stress response, promoting mental clarity and reducing anxiety.

Skin Health and Aging

Skin health is closely tied to lifestyle factors and environmental exposure. Chronic stress, poor diet, and exposure to pollutants can lead to premature aging, wrinkles, and skin conditions such as acne, eczema, and psoriasis. High levels of cortisol lead to collagen breakdown, reducing skin elasticity and increasing the appearance of fine lines.

Dehydration and nutrient deficiencies also impact skin health. Essential vitamins and minerals like vitamins A, C, and E, and omega-3 fatty acids play vital roles in maintaining skin elasticity, hydration, and overall radiance. A lack of these nutrients can make the skin more susceptible to environmental damage and accelerate aging.

- **Daily Skin Care**: A skincare routine that includes hydration, sun protection, and a balanced diet rich in antioxidants supports skin health. Natural oils like jojoba and rosehip provide moisture and help repair skin cells, while green tea and aloe vera can soothe inflammation and support skin resilience.

Muscular and Skeletal Pain from Sedentary Lifestyles

With the rise of desk jobs and digital technology, many individuals spend hours sitting each day. Prolonged sitting and poor posture contribute to musculoskeletal issues, including back pain, neck stiffness, and carpal tunnel syndrome. The body is not designed for extended periods of inactivity, and lack of movement can lead to muscle weakness, imbalances, and chronic pain.

To mitigate these risks, incorporating regular movement breaks, stretching exercises, and ergonomic adjustments to workspaces is essential. Simple practices, such as standing up every hour, walking around, and performing stretching exercises, can alleviate muscular discomfort and reduce the risk of chronic pain.

- **Natural Relief**: For those experiencing musculoskeletal pain, natural remedies like turmeric and ginger, which possess anti-inflammatory properties, can be beneficial.

Massage therapy and physical therapies that focus on muscle relaxation and alignment can also provide relief.

By understanding these various physical health risks and adopting preventive and supportive measures, individuals can significantly reduce their chances of developing chronic health conditions and maintain a healthier, more balanced life.

Chapter 2: Techniques for Managing Stress

In an increasingly fast-paced world, mindfulness and meditation have become essential tools for grounding oneself, enhancing mental clarity, and promoting overall well-being. These practices are rooted in ancient traditions, yet their relevance is timeless, particularly in managing modern stressors and fostering a balanced lifestyle.

Mindfulness and Meditation Practices

Mindfulness and meditation are not only beneficial for mental health; they have profound physical effects that can improve overall health, reduce chronic pain, lower blood pressure, and even enhance immunity. This section explores various mindfulness and meditation practices, their benefits, and how to integrate them into daily life.

Understanding Mindfulness: The Basics and Its Importance

Mindfulness is the practice of being fully present and engaged in the current moment without judgment. It involves observing one's thoughts, emotions, and bodily sensations as they arise, fostering a deep sense of self-awareness. By focusing on the present, mindfulness reduces overthinking and cultivates calm, enhancing the ability to respond rather than react to life's challenges.

Studies have shown that mindfulness can significantly reduce stress by activating the body's relaxation response, which counters the stress-induced "fight or flight" reaction. Practicing mindfulness helps lower cortisol levels, which are often elevated by chronic stress. Cortisol, a hormone produced by the adrenal glands, can impair immune function, increase inflammation, and lead to health issues when chronically elevated.

The Science Behind Mindfulness

Research has demonstrated that mindfulness impacts the brain in several powerful ways. Regular mindfulness practice is associated with increased gray matter density in areas of the brain related to memory, sense of self, empathy, and stress regulation. Additionally, mindfulness can improve neuroplasticity, or the brain's ability to form and reorganize synaptic connections. This adaptability allows individuals to manage stress better, develop resilience, and adapt to new circumstances.

For example, studies using brain imaging have shown that the amygdala, the area of the brain associated with stress and anxiety, actually shrinks in individuals who practice mindfulness regularly. Simultaneously, the prefrontal cortex—the part of the brain responsible for higher-order functions such as awareness, concentration, and decision-making—grows stronger.

Meditation: Different Techniques and Their Benefits

Meditation is a core component of mindfulness and involves training the mind to focus, redirect thoughts, and achieve mental clarity. There are various types of meditation, each with unique benefits and approaches. Below are some popular meditation practices that support mindfulness and mental well-being.

1. Focused Attention Meditation

Focused attention meditation is one of the simplest and most commonly practiced forms of meditation. It involves focusing on a single point of reference, such as the breath, a mantra, or an object. The goal is to gently bring the mind back to the chosen point of focus whenever it wanders. This technique is ideal for beginners as it builds concentration and awareness.

- **Scenario**: An individual feeling overwhelmed at work might take five minutes to focus on their breathing, noticing each inhale and exhale. As they do so, they feel their heart rate slow down and their mind clear, enabling them to return to their tasks with renewed focus.

2. Body Scan Meditation

Body scan meditation is a mindfulness technique that involves systematically directing attention to different parts of the body, from head to toe. Practitioners observe any sensations, tensions, or discomforts in each area without judgment. This meditation fosters a strong mind-body connection, heightens bodily awareness, and can relieve tension.

Body scan meditation is particularly helpful for those experiencing chronic pain, as it encourages the mind to focus on each body part, relaxing muscles and reducing pain perception over time.

3. Loving-Kindness Meditation (Metta)

Loving-kindness meditation, or Metta, involves cultivating feelings of love, compassion, and kindness towards oneself and others. The practice begins by directing loving thoughts towards oneself, then gradually expanding to include loved ones, acquaintances, and eventually all beings.

This form of meditation enhances emotional resilience, increases empathy, and reduces feelings of anger or resentment. Studies have shown that individuals who practice loving-kindness meditation regularly experience increased positive emotions and improved interpersonal relationships.

4. Transcendental Meditation (TM)

Transcendental Meditation (TM) is a technique that involves silently repeating a mantra for 15-20 minutes, twice daily. TM aims to reach a state of pure consciousness, a state of restful alertness where the mind transcends all mental activity.

TM has been shown to reduce stress significantly, lower blood pressure, and improve overall mental health. It is especially popular among those seeking a structured practice with specific guidelines.

5. Guided Visualization

Guided visualization involves visualizing a peaceful scene or positive outcome. It encourages the mind to use its creative powers to evoke calm and relaxation. Visualization is often led by an instructor or a recording, making it accessible to those new to meditation.

- **Example**: Someone preparing for a stressful presentation might visualize themselves confidently speaking in front of an audience, projecting calm and clarity. By repeatedly visualizing a positive outcome, they become more relaxed and prepared.

Incorporating Mindfulness into Daily Life

One of the strengths of mindfulness is its versatility; it can be practiced almost anywhere, from a quiet room to a busy subway. Integrating mindfulness into daily routines does not require large time commitments, making it accessible to even the busiest individuals.

Mindful Eating

Mindful eating is the practice of paying full attention to the experience of eating and savoring each bite. It involves noticing the colors, textures, flavors, and aromas of food, as well as being aware of hunger and fullness cues. This approach can help prevent overeating, promote healthier food choices, and enhance enjoyment.

For example, someone might take a few minutes to enjoy a meal without distractions, savoring each bite and appreciating the flavors. Mindful eating can also reduce the tendency to reach for food when stressed, as it helps individuals identify true hunger versus emotional hunger.

Mindful Walking

Mindful walking involves focusing on the physical sensations of walking, such as the feeling of the feet hitting the ground, the rhythm of breathing, and the movement of the body. Practiced regularly, mindful walking can bring a sense of calm and rejuvenation to daily life. Whether walking in nature or navigating a city sidewalk, taking a few minutes to practice mindful walking can help to break up long periods of sitting and bring clarity to the mind. Engaging in nature walks is particularly beneficial, as nature itself has a calming effect on the nervous system, enhancing the benefits of mindfulness.

Mindful Listening

Mindful listening involves fully focusing on the speaker without interruptions or judgments. This practice enhances relationships by allowing for more genuine connections and reducing misunderstandings. It requires setting aside distractions, such as phones or computers, and giving full attention to the person speaking.

Incorporating mindful listening into daily interactions can improve relationships and create a greater sense of empathy and understanding. It also helps to reduce stress in social settings by alleviating the pressure to constantly prepare a response.

Practical Tips for Building a Mindfulness and Meditation Routine

Starting a mindfulness and meditation routine does not require a significant time commitment. Practicing even a few minutes daily can yield substantial benefits over time. Here are some practical tips to build a routine:

1. **Start Small**: Begin with just 5–10 minutes per day, gradually increasing the duration as you become more comfortable. Short, consistent practice is more effective than sporadic, long sessions.
2. **Set a Consistent Time**: Establishing a regular time for mindfulness or meditation, such as in the morning or before bed, helps build a habit. Consistency reinforces the practice and makes it part of the daily routine.

3. **Create a Peaceful Space**: Designate a quiet, comfortable space for meditation. A designated space helps signal the mind that it's time to relax and focus.

4. **Use Guided Meditation Apps**: For beginners, apps like Headspace, Calm, or Insight Timer offer guided meditations, making it easy to start a meditation routine without feeling overwhelmed.

5. **Practice Patience and Self-Compassion**: It's normal for the mind to wander during meditation. Practicing patience and gently redirecting focus back to the breath or mantra is part of the process. Self-compassion is essential, as meditation is a skill that improves with time and consistency.

The Long-Term Benefits of Mindfulness and Meditation

Regular mindfulness and meditation practice offers a wealth of long-term benefits that extend far beyond relaxation. Over time, individuals often notice improvements in mental clarity, emotional stability, and resilience in the face of stress. These benefits contribute to a higher quality of life and can even slow the effects of aging on the brain.

Improved Emotional Regulation

Mindfulness and meditation enhance emotional regulation by fostering self-awareness and reducing impulsive reactions. With regular practice, individuals can respond to stressful situations with greater calm and clarity rather than reacting emotionally.

Enhanced Focus and Productivity

Mindfulness strengthens focus and concentration, making it easier to handle complex tasks and make sound decisions. These qualities are particularly valuable in professional settings where multitasking and constant demands can easily overwhelm.

Reduced Symptoms of Anxiety and Depression

Numerous studies have shown that mindfulness and meditation can reduce symptoms of anxiety and depression. By teaching individuals to observe their thoughts without attachment, these practices help mitigate negative thought patterns that contribute to mental health challenges.

Support for Physical Health

The mind-body connection means that mental wellness often translates to physical health. Mindfulness has been shown to lower blood pressure, reduce inflammation, and even enhance immune function. Meditation promotes relaxation, which counteracts the body's stress response, protecting against conditions exacerbated by chronic stress, such as cardiovascular disease.

Integrating Natural Remedies with Mindfulness Practices

Mindfulness and meditation complement natural remedies by creating a holistic approach to health. For example, individuals seeking to reduce anxiety might combine mindfulness practices with herbal supplements like chamomile, valerian, or lavender, which promote calm and relaxation. Similarly, anti-inflammatory herbs like turmeric and ginger can be combined with mindfulness techniques to address chronic pain or inflammation.

Embracing mindfulness and meditation as part of a daily routine provides a powerful foundation for managing stress, improving mental and physical health, and enhancing quality of life. With patience and dedication, these practices become transformative tools that enrich every aspect of well-being.

Physical Activity

Physical activity is a cornerstone of health and well-being, contributing not only to physical fitness but also to mental and emotional resilience. Exercise triggers a cascade of positive effects within the body, ranging from improved cardiovascular health to enhanced cognitive function. For those interested in natural remedies and holistic health, incorporating regular physical activity is one of the most powerful steps toward a balanced, vibrant life. This section explores how physical activity supports various aspects of health, delves into different types of exercises, and provides practical strategies for incorporating movement into daily routines.

The Physiological Benefits of Physical Activity

Physical activity offers a multitude of physiological benefits that support the body's ability to function optimally. These benefits encompass cardiovascular health, muscle and bone strength, immune support, and metabolic efficiency, creating a foundation for longevity and vitality. Understanding how exercise influences specific systems in the body can help individuals tailor their fitness routines to meet their health goals.

1. **Cardiovascular Health**: Regular physical activity strengthens the heart and enhances circulation, which helps maintain healthy blood pressure and reduces the

risk of cardiovascular disease. Aerobic exercises, such as walking, running, and swimming, improve heart health by increasing the heart rate and promoting efficient blood flow. When the cardiovascular system is strong, it can better support other bodily functions, ensuring nutrients and oxygen reach organs and tissues efficiently.

2. **Bone and Muscle Strength**: Weight-bearing activities, including strength training, walking, and dancing, stimulate bone formation and reduce the risk of osteoporosis. Building muscle strength is equally important, as it supports joint stability, enhances mobility, and reduces the risk of injury. Additionally, strong muscles are essential for maintaining good posture and preventing musculoskeletal issues, especially as the body ages.

3. **Immune Support**: Moderate, regular physical activity has been shown to boost the immune system. Exercise promotes circulation, which allows immune cells to move more freely throughout the body, enhancing the immune system's ability to detect and respond to pathogens. However, it is worth noting that excessive, intense exercise without adequate rest can temporarily suppress immune function.

4. **Metabolic Health**: Physical activity boosts metabolism by promoting insulin sensitivity, which helps regulate blood sugar levels. It also enhances the body's ability to burn fat and maintain a healthy weight. When metabolism is functioning optimally, it supports energy levels, reducing the risk of fatigue and improving overall vitality.

5. **Mental Health and Cognitive Function**: Exercise releases endorphins, which act as natural mood lifters, reducing symptoms of anxiety and depression. Physical activity also increases blood flow to the brain, promoting cognitive function, improving memory, and enhancing focus. Exercise can even stimulate the production of new brain cells, particularly in the hippocampus, an area associated with memory and learning.

The Mental and Emotional Benefits of Physical Activity

The mental and emotional benefits of physical activity are as significant as the physical benefits. Regular exercise acts as a natural remedy for stress, anxiety, and even depression, improving mental resilience and emotional stability. For many people, exercise provides a break from daily stresses, offering a mental reset that enhances clarity, focus, and mood.

1. **Stress Relief**: Physical activity is one of the most effective natural stress relievers. Exercise reduces the body's levels of cortisol, a primary stress hormone, while

promoting the release of endorphins, known as "feel-good" hormones. Engaging in regular physical activity helps individuals develop resilience to stress, reducing the negative impact of life's challenges on mental well-being.

2. **Enhanced Mood and Emotional Stability**: Exercise is often recommended as a complementary approach to treating mild depression and anxiety. The mood-enhancing effects of physical activity are immediate, as exercise promotes the release of serotonin and dopamine, neurotransmitters that support feelings of happiness and relaxation. Regular exercise also creates a sense of accomplishment, which can enhance self-esteem and contribute to emotional stability.

3. **Improved Cognitive Function**: Exercise enhances brain function by increasing blood flow to the brain, which delivers oxygen and nutrients to support cognitive processes. Physical activity has been shown to improve memory, focus, and problem-solving skills, making it especially valuable for those seeking mental clarity and cognitive longevity.

4. **Better Sleep Quality**: Quality sleep is essential for both physical and mental health, and regular exercise can improve sleep patterns. Physical activity helps regulate circadian rhythms, making it easier to fall asleep and enjoy deeper, more restorative rest. Improved sleep quality further supports mental health, as well as physical energy and recovery.

Types of Physical Activity and Their Unique Benefits

Physical activity can take many forms, each offering unique benefits. A well-rounded fitness routine typically includes a mix of aerobic, strength, flexibility, and balance exercises. Understanding the benefits of each type can help individuals create a balanced program that supports comprehensive health.

1. **Aerobic Exercise**: Aerobic activities, also known as cardiovascular or endurance exercises, include activities like brisk walking, running, cycling, and swimming. These exercises elevate the heart rate and improve cardiovascular fitness, making them essential for heart health, stamina, and calorie burning.

2. **Strength Training**: Strength training, or resistance exercise, involves using weights, resistance bands, or body weight to build muscle mass and improve strength. This type of exercise is critical for bone density, metabolic health, and muscle tone. It also

enhances functional strength, making daily activities easier and reducing the risk of injury.

3. **Flexibility Exercises**: Flexibility exercises, such as stretching and yoga, improve the range of motion in the joints and increase muscle flexibility. Enhanced flexibility reduces the risk of strains and sprains, supports better posture, and improves overall movement quality. Flexibility exercises are particularly beneficial for those who engage in strength training, as they help prevent tightness and maintain muscle balance.

4. **Balance and Stability**: Balance exercises, like tai chi and certain yoga poses, help improve stability and coordination. These exercises are especially valuable for older adults, as they reduce the risk of falls and enhance body awareness. Balance and stability exercises engage the core muscles, which play a key role in overall movement and injury prevention.

Practical Strategies for Incorporating Physical Activity into Daily Life

For those new to exercise or struggling to maintain a routine, incorporating physical activity into daily life doesn't have to be challenging. Small, consistent steps can make a significant difference in overall health and well-being.

1. **Set Realistic Goals**: Start with achievable goals, such as a daily 10-minute walk, and gradually increase the time and intensity. Setting realistic goals prevents burnout and creates a sense of accomplishment, encouraging long-term consistency.

2. **Find Enjoyable Activities**: Choosing activities that are enjoyable is key to maintaining motivation. Dancing, hiking, gardening, and even playing with pets are all forms of physical activity that don't feel like exercise but offer substantial health benefits.

3. **Incorporate Movement into Routine**: Simple changes, like taking the stairs instead of the elevator, parking further away, or standing up to stretch during breaks, can help incorporate movement throughout the day. For desk-bound workers, standing desks or periodic walking breaks are excellent ways to stay active.

4. **Schedule Exercise**: Treat exercise as an important appointment, blocking time in the schedule for physical activity. Whether it's a morning walk, an afternoon yoga session, or an evening workout, scheduling exercise increases the likelihood of consistency.

5. **Practice Mind-Body Connection**: Mindful movement practices like yoga, tai chi, and Pilates encourage awareness of the body and breath, fostering a mind-body connection that supports mental and physical health. These practices not only enhance flexibility and strength but also provide a meditative experience that reduces stress.

Overcoming Barriers to Physical Activity

For many, barriers such as lack of time, motivation, or physical limitations can make it difficult to engage in regular physical activity. Recognizing these barriers and developing strategies to overcome them can help individuals cultivate a lasting exercise routine.

1. **Time Constraints**: For those with busy schedules, short bursts of activity can be just as effective as longer sessions. High-intensity interval training (HIIT), for example, provides an effective workout in a short time. Additionally, finding ways to integrate movement into daily routines, such as walking during lunch breaks, can help overcome time barriers.

2. **Lack of Motivation**: To stay motivated, it's helpful to focus on the immediate benefits of exercise, such as mood improvement and stress relief. Setting small, achievable goals and tracking progress can also build momentum and motivation. For social individuals, joining a group class or finding an exercise buddy can provide accountability and make exercise more enjoyable.

3. **Physical Limitations or Health Conditions**: For those with physical limitations, low-impact activities like swimming, cycling, and chair exercises offer safe alternatives. Consulting a healthcare provider or physical therapist can help tailor exercises to specific needs, ensuring a safe and beneficial fitness routine.

Physical Activity as a Component of Holistic Health

In holistic health, physical activity is viewed not only as a way to improve physical strength and endurance but also as a means to support mental, emotional, and spiritual well-being. Practices like yoga, tai chi, and mindful walking are excellent examples of exercises that bridge the gap between physical activity and mental health. They encourage individuals to connect with their bodies, foster gratitude, and develop a deeper sense of self-awareness.

1. **Yoga and Mindfulness**: Yoga combines movement, breath control, and meditation, offering both physical and mental benefits. Beyond enhancing flexibility and strength, yoga promotes mindfulness, which can reduce stress and foster a positive mindset.

2. **Nature Walks**: Walking in nature, often referred to as "green exercise," provides mental and physical benefits. Time spent in nature has been shown to lower stress levels, reduce anxiety, and improve mood. Walking outside also encourages exposure to sunlight, which helps the body produce vitamin D, essential for immune and mental health.

3. **Dance as Expression**: Dance is not only a form of exercise but also a creative outlet that allows for emotional expression. Moving rhythmically to music can improve coordination, balance, and flexibility while providing an uplifting experience that boosts mental well-being.

Incorporating physical activity as a daily habit transforms it from a task into a lifestyle, promoting comprehensive well-being and enhancing the effectiveness of other natural remedies. A well-rounded approach to physical activity aligns seamlessly with the principles of holistic health, offering a sustainable path toward improved health, vitality, and resilience.

Walking for Stress Relief

Walking is one of the simplest and most accessible forms of exercise, yet it offers powerful benefits for both mental and physical well-being. As a natural stress reliever, walking has become an essential practice for those seeking to reduce anxiety, manage stress, and boost their overall health. Whether it's a brisk walk in the park, a leisurely stroll around the neighborhood, or a more challenging hike in nature, walking provides a holistic approach to managing stress and improving quality of life. This section delves into the science behind walking for stress relief, different techniques, and practical tips for incorporating this practice into daily routines.

The Science Behind Walking and Stress Relief

When we experience stress, our body's natural "fight or flight" response is activated, releasing stress hormones like cortisol and adrenaline. These hormones can cause increased heart rate, muscle tension, and a sense of alertness. While these reactions are useful in short bursts, chronic activation of the stress response can lead to physical and mental health issues. Walking, however, can help counteract these effects by promoting the release of endorphins—natural mood boosters that enhance feelings of relaxation and reduce anxiety.

The Role of Endorphins

Endorphins, often referred to as the body's "feel-good" chemicals, are released during physical activity. These neurotransmitters interact with receptors in the brain to reduce the perception of pain and induce feelings of pleasure. Regular walking triggers endorphin release, which helps counteract stress, improve mood, and create a sense of well-being. Studies have shown that even short walks can lead to a notable increase in endorphin levels, making walking a powerful, natural mood enhancer.

Reducing Cortisol Levels Through Walking

Chronic stress keeps cortisol levels elevated, leading to various health issues such as weakened immunity, increased blood pressure, and weight gain. Walking, especially in natural settings, has been shown to lower cortisol levels significantly. This reduction in cortisol not only helps to calm the body's stress response but also promotes better physical health by reducing inflammation and improving cardiovascular function. Research has demonstrated that those who engage in regular walking routines tend to have lower resting cortisol levels, which contributes to an overall sense of calm and resilience.

Walking Techniques for Enhanced Stress Relief

Different walking techniques can provide varying levels of relaxation and mental clarity. Here are some approaches to maximize the stress-relieving benefits of walking:

1. Mindful Walking

Mindful walking involves paying full attention to the present moment, focusing on each step and observing the environment without judgment. By directing attention to the sensations of walking—such as the feeling of feet hitting the ground, the rhythm of breathing, and the movement of the body—mindful walking allows individuals to disconnect from stressors and enter a state of calm. This technique is particularly useful for those prone to overthinking, as it fosters mental clarity and encourages a sense of grounding.

- **Example**: During a mindful walk, someone may focus on the crunch of leaves beneath their feet or the sound of birds in the trees. As they pay attention to these details, their mind becomes less preoccupied with daily worries, promoting a sense of peace and presence.

2. Nature Walking

Walking in natural surroundings, such as parks, forests, or by the ocean, enhances stress relief due to the calming effect of nature. Studies have shown that spending time in green spaces reduces cortisol levels more effectively than urban environments. Nature walking allows individuals to benefit from "biophilia," the innate human affinity for nature, which has been shown to improve mood, reduce anxiety, and enhance overall well-being.

Research suggests that individuals who engage in regular nature walks have lower levels of stress and anxiety compared to those who walk in urban areas. This is partly due to the exposure to natural stimuli, which promotes relaxation and reduces cognitive fatigue.

3. Walking Meditation

Walking meditation combines the calming effects of walking with the mental focus of meditation. Practiced by various spiritual traditions, walking meditation involves walking slowly and mindfully while focusing on each step. The practice often includes synchronizing breathing with the rhythm of walking, which enhances relaxation and mindfulness. Walking meditation can be particularly beneficial for those who struggle to sit still in traditional meditation, as it provides a way to achieve mental clarity while remaining physically active.

4. Interval Walking

For those who prefer a more dynamic approach, interval walking—alternating between brisk and moderate paces—can be highly effective. Interval walking elevates the heart rate, leading to increased endorphin release and improved physical fitness. This type of walking also adds variety, making the exercise more engaging. By incorporating intervals, individuals can experience both the energizing effects of brisk walking and the calming effects of slower-paced walking, creating a balanced exercise that relieves stress.

5. Social Walking

Walking with friends, family, or a pet can also serve as a powerful stress reliever. Social walking not only provides the physical benefits of walking but also promotes social interaction, which has been shown to enhance mood and reduce stress. The act of sharing time with loved ones or connecting with a pet creates a sense of community and support, which can mitigate feelings of loneliness and improve emotional resilience.

- **Example**: A person who walks with a friend regularly can enjoy the therapeutic benefits of companionship, laughter, and shared conversation, all of which contribute to stress reduction and overall happiness.

Practical Tips for Incorporating Walking into Daily Life

Incorporating regular walks into daily routines can be both easy and enjoyable, even for those with busy schedules. Here are some practical tips to make walking a consistent part of daily life:

1. **Set a Goal**: Begin with a realistic goal, such as walking for 10–15 minutes per day, and gradually increase the duration as the habit becomes more established. Setting goals provides motivation and a sense of accomplishment, making it easier to maintain a routine.

2. **Choose an Enjoyable Route**: Find a route that brings enjoyment, whether it's a neighborhood park, a scenic trail, or a city street with vibrant surroundings. Enjoying the scenery enhances the experience and makes walking more appealing.

3. **Wear Comfortable Footwear**: Investing in comfortable, supportive shoes is essential for enjoyable walking. Proper footwear not only prevents discomfort but also supports the body's alignment, reducing the risk of strain.

4. **Bring Music or Podcasts**: Listening to calming music, podcasts, or audiobooks can make walking more enjoyable and provide an opportunity for relaxation or learning. However, if practicing mindful walking, it's recommended to forgo audio distractions to fully engage with the present moment.

5. **Schedule Walking Breaks**: For individuals with busy schedules, setting aside short walking breaks throughout the day can make a significant difference. Even a five-minute walk during a lunch break or between tasks can boost energy, reduce stress, and improve productivity.

The Long-Term Benefits of Regular Walking for Mental Health

Engaging in regular walking has a wide range of long-term benefits for mental and physical health. By consistently incorporating walking into daily life, individuals can cultivate resilience, improve their mood, and achieve better overall well-being.

Enhanced Emotional Resilience

Regular walking promotes emotional resilience by reducing baseline stress levels and improving mood. Over time, individuals who walk regularly may notice that they respond to stressful situations with greater calm and control, as walking strengthens the body's ability to handle stress.

Improved Sleep Quality

Walking, especially in the morning, helps regulate the body's circadian rhythm, promoting better sleep quality. Quality sleep is essential for stress management, as it allows the body to recover and maintain healthy cortisol levels. Those who walk regularly often experience more restful sleep, which further contributes to emotional well-being and reduced stress.

Boosted Immune Function

By reducing stress and supporting physical health, walking also enhances immune function. Regular physical activity has been shown to increase the circulation of immune cells, which helps the body fight off illness. Walking, therefore, not only alleviates stress but also contributes to overall health by supporting immune resilience.

Weight Management and Cardiovascular Health

Walking is an effective way to maintain a healthy weight and improve cardiovascular health. These physical benefits, in turn, support mental well-being by reducing the physical toll of stress on the body. Improved cardiovascular function means better blood flow, which supports brain health and mental clarity.

Combining Walking with Natural Remedies for Optimal Stress Relief

For those interested in a holistic approach, walking can be combined with natural remedies to further support stress relief. Herbal supplements like chamomile, valerian root, and lavender are known for their calming effects and can be used in conjunction with a walking routine. For instance, a person might take chamomile tea before a relaxing evening walk, creating a peaceful prelude to bedtime.

Aromatherapy can also be integrated with walking by using essential oils like lavender or eucalyptus. Some individuals apply a small amount of essential oil to a cotton ball and carry it in their pocket during a walk. As they breathe in the calming aroma, they enhance the relaxation benefits of their walk.

Walking as a Gateway to Other Mindfulness Practices

Walking can serve as an accessible gateway to other mindfulness practices. Those who find peace and clarity through walking may be inspired to explore other forms of meditation, yoga, or breathing exercises. Walking instills a sense of presence and mindfulness, which can lay the foundation for a broader mindfulness practice.

Additionally, regular walkers often find that they begin to naturally observe their surroundings and appreciate the details of daily life. This heightened awareness can lead to a more mindful approach in all areas of life, from eating to interacting with others.

A Practical and Accessible Tool for Stress Relief

Walking offers a simple, effective, and accessible tool for managing stress and enhancing well-being. Unlike more complex exercise routines, walking does not require special skills or equipment, making it suitable for people of all ages and fitness levels. It can be adapted to fit any lifestyle, whether as a solitary practice for self-reflection or a social activity for connecting with others.

By incorporating regular walking into daily life, individuals can enjoy a holistic approach to stress relief, supporting their physical, mental, and emotional health in a balanced and sustainable way

Yoga Poses for Relaxation

Incorporating yoga into daily life can be an immensely effective way to promote relaxation, reduce stress, and cultivate a calm state of mind. For centuries, yoga has been celebrated for its power to connect the body and mind, fostering a sense of peace that radiates into everyday life. In this section, we will explore specific yoga poses that are particularly effective for relaxation. Whether you are a beginner or an experienced yogi, these poses are accessible, gentle, and designed to help release tension in the body and calm the mind.

Understanding the Benefits of Relaxation Poses in Yoga

Yoga for relaxation targets the parasympathetic nervous system, also known as the "rest and digest" system. By activating this system, relaxation poses can lower heart rate, reduce blood pressure, and encourage deep, restorative breathing. When practiced regularly, these poses can help manage chronic stress, improve sleep quality, and even reduce symptoms of anxiety and depression. Relaxation yoga poses work on multiple levels:

1. **Physically**, they help release tight muscles, especially in areas where we commonly store tension, like the shoulders, neck, and lower back.
2. **Mentally**, these poses encourage mindfulness, allowing the mind to detach from stressors and find clarity.
3. **Emotionally**, yoga supports a sense of self-acceptance and compassion, fostering resilience and emotional balance.

Let's delve into some of the most effective yoga poses for relaxation, each offering unique benefits and accessible modifications.

1. Child's Pose (Balasana)

Child's Pose is a gentle, grounding posture that provides a sense of safety and release. It's often used as a resting position in yoga, allowing the body to reset between more intense poses.

- **How to Practice**: Begin on your hands and knees, with your big toes touching and your knees either together or apart, depending on what feels comfortable. Sit back on your heels and extend your arms forward, lowering your forehead to the mat. Allow your body to relax as you sink deeper into the stretch.
- **Benefits**: This pose stretches the lower back, hips, and thighs while calming the mind. The gentle forward fold encourages introspection and relaxation, making it a great choice for winding down.
- **Modifications**: If sitting back on your heels is uncomfortable, place a folded blanket between your calves and thighs for extra support. You can also rest your head on a block if your forehead doesn't comfortably reach the floor.

2. Legs Up the Wall (Viparita Karani)

Legs Up the Wall is a gentle inversion that allows gravity to aid in circulation and relaxation. This pose is especially helpful for relieving tired legs and feet while gently stretching the lower back and hamstrings.

- **How to Practice**: Sit sideways next to a wall, then lie back and swing your legs up against the wall. Adjust so that your hips are close to the wall, and your legs are extended vertically. Relax your arms at your sides, palms facing up, and focus on breathing deeply.

- **Benefits**: This pose reverses blood flow, reducing swelling in the legs and encouraging lymphatic drainage. It also soothes the nervous system and promotes relaxation by slowing down the heart rate.
- **Modifications**: Place a folded blanket or bolster under your hips for a slight lift, which can enhance the relaxation effect. If hamstring tightness makes this pose challenging, move a few inches away from the wall.

3. Reclining Bound Angle Pose (Supta Baddha Konasana)

This pose opens the hips and stretches the inner thighs, providing a deep sense of release and relaxation. The reclining posture also allows for a passive stretch in the chest, encouraging deep breathing.

- **How to Practice**: Lie on your back and bring the soles of your feet together, allowing your knees to fall open. Place your arms by your sides or overhead, depending on what feels most comfortable. Close your eyes and focus on relaxing every muscle.
- **Benefits**: This pose gently stretches the inner thighs and hips, areas that commonly hold tension. By opening the chest, it also encourages deep breathing, which can activate the parasympathetic nervous system.
- **Modifications**: Place blankets or blocks under your knees for support, especially if the stretch in your hips is too intense. A bolster under the spine can provide additional support and elevate the chest, making breathing even easier.

4. Cat-Cow Stretch (Marjaryasana-Bitilasana)

The Cat-Cow sequence is a flowing movement that gently stretches the spine, shoulders, and neck, relieving tension in the upper body. It's an excellent pose for calming the mind while loosening tight muscles.

- **How to Practice**: Start on your hands and knees with your wrists under your shoulders and knees under your hips. Inhale as you drop your belly and lift your head and tailbone into Cow Pose. Exhale as you round your spine, drawing your navel toward your spine, and tuck your chin into Cat Pose. Repeat this movement in sync with your breath.
- **Benefits**: This dynamic stretch warms up the spine, reduces stiffness, and encourages flexibility. It's also a grounding movement that connects breath with body, promoting relaxation.

- **Modifications**: If you have sensitive wrists, try making fists with your hands or placing a folded blanket under them for extra padding. Move slowly and with intention, focusing on the rhythm of your breath.

5. Standing Forward Fold (Uttanasana)

A forward fold stretches the entire back body and encourages the release of tension in the neck and shoulders. By allowing the head to hang, this pose can provide a soothing effect on the nervous system.

- **How to Practice**: Stand with feet hip-width apart, then slowly hinge at your hips to fold forward, allowing your head to hang toward the ground. Keep your knees slightly bent if needed, and let your arms relax toward the floor.
- **Benefits**: This pose stretches the hamstrings, calves, and lower back, while also calming the mind. The inversion aspect of Uttanasana helps soothe the nervous system and relieve stress.
- **Modifications**: Use a yoga block under your hands if you cannot reach the floor comfortably. You can also bend your knees more deeply, especially if your hamstrings are tight.

6. Corpse Pose (Savasana)

Often practiced at the end of a yoga session, Savasana is the ultimate relaxation pose. It allows the body to rest, the mind to release tension, and the breath to deepen naturally.

- **How to Practice**: Lie on your back with your arms by your sides, palms facing up, and legs extended. Close your eyes and focus on your breathing, allowing each muscle in your body to relax completely.
- **Benefits**: Savasana offers deep relaxation and helps integrate the benefits of your practice. It's also an opportunity to practice mindfulness, observing thoughts without attachment and allowing stress to melt away.
- **Modifications**: Place a bolster under your knees to reduce strain on the lower back. You can also cover yourself with a blanket to stay warm as your body cools down during relaxation.

Creating a Relaxing Yoga Routine

Combining these poses into a routine can offer profound relaxation benefits. Here's a suggested sequence that incorporates each pose:

1. Begin with **Cat-Cow Stretch** to gently warm up the spine.

2. Transition into **Child's Pose** to ground yourself and connect with your breath.

3. Move to **Standing Forward Fold** to release tension in the back and shoulders.

4. Gently shift into **Reclining Bound Angle Pose** to open the hips and deepen the breath.

5. Follow with **Legs Up the Wall** for circulatory benefits and additional relaxation.

6. Conclude with **Savasana**, allowing the body to fully relax and absorb the practice.

This routine, practiced in a quiet, comfortable space, can help promote relaxation and reduce stress in just 20-30 minutes. Aim to hold each pose for several minutes, focusing on slow, mindful breathing.

Practical Tips for a Relaxing Yoga Practice

To enhance the calming effects of these poses, consider the following tips:

1. **Create a Peaceful Environment**: Dim the lights, play soft music, or use a diffuser with calming essential oils like lavender or chamomile.

2. **Focus on Breathing**: Deep, intentional breathing is essential for relaxation. Practice inhaling deeply and exhaling fully, allowing each breath to guide your movement.

3. **Practice Mindfulness**: Try to stay present in each pose, observing any sensations in the body without judgment. Notice where tension may be held, and visualize it releasing with each exhale.

4. **Use Props for Comfort**: Props such as bolsters, blankets, and blocks can make relaxation poses more accessible and comfortable. They help you find a supportive position, so you can relax more fully into each stretch.

5. **Set an Intention for Relaxation**: At the beginning of your practice, set an intention to relax and let go. This can help you focus and fully embrace the benefits of each pose.

Incorporating Relaxation Yoga into Daily Life

In addition to practicing yoga poses on a mat, consider how elements of relaxation yoga can be applied to everyday life. Small practices, such as mindful breathing, gentle stretches, and setting aside moments of stillness, can bring the calmness cultivated on the mat into your daily routine. With consistent practice, yoga becomes more than just exercise; it becomes a way of fostering inner peace and resilience that support your holistic well-being.

Chapter 3: Nutrition for Mental Wellness

A healthy, well-functioning brain is essential to enjoying a high quality of life, achieving goals, and managing stress effectively. The food we eat plays a vital role in supporting cognitive function, memory, and overall mental well-being. Research has shown that certain foods, rich in essential nutrients, antioxidants, and fatty acids, can significantly enhance brain health.

Foods that Support Brain Health

This section explores a range of foods known to benefit cognitive function, improve mood, and protect against age-related cognitive decline, offering a roadmap to a diet that supports both the brain and body.

The Link Between Diet and Brain Health

The brain is one of the most metabolically active organs, requiring a steady supply of nutrients to function at its best. Every aspect of brain health, from neurogenesis (the creation of new neurons) to neurotransmitter synthesis and cellular protection, depends on the availability of specific nutrients. An optimal diet supports memory, decision-making, and even emotional resilience, while a poor diet can increase the risk of mental fatigue, mood disorders, and cognitive decline.

Antioxidants and Brain Protection

Antioxidants are essential for brain health as they protect brain cells from oxidative stress and damage caused by free radicals. Free radicals are unstable molecules that can cause cell damage and contribute to aging and neurodegenerative diseases. Antioxidants found in various foods help neutralize these harmful molecules, reducing inflammation and promoting long-term brain health.

Omega-3 Fatty Acids for Cognitive Function

Omega-3 fatty acids, particularly DHA (docosahexaenoic acid) and EPA (eicosapentaenoic acid), are vital for brain health. These essential fats contribute to the structure of brain cell membranes, support communication between neurons, and play a role in neuroplasticity (the brain's ability to adapt and form new connections). Omega-3s are also linked to reduced risk of cognitive decline, making them a critical component of a brain-healthy diet.

Top Foods That Boost Brain Health

Several foods are known to support brain function and protect against cognitive decline. Here's a closer look at some of the best foods to include in a diet aimed at maintaining brain health.

1. Blueberries

Blueberries are rich in antioxidants, particularly anthocyanins, which give them their deep blue color. Anthocyanins have been shown to improve brain function by reducing oxidative stress and inflammation. Studies have demonstrated that regular blueberry consumption is associated with improved memory and cognitive function, particularly in older adults.

- **Example**: A daily handful of blueberries, either fresh or frozen, can provide a potent dose of brain-protecting antioxidants.

2. Walnuts

Walnuts are a particularly beneficial nut for brain health due to their high levels of DHA, a type of omega-3 fatty acid. Walnuts also contain antioxidants and polyphenols that reduce inflammation and support cognitive function. Research suggests that walnut consumption is linked to improved memory and cognitive performance, making them an ideal snack for brain health.

- **Example**: Incorporate a small handful of walnuts into your daily diet, whether in oatmeal, salads, or as a snack, to benefit from their brain-boosting properties.

3. Fatty Fish

Fatty fish such as salmon, trout, and sardines are excellent sources of omega-3 fatty acids, particularly DHA and EPA, which are essential for brain health. Omega-3s from fish have been linked to slower cognitive decline in aging and may reduce the risk of Alzheimer's disease. Fatty fish also promote neuroplasticity, allowing the brain to adapt and form new neural connections, which is crucial for learning and memory.

- **Example**: Aim to consume fatty fish at least twice a week to meet the recommended intake of omega-3s and support brain function.

4. Turmeric

Turmeric, a spice commonly used in Indian cuisine, contains curcumin, a powerful antioxidant with anti-inflammatory effects. Curcumin has been shown to cross the blood-brain barrier, allowing it to exert its benefits directly in the brain. Research suggests that curcumin may help improve mood, enhance memory, and stimulate the growth of new brain cells.

- **Example**: Adding turmeric to soups, stews, or smoothies, or even consuming it in supplement form, can provide daily curcumin benefits for brain health.

5. Broccoli

Broccoli is a cruciferous vegetable that contains a range of beneficial nutrients for brain health, including vitamin K, choline, and antioxidants. Vitamin K is essential for forming sphingolipids, a type of fat that is highly abundant in brain cells. Broccoli also contains compounds that have been shown to promote cognitive health and protect the brain from oxidative damage.

- **Example**: Including broccoli in meals a few times a week, whether steamed, roasted, or raw, can help support cognitive health.

6. Pumpkin Seeds

Pumpkin seeds are rich in antioxidants and provide a good source of magnesium, iron, zinc, and copper—minerals crucial for brain health. Zinc plays a vital role in nerve signaling, while magnesium is essential for learning and memory. Iron supports oxygen transport to the brain, and copper helps with brain cell communication.

- **Example**: A small daily serving of pumpkin seeds, either alone or sprinkled on salads or yogurt, can contribute to daily mineral intake for optimal brain function.

7. Oranges

Oranges are an excellent source of vitamin C, an antioxidant that is vital for preventing oxidative stress in the brain. Vitamin C is also essential for producing neurotransmitters, which play a critical role in mood and cognitive function. Studies suggest that higher vitamin C intake is associated with better memory and mental clarity.

- **Example**: Enjoy an orange daily or add slices to salads to support brain health with vitamin C.

8. Eggs

Eggs are a rich source of several nutrients linked to brain health, including choline, B vitamins, and folate. Choline is essential for producing acetylcholine, a neurotransmitter involved in memory and learning. B vitamins help slow the progression of cognitive decline by lowering levels of homocysteine, an amino acid associated with cognitive impairment.

- **Example**: Including eggs in your diet a few times a week, such as in breakfast scrambles or salads, can enhance cognitive health.

9. Dark Chocolate

Dark chocolate contains flavonoids, caffeine, and antioxidants, all of which contribute to brain health. Flavonoids in dark chocolate have been shown to enhance memory and boost mood. The moderate amount of caffeine in dark chocolate can improve focus and mental alertness.

- **Example**: Choosing a small portion of dark chocolate with a high cocoa content as a daily treat can support cognitive function.

Practical Tips for Incorporating Brain-Boosting Foods

While it's beneficial to know which foods support brain health, incorporating them into a daily diet is key to reaping the benefits. Here are some practical tips for making brain-healthy eating a regular part of life:

1. **Create Balanced Meals**: Aim to include a variety of brain-boosting foods in each meal, such as adding berries to morning oatmeal, incorporating broccoli into lunch, and having salmon for dinner.
2. **Snack Smart**: Replace processed snacks with brain-friendly options like a handful of walnuts, pumpkin seeds, or a piece of dark chocolate.
3. **Use Herbs and Spices**: Incorporate turmeric, rosemary, and other brain-healthy spices into cooking. These add flavor and antioxidants to meals without extra calories.
4. **Opt for Whole Foods**: Whenever possible, choose whole, nutrient-dense foods rather than processed options to ensure the highest nutritional value.

Long-Term Benefits of a Brain-Healthy Diet

Adopting a diet rich in brain-supportive foods offers a variety of long-term benefits. Regular consumption of these foods not only improves cognitive function and mood but also protects against age-related cognitive decline and neurodegenerative diseases.

Enhanced Cognitive Resilience

Eating a diet rich in antioxidants, healthy fats, and essential nutrients supports the brain's natural resilience to aging and environmental stressors. As the body and brain face oxidative stress from free radicals, antioxidants in foods like berries, dark chocolate, and nuts help neutralize these damaging molecules.

Better Memory and Learning Capacity

Foods rich in choline, B vitamins, and omega-3 fatty acids support memory formation and learning capacity. By maintaining healthy brain cell membranes and supporting neurotransmitter production, these nutrients enhance cognitive abilities over time.

Mood Stabilization

Certain foods, such as those rich in omega-3 fatty acids, antioxidants, and B vitamins, have mood-stabilizing effects. Omega-3s, for example, have been shown to reduce symptoms of depression, while antioxidant-rich foods reduce oxidative stress, which is linked to anxiety and mood disorders.

Protection Against Cognitive Decline

A diet rich in foods that support brain health can slow the progression of cognitive decline associated with aging. Studies have shown that individuals who consume antioxidant-rich fruits, vegetables, and fish regularly have a lower risk of developing Alzheimer's disease and other forms of dementia.

Brain-Boosting Meal Examples

Incorporating brain-healthy foods into meals can be simple and enjoyable. Here are a few meal ideas that combine multiple brain-supportive ingredients:

1. **Breakfast**: A bowl of oatmeal topped with blueberries, walnuts, and a sprinkle of cinnamon provides antioxidants, omega-3s, and brain-supportive vitamins.
2. **Lunch**: A spinach and broccoli salad with slices of boiled egg, pumpkin seeds, and a dressing made from olive oil and lemon juice offers a balanced blend of brain-healthy nutrients.
3. **Dinner**: Baked salmon with a side of roasted sweet potatoes and steamed green vegetables such as broccoli and kale provides a satisfying, omega-3-rich meal that supports cognitive health.
4. **Snack**: Greek yogurt with orange slices and a few pieces of dark chocolate offers a balanced, nutrient-rich snack that satisfies while nourishing the brain.

By incorporating these foods into a daily diet, individuals can naturally support cognitive health, improve memory, and enjoy a stronger, healthier mind.

In a world where sugary foods and beverages are marketed at every turn, avoiding sugar can feel like a monumental task. But cutting down on sugar is not only achievable but also profoundly beneficial for your mental and physical stability. High sugar intake has been linked to various health issues, from unstable blood sugar levels and mood swings to inflammation and cognitive challenges. In this section, we will explore the ways in which reducing or eliminating sugar from your diet can support a balanced and stable life. We'll look into how sugar impacts mental and physical health, strategies for cutting back, and practical tips for stabilizing energy and mood without relying on sugar.

The Physical and Emotional Impact of Sugar

Sugar is found naturally in many foods, but the added sugars that infiltrate our diets in processed foods and sugary drinks create the most concern. When you consume added sugars, your body quickly absorbs the glucose into the bloodstream, causing a sharp spike in blood sugar. This spike is usually followed by a rapid drop, which can make you feel tired, irritable, and crave more sugar, creating a rollercoaster of energy and mood swings.

1. **Blood Sugar Instability**: When you eat sugar, your blood sugar level rises rapidly. In response, your body releases insulin to help process the glucose and bring your blood sugar back down. However, excessive sugar consumption can lead to large insulin spikes, followed by sudden blood sugar drops. These fluctuations can leave you feeling fatigued and moody.

2. **Insulin Resistance and Weight Gain**: Chronic high blood sugar and insulin levels can lead to insulin resistance, a condition where cells become less responsive to insulin's effects. Over time, this resistance can lead to weight gain and an increased risk of type 2 diabetes.

3. **Mood and Mental Health**: The blood sugar rollercoaster doesn't only affect energy; it can also impact your mood and mental clarity. Studies have shown that diets high in sugar are associated with a greater risk of anxiety and depression. This is partly because sugar can disrupt neurotransmitter balance, including dopamine and serotonin, both of which are crucial for mood stability.

4. **Inflammation**: Sugar is known to trigger inflammation in the body, a contributing factor in chronic diseases such as heart disease, arthritis, and even certain cancers. Chronic inflammation also affects the brain, which can further complicate mental health and cognitive stability.

Understanding these impacts is essential for building the motivation to reduce sugar intake, but managing cravings and rebalancing your diet are key steps in maintaining this change.

The Cycle of Sugar Cravings

The craving cycle is a challenge many people face when reducing sugar. Eating sugar triggers the release of dopamine, a neurotransmitter that creates feelings of pleasure and reward. This response can make sugar seem addictive, as the brain begins to associate sugary foods with comfort and pleasure. Breaking this cycle is essential for achieving a more balanced state of health. Here's how to start:

1. **Identify Triggers**: Notice what causes you to reach for sugar. Is it stress, fatigue, boredom, or a need for comfort? By identifying these triggers, you can begin to create alternative strategies for coping.

2. **Balanced Meals**: Sugar cravings are often a response to unbalanced meals. When you eat meals that are low in protein, healthy fats, and fiber, your body digests them quickly, leaving you hungry sooner and more likely to crave sugary snacks. Aim for balanced meals that include a source of lean protein, healthy fats, and complex carbohydrates to keep you full and satisfied.

3. **Stay Hydrated**: Dehydration can sometimes feel like hunger or cravings, leading you to eat sugar when what you actually need is water. Drinking enough water throughout the day can help reduce the chances of confusing thirst with cravings.

4. **Sleep and Stress Management**: Poor sleep and high stress levels can increase sugar cravings. Lack of sleep disrupts hunger-regulating hormones, making it harder to resist sugary foods. Stress can lead to emotional eating, as people often turn to sugar for comfort. Prioritizing good sleep and managing stress can support your efforts to avoid sugar.

Replacing Sugar with Healthier Alternatives

If giving up sugar seems overwhelming, remember that there are plenty of natural, lower-glycemic options to satisfy your sweet tooth without the same dramatic effects on blood sugar. Replacing refined sugar with alternatives can provide sweetness without triggering the same insulin spikes.

1. **Natural Sweeteners**: Options like stevia, monk fruit, and erythritol are low-calorie and low-glycemic sweeteners that don't spike blood sugar. They are ideal for baking, beverages, and any recipe where you would typically use sugar.

2. **Whole Fruits**: Fresh fruits contain natural sugars, but they also come with fiber, vitamins, and minerals. The fiber in fruit slows down sugar absorption, providing a steadier release of energy. Berries, apples, and citrus fruits are excellent choices for those looking to reduce sugar but still want a touch of sweetness.

3. **Spices**: Cinnamon, nutmeg, and vanilla extract add flavor and sweetness without sugar. Cinnamon, in particular, has been shown to improve insulin sensitivity and help stabilize blood sugar levels, making it a valuable tool in reducing sugar reliance.

4. **Healthy Fats**: Incorporating healthy fats like avocado, nuts, and seeds can help reduce sugar cravings by keeping you fuller for longer. Fats slow down digestion, providing sustained energy and helping prevent blood sugar fluctuations.

Stabilizing Energy without Sugar

Achieving stable energy levels without relying on sugar is a transformative shift. This balance not only helps you avoid the energy crash that comes after consuming sugar but also supports better concentration, mood, and productivity throughout the day.

1. **Complex Carbohydrates**: Instead of reaching for sugary snacks, choose complex carbohydrates like whole grains, legumes, and vegetables. These foods are high in fiber, which slows digestion and stabilizes blood sugar.

2. **Protein-Packed Foods**: Incorporate protein into every meal, as it provides a steady source of energy without spiking blood sugar. Lean meats, fish, eggs, and plant-based proteins like beans and lentils are excellent sources.

3. **Fiber-Rich Vegetables**: Vegetables like leafy greens, carrots, and bell peppers offer fiber, vitamins, and minerals. Fiber slows down the absorption of sugar in the bloodstream, promoting steady energy.

4. **Healthy Fats**: Healthy fats like those found in olive oil, coconut oil, nuts, and seeds are essential for maintaining stable blood sugar. They provide a steady energy source that doesn't rely on sugar spikes.

Practical Tips for Reducing Sugar Intake

Reducing sugar intake doesn't require drastic changes overnight. Gradual steps can help make the transition more manageable and sustainable.

1. **Read Labels Carefully**: Sugar is hidden in many processed foods under different names, such as high fructose corn syrup, sucrose, maltose, and dextrose. Reading ingredient labels can help you avoid unexpected sources of added sugars.

2. **Swap Sugary Drinks for Water or Herbal Tea**: Beverages like soda and juice contain high amounts of sugar. Opt for water, sparkling water with a splash of lemon, or herbal tea. Unsweetened beverages provide hydration without the added sugars.

3. **Reduce Sugar in Recipes**: When cooking or baking, try reducing the sugar amount in your recipes. You might find that you enjoy the natural flavors of foods without as much added sweetness.

4. **Focus on Whole Foods**: Processed foods are often high in sugar and low in nutrients. Whole foods like vegetables, fruits, lean proteins, and whole grains offer natural flavors and better satiety without added sugars.

5. **Make Desserts a Treat, Not a Staple**: Save sugary desserts for special occasions instead of daily indulgences. When you do have dessert, enjoy it mindfully, savoring each bite.

Building a Sugar-Free Lifestyle

Creating a low-sugar lifestyle is about making choices that prioritize long-term stability over short-term gratification. Here's how to make sugar-free habits a sustainable part of your life:

1. **Find New Comfort Foods**: If you typically turn to sugar for comfort, identify other foods or activities that provide the same feeling. Healthy comfort foods like a warm bowl of oatmeal, a handful of nuts, or a cup of herbal tea can be just as satisfying without the sugar crash.

2. **Meal Prep for Success**: Plan your meals and snacks in advance to avoid reaching for sugary convenience foods. Keep a stock of low-sugar snacks like sliced vegetables, nuts, or Greek yogurt to satisfy hunger between meals.

3. **Stay Motivated with Your "Why"**: Remind yourself why you're reducing sugar. Whether it's for mental clarity, stable energy, or long-term health, keeping your motivation in mind can help you resist cravings.

4. **Celebrate Progress, Not Perfection**: Reducing sugar doesn't mean you have to eliminate it entirely or be perfect. Celebrate small victories, like choosing fruit over a candy bar or cutting back on sugary drinks. These steps add up over time.

Long-Term Health Benefits of Reducing Sugar

Avoiding sugar for stability offers benefits that extend beyond daily energy and mood. Here are some long-term advantages:

- **Improved Cardiovascular Health**: High sugar intake has been linked to high blood pressure, inflammation, and other cardiovascular risks. Reducing sugar can support heart health by lowering these risk factors.

- **Enhanced Immune Function**: Sugar can suppress the immune system, making the body more susceptible to illness. Cutting back can support stronger immunity.

- **Better Cognitive Function**: High sugar diets are linked to cognitive decline and memory issues. A diet low in sugar helps protect brain health and supports mental clarity.

- **Weight Management**: Reducing sugar helps with weight loss or maintenance by lowering empty calorie intake and reducing the cycle of insulin spikes and crashes.

- **Longevity and Quality of Life**: Many chronic diseases, including diabetes, cancer, and heart disease, are linked to high sugar consumption. By limiting sugar, you support a longer, healthier life.

Avoiding sugar is a powerful choice for those seeking a stable, balanced lifestyle. With the right strategies, healthier alternatives, and a focus on whole foods, it's possible to reduce sugar without feeling deprived, all while building a foundation for lasting health and well-being.

Chapter 4: Stress-Relief Herbal Recipes

A bath soak with lavender and chamomile is a time-honored way to relieve stress, relax muscles, and promote restful sleep. Lavender and chamomile, two powerful herbs known for their soothing properties, work synergistically to create a calming bath experience that nourishes both the body and mind.

Lavender and Chamomile Bath Soak

This section delves into the specific benefits of lavender and chamomile, the science behind their calming effects, and the practical steps to prepare an effective bath soak at home.

The Benefits of a Lavender and Chamomile Bath Soak

Herbal bath soaks have been used for centuries as part of self-care rituals to relieve stress and restore energy. The warm water combined with herbs like lavender and chamomile offers a natural way to relax, making it easier to unwind and achieve restful sleep. Both lavender and chamomile are packed with bioactive compounds that work directly on the body's central nervous system to promote a sense of calm. Additionally, a warm bath naturally raises the body's core temperature, which then drops upon exiting the bath, preparing the body for restful sleep.

Lavender: The Herb of Calm

Lavender (Lavandula angustifolia) is renowned for its calming aroma, which is often used in aromatherapy to reduce stress and promote relaxation. Lavender oil is rich in linalool and linalyl acetate, compounds that have been shown to interact with the body's central nervous system. These compounds bind to neurotransmitter receptors in the brain, promoting relaxation and reducing anxiety levels. Lavender's unique chemical composition also has mild sedative effects, making it particularly beneficial for people who struggle with insomnia or stress-induced tension.

- **Example Scenario**: Imagine coming home after a long, stressful day. Adding lavender to a bath soak not only infuses the bathroom with a calming scent but also provides physical relaxation as its compounds are absorbed through the skin.

Chamomile: Nature's Tranquilizer

Chamomile (Matricaria chamomilla or Chamaemelum nobile) is another herb famous for its relaxing and anti-inflammatory properties. Chamomile contains flavonoids and terpenoids, especially apigenin, which bind to GABA receptors in the brain. This action promotes a mild sedative effect, making chamomile highly effective in reducing anxiety and improving sleep quality. Additionally, chamomile has anti-inflammatory properties, which can help soothe sore muscles and irritated skin.

- **Example Scenario**: A chamomile-infused bath soak is ideal after physical activity or on days when your muscles feel tense and need extra relaxation.

How Lavender and Chamomile Work Together in a Bath Soak

When used together in a bath soak, lavender and chamomile create a powerful synergy. Lavender provides the calming aroma that reduces stress, while chamomile works to relax muscles and encourage a restful mind. Together, they enhance each other's effects, creating a therapeutic experience that addresses both physical and mental tension.

Preparing a Lavender and Chamomile Bath Soak

Creating a lavender and chamomile bath soak at home is straightforward and does not require expensive ingredients. Here is a step-by-step guide to making a basic herbal bath soak that can be customized with other natural ingredients to enhance its benefits.

Ingredients

1. **Dried Lavender Buds**: These release lavender's essential oils into the water, offering aromatherapeutic benefits and skin-soothing properties.
2. **Dried Chamomile Flowers**: Chamomile adds a gentle, sweet aroma and releases apigenin, which promotes relaxation.
3. **Epsom Salt or Sea Salt**: These salts help soothe muscle tension and soften the skin. Epsom salt, in particular, provides magnesium, which aids in muscle relaxation.
4. **Baking Soda**: Adding baking soda to the soak can soften the skin and improve the bath's soothing properties.
5. **Lavender Essential Oil**: For a stronger scent, add a few drops of lavender essential oil, which enhances the aromatherapy experience.

Instructions

1. **Prepare the Herbs**: Use about ½ cup of dried lavender buds and ½ cup of dried chamomile flowers. If you don't have access to dried herbs, you can use pre-made tea bags containing lavender or chamomile.

2. **Combine with Epsom Salt and Baking Soda**: Mix the dried herbs with 1 cup of Epsom salt and ½ cup of baking soda in a bowl.

3. **Add Essential Oils**: For an enhanced scent, add 5–10 drops of lavender essential oil to the mixture.

4. **Store the Mixture**: Store your bath soak mixture in an airtight container, like a glass jar. This mixture can be kept for several weeks if stored in a cool, dry place.

5. **Add to Bath**: When you're ready for a bath, add 1 cup of the mixture to warm bathwater. Stir the water to help dissolve the salts and release the aroma of the herbs.

6. **Soak and Relax**: Soak in the bath for at least 20 minutes to allow your skin to absorb the herbs and salts fully.

Additional Tips for Enhancing Your Bath Soak Experience

While the lavender and chamomile bath soak is highly beneficial on its own, there are several ways to make the experience even more enjoyable and tailored to specific needs.

Add Other Herbs

Lavender and chamomile work well with other calming herbs. For example, adding a handful of dried rose petals can create a more luxurious, skin-softening bath. Alternatively, adding dried peppermint leaves can create a refreshing sensation, perfect for soothing tired feet after a long day.

Use an Herbal Infusion Bag

If you prefer not to have loose herbs floating in the bath, you can place the mixture in a muslin or cotton bag. This keeps the herbs contained while still allowing them to infuse into the water. After the bath, you can squeeze any remaining water out of the bag and compost the herbs.

Adjusting the Temperature

The temperature of the bath can impact the bath soak's effectiveness. A warm bath (not too hot) is ideal for relaxation and stress relief, as overly hot water can dry out the skin. Aim for a temperature that feels comfortably warm to encourage muscle relaxation.

Set the Mood with Lighting and Music

Creating a calming environment enhances the effects of a lavender and chamomile bath soak. Dim the lights, light a candle, and consider playing soft, relaxing music. These additions help activate the body's relaxation response, making the bath soak even more therapeutic.

Health Benefits of a Lavender and Chamomile Bath Soak

Beyond the immediate relaxation, using a lavender and chamomile bath soak regularly can offer numerous health benefits, from improved sleep quality to relief from minor aches and pains. Here are some of the key benefits:

Improved Sleep Quality

Both lavender and chamomile are well-known sleep aids, and a warm bath with these herbs can promote a smoother transition to sleep. The warmth of the bath, combined with the calming effects of the herbs, helps lower cortisol levels, the body's primary stress hormone. This relaxation effect allows for deeper, more restful sleep.

Stress and Anxiety Reduction

Studies have shown that lavender, in particular, has significant anxiolytic (anxiety-reducing) properties. A bath soak with lavender and chamomile provides an opportunity for mindfulness and relaxation, helping to lower stress levels and reduce symptoms of anxiety.

Relief from Muscle Tension

The Epsom salt in the bath soak provides magnesium, which helps relax tense muscles. Combined with the anti-inflammatory properties of chamomile, this bath soak is an ideal solution for sore muscles, making it a perfect choice after exercise or a physically demanding day.

Skin-Soothing Properties

Both lavender and chamomile contain anti-inflammatory compounds that can soothe irritated or inflamed skin. Chamomile, in particular, has been used for centuries to treat skin conditions, including eczema and minor irritations. Lavender also has mild antiseptic properties, which can be beneficial for maintaining healthy skin.

Enhanced Respiratory Health

The steam from a hot bath, infused with lavender and chamomile, can help open airways and soothe minor respiratory discomfort. The aroma of lavender and chamomile has a gentle, decongesting effect, which is especially helpful during cold and flu season.

Customizing Your Bath Soak for Specific Needs

Depending on your unique health needs or personal preferences, a lavender and chamomile bath soak can be modified. Here are some ideas for enhancing the bath soak to address specific wellness goals:

- **For Extra Relaxation**: Add a few drops of cedarwood essential oil, which pairs well with lavender and chamomile for an earthy, grounding scent that promotes relaxation.
- **For Skin Hydration**: Mix in a tablespoon of almond or coconut oil, which will dissolve in the warm bathwater and provide a moisturizing effect on the skin.
- **For Respiratory Relief**: Add eucalyptus essential oil to the bath soak mixture. The eucalyptus scent can help open airways, making it easier to breathe and relieving mild congestion.
- **For Enhanced Circulation**: A pinch of ginger powder in the bath soak can help stimulate circulation. Ginger creates a warming sensation on the skin, which can be particularly soothing during colder months.

Regular Use and Long-Term Benefits

Incorporating a lavender and chamomile bath soak into your regular self-care routine offers both short- and long-term benefits. Regular baths with this blend can help maintain healthy sleep patterns, reduce stress levels, and contribute to a general sense of well-being.

Valerian Root Tea

Valerian root tea is a renowned herbal remedy used for centuries, primarily known for its calming effects and ability to promote relaxation and sleep. Originating from the root of the Valeriana officinalis plant, valerian has been used in both traditional European and Asian medicine for its sedative qualities. While other herbal remedies can offer similar benefits, valerian root tea has a unique compound profile that makes it particularly effective for relaxation and addressing mild to moderate insomnia, stress, and anxiety. This section will explore the benefits, usage, preparation, and considerations around valerian root tea, highlighting its importance in natural remedies for mental and physical well-being.

Historical Context of Valerian Root

The medicinal use of valerian dates back to ancient Greece and Rome, where Hippocrates and Galen, two pioneers of early medicine, recognized its value in treating ailments like insomnia and anxiety. In Medieval Europe, valerian was even known as "all-heal" due to its wide range of applications, from soothing headaches to relieving digestive problems. Its use has evolved over time, but valerian root continues to be a key component in many herbal traditions, especially for those seeking a natural solution to stress and sleep issues.

Valerian's reputation as a sedative herb grew in the 18th century when it was commonly used to treat "nervousness," a term that broadly covered anxiety, mood swings, and other symptoms of emotional imbalance. Its effectiveness has stood the test of time, and today, valerian root tea remains a popular choice for individuals seeking a gentle, non-habit-forming remedy for improved mental health and relaxation.

How Valerian Root Tea Works

The effectiveness of valerian root tea lies in its unique combination of active compounds, including valerenic acid, isovaleric acid, and various antioxidants. These compounds interact with the brain and central nervous system to produce a relaxing effect, often compared to mild sedatives without the potential side effects of prescription medications.

1. **Interaction with GABA**: One of the primary ways valerian root works is by increasing levels of gamma-aminobutyric acid (GABA) in the brain. GABA is a neurotransmitter that reduces nerve transmission in the brain, calming nervous activity. Many prescription medications for anxiety, such as benzodiazepines, work by enhancing GABA levels. Valerian root naturally encourages higher GABA production, promoting relaxation without the addictive properties often associated with pharmaceuticals.

2. **Valerenic Acid and Anxiety Relief**: Valerenic acid is one of the main compounds in valerian root and is particularly effective for its anti-anxiety properties. It helps inhibit the breakdown of GABA in the brain, allowing this calming neurotransmitter to remain active longer, thereby reducing stress and anxiety levels.

3. **Other Sedative Compounds**: Valerian root contains other compounds, like flavonoids and alkaloids, that contribute to its overall sedative and relaxing effects. These compounds work synergistically with valerenic acid to promote calmness, reduce overactivity in the nervous system, and support better sleep.

4. **Antioxidants and Anti-inflammatory Effects**: In addition to its sedative qualities, valerian root also contains antioxidants that help protect the body from oxidative stress. This property is beneficial because stress and anxiety can increase oxidative damage in the body, and the antioxidants in valerian root tea can counteract some of these negative effects.

Preparing and Using Valerian Root Tea

To experience the benefits of valerian root, many people prefer tea as a soothing, warm beverage that can easily be incorporated into an evening relaxation routine. Preparing valerian root tea at home is simple, but there are specific considerations to keep in mind for the best results.

1. **Choosing the Right Valerian Root**: For tea, it's best to use dried valerian root, which can be purchased at health food stores, herbal apothecaries, or online. Make sure to buy from a reputable source, as the quality of valerian root can vary.

2. **Preparation Process**: Preparing valerian root tea requires simmering rather than steeping, as valerian's compounds are best extracted at a slightly higher temperature than regular tea.
   - **Ingredients**:
     - 1–2 teaspoons of dried valerian root (adjust to preference)
     - 1 cup of water
   - **Instructions**:
     - Place the valerian root in a small pot and add water.
     - Heat the mixture until it starts to simmer, then reduce heat and allow it to simmer gently for 10–15 minutes.
     - Strain the tea and drink it warm.

3. **Best Time to Drink**: Valerian root tea is most effective when taken 30–60 minutes before bedtime. Drinking it too early or too late may not yield the desired effects. Some people find that it works best as part of a nightly wind-down routine, combined with calming activities such as reading or meditating.

4. **Adding Flavor**: Valerian root has a unique, somewhat earthy taste that some may find unpleasant at first. Adding a natural sweetener, like honey, or blending it with other calming herbs, like chamomile or lemon balm, can enhance the flavor without diminishing its effects.

Benefits of Valerian Root Tea

Valerian root tea offers a variety of health benefits that make it an ideal choice for those looking to manage stress, anxiety, and sleep issues naturally.

1. **Improved Sleep Quality**: One of the main uses of valerian root tea is to improve sleep. Unlike some sleep aids, valerian root doesn't induce sleepiness but instead calms the nervous system, making it easier to drift off. Many people report fewer night-time awakenings and more restful sleep after drinking valerian tea regularly.

2. **Anxiety Relief**: Because valerian root increases GABA levels, it's effective in managing mild to moderate anxiety. This is particularly beneficial for those who experience anxiety-related sleep issues, as valerian can address both at once. It's a natural alternative for those who want to avoid the side effects of pharmaceutical anxiety medications.

3. **Reduced Stress and Tension**: Valerian's sedative qualities also help reduce physical manifestations of stress, such as muscle tension, headaches, and an elevated heart rate. Drinking valerian root tea during high-stress periods can serve as a preventive measure against these symptoms.

4. **Menstrual Symptom Relief**: Valerian root has antispasmodic properties, which can help relieve muscle cramps and spasms, particularly those associated with menstrual cycles. Women experiencing menstrual discomfort may find that drinking valerian root tea provides some relief.

5. **Neuroprotective Effects**: The antioxidants in valerian root help protect the brain from oxidative stress, which is beneficial for long-term mental health. Chronic stress and anxiety can increase oxidative damage in the brain, and valerian root's antioxidant properties offer protective benefits.

Considerations and Precautions

While valerian root tea is generally safe for most people, there are some considerations and precautions to be aware of to ensure safe and effective use.

1. **Potential Grogginess**: Valerian root can cause grogginess in some people, especially if consumed in large quantities. Start with a small amount (around 1 teaspoon) and adjust the dose gradually as you become accustomed to it.

2. **Pregnancy and Breastfeeding**: Valerian root is not recommended for pregnant or breastfeeding women due to limited research on its safety during these stages. Consult with a healthcare professional before using valerian if you are pregnant or nursing.

3. **Interactions with Medications**: Valerian root can interact with certain medications, particularly those with sedative effects, such as benzodiazepines, barbiturates, and sleep medications. Always consult your doctor if you are on medication and want to incorporate valerian root into your routine.

4. **Long-Term Use**: Although valerian root is considered safe for short-term use, it's best to avoid extended use without breaks. Taking valerian root tea daily for several weeks, followed by a break, can help prevent potential dependence and maintain its effectiveness.

5. **Individual Reactions**: Every individual may respond differently to valerian root. While many find it beneficial for sleep and relaxation, others may experience digestive discomfort or mild headaches. Listen to your body and discontinue use if you notice any adverse effects.

Enhancing Valerian Root Tea's Effects

Valerian root tea can be combined with other calming herbs to enhance its effects. Blending valerian with other herbs offers a more rounded flavor and can create a synergistic calming effect.

1. **Chamomile**: Adding chamomile to valerian root tea is a common choice for enhanced relaxation. Chamomile has mild sedative effects and adds a gentle floral note to the tea, which can make valerian's earthy taste more pleasant.

2. **Lemon Balm**: Known for its anxiety-relieving properties, lemon balm can enhance the calming effects of valerian. It has a pleasant lemony flavor that pairs well with valerian root, providing additional support for stress and sleep.

3. **Lavender**: Adding a pinch of dried lavender flowers can create an aromatic, floral tea with extra calming effects. Lavender is known to promote relaxation and may help enhance the sleep-promoting qualities of valerian root.

4. **Passionflower**: Passionflower is another herb that works well with valerian root. It has calming effects similar to valerian and can support anxiety reduction, making it an excellent choice for those with sleep disturbances related to stress or overthinking.

Incorporating Valerian Root Tea into a Relaxation Routine

For the best results, valerian root tea should be part of a broader relaxation routine. By pairing valerian tea with other calming practices, you can create a more peaceful transition into restful sleep.

1. **Create a Wind-Down Environment**: Dim the lights, put away screens, and engage in quiet activities such as reading or journaling. Valerian root tea complements these activities, reinforcing the body's natural signals to prepare for sleep.

2. **Deep Breathing Exercises**: Practicing deep breathing or mindfulness while sipping valerian root tea can increase its calming effects. Deep breathing reduces stress, while valerian root tea soothes the nervous system, working together to promote relaxation.

3. **Set a Regular Bedtime**: Valerian root tea is most effective when consumed consistently around the same time each night.

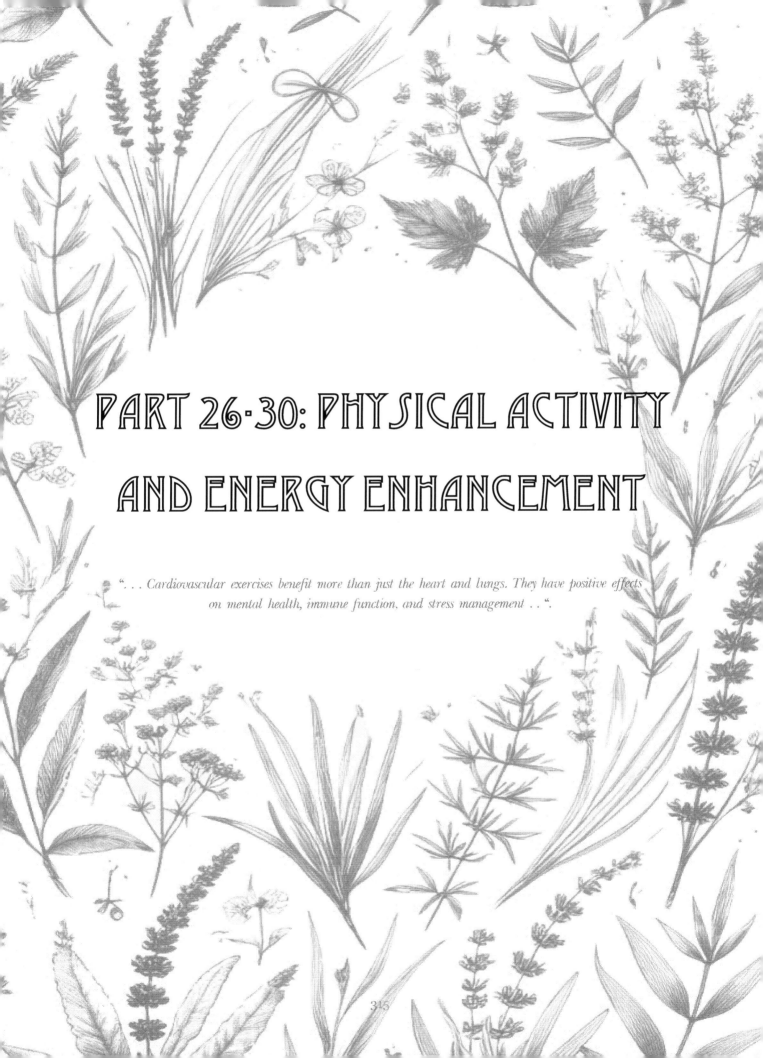

PART 26-30: PHYSICAL ACTIVITY AND ENERGY ENHANCEMENT

". . . Cardiovascular exercises benefit more than just the heart and lungs. They have positive effects on mental health, immune function, and stress management . . ".

Chapter 1: Role of Movement in Health

Engaging in various types of physical activities is essential for maintaining holistic wellness. Physical activity goes beyond just enhancing physical fitness; it also contributes to mental well-being, stress relief, and overall life quality.

Types of Physical Activities

From cardiovascular workouts to flexibility exercises, each type of physical activity offers unique benefits for the body and mind. In this section, we'll explore the main categories of physical activities, their benefits, and practical ways to incorporate them into daily routines, particularly to support natural wellness practices.

Cardiovascular Activities: Boosting Heart Health and Stamina

Cardiovascular activities, also known as aerobic exercises, involve continuous movement that elevates the heart rate. These activities improve cardiovascular health by strengthening the heart, lungs, and circulatory system. When performed consistently, aerobic exercises increase stamina, reduce blood pressure, and aid in weight management.

Some common cardiovascular exercises include brisk walking, jogging, running, swimming, cycling, and dancing. These activities vary in intensity, from low to high, making it easy to find one that suits individual fitness levels.

- **Example Scenario**: If you're new to aerobic exercise, start with brisk walking for 20–30 minutes daily. This low-impact activity is gentle on the joints and helps improve endurance over time. As you build stamina, you can progress to jogging or other high-intensity exercises.

Benefits of Cardiovascular Activities

Cardiovascular exercises benefit more than just the heart and lungs. They have positive effects on mental health, immune function, and stress management. When we engage in cardio, the body releases endorphins, often referred to as "feel-good" hormones. These chemicals reduce stress and anxiety, providing a natural way to uplift mood and reduce symptoms of depression.

Aerobic exercise also enhances immune function by promoting efficient circulation. This allows white blood cells, which help fight off infections, to travel more freely throughout the body. Additionally, aerobic activity can help regulate blood sugar levels, reduce the risk of chronic diseases, and support brain health by boosting blood flow to the brain.

Strength Training: Building Muscle and Bone Health

Strength training, or resistance training, involves exercises that strengthen muscles by working against resistance. This type of exercise is crucial for maintaining muscle mass, improving bone density, and supporting metabolic health. Strength training can be done using weights, resistance bands, or even one's body weight in exercises like push-ups, squats, and lunges.

- **Example Scenario**: If you're new to strength training, consider starting with bodyweight exercises, such as lunges and planks, before progressing to weights. Begin with light weights to learn proper form and gradually increase resistance as you become more comfortable.

Benefits of Strength Training

Strength training is beneficial for individuals of all ages, especially as it helps combat the natural decline in muscle mass that occurs with aging. By building lean muscle, strength training supports metabolic health, as muscles burn more calories at rest than fat. This makes it easier to manage body weight and reduces the risk of obesity-related health issues. Additionally, resistance exercises are known to improve bone density, which is essential for preventing osteoporosis, particularly in older adults. Strength training has also been linked to better insulin sensitivity, which is beneficial for those at risk of diabetes. Regular strength training helps improve posture, reduces the risk of injury, and enhances overall physical resilience, making daily tasks easier to accomplish.

Flexibility and Stretching: Enhancing Range of Motion

Flexibility exercises are often overlooked but are essential for maintaining a full range of motion in the joints. These exercises primarily focus on stretching the muscles, tendons, and ligaments, which helps improve flexibility and reduce stiffness. Popular flexibility activities include yoga, Pilates, and specific stretching routines targeting different muscle groups.

- **Example Scenario**: A simple stretching routine can be done in the morning to wake up the muscles and joints. Start by stretching the arms overhead, then move to shoulder, hamstring, and calf stretches. Hold each stretch for 20–30 seconds to maximize flexibility benefits.

Benefits of Flexibility and Stretching Exercises

Improving flexibility has numerous benefits for physical health and functionality. Stretching exercises help reduce muscle stiffness, improve blood flow to the muscles, and relieve stress. A flexible body is less prone to injuries, as the muscles and joints can handle a broader range of movements without strain.

Flexibility training is particularly beneficial for individuals with sedentary lifestyles or those who experience muscle stiffness. Regular stretching can reduce muscle imbalances, correct posture, and relieve tension, especially in areas that tend to become tight, like the shoulders and lower back. Furthermore, flexibility exercises support mobility, making everyday tasks easier and more comfortable.

Balance and Stability: Supporting Core Strength and Coordination

Balance and stability exercises are essential for maintaining proper posture, reducing the risk of falls, and supporting core strength. These exercises typically engage the muscles in the abdomen, back, and legs, which contribute to better overall stability. Activities such as tai chi, yoga, and specific balance exercises like standing on one foot or using a balance board are effective in improving balance.

- **Example Scenario**: Practicing yoga poses like the tree pose can enhance balance and engage the core. Beginners can start with shorter holds and progress to holding the pose for longer durations as their stability improves.

Benefits of Balance and Stability Exercises

Good balance and stability are vital for performing daily tasks and preventing falls, especially in older adults. By engaging the core and lower body muscles, balance exercises strengthen the muscles around the spine, supporting better posture and alignment. Improved balance also aids in coordination and reduces the likelihood of injury during other forms of exercise.

Engaging in balance exercises can be particularly beneficial for athletes and those recovering from injuries, as these exercises help build proprioception, or the body's awareness of its position in space. Better proprioception enhances agility, coordination, and overall physical control, which is valuable in various sports and physical activities.

Mind-Body Exercises: Promoting Relaxation and Mental Clarity

Mind-body exercises like yoga, tai chi, and qigong emphasize the connection between the body and the mind. These activities involve slow, deliberate movements combined with focused breathing, which promotes relaxation, mindfulness, and mental clarity. Mind-body exercises are known for their stress-relieving benefits and are often incorporated into holistic wellness practices.

- **Example Scenario**: A gentle yoga session in the morning or before bed can serve as a natural way to start or wind down the day. Practicing deep breathing during each pose promotes relaxation, while the slow movements engage the muscles and improve flexibility.

Benefits of Mind-Body Exercises

Mind-body exercises are highly beneficial for reducing stress, improving focus, and promoting emotional well-being. Practices like yoga and tai chi have been shown to lower cortisol levels, the body's primary stress hormone. This makes these exercises ideal for those dealing with high levels of stress or anxiety.

In addition to mental benefits, mind-body exercises improve physical flexibility, balance, and strength. For individuals seeking a low-impact, holistic approach to physical activity, mind-body exercises offer a comprehensive solution that addresses both physical and emotional health.

Combining Different Types of Physical Activities

While each type of physical activity offers unique benefits, a well-rounded fitness routine often combines various types to maximize health and wellness. For example, a weekly fitness regimen might include aerobic exercises for cardiovascular health, strength training to build muscle, stretching for flexibility, and mind-body practices for mental clarity and relaxation.

- **Example Scenario**: A balanced fitness routine could involve cardio sessions on Mondays and Wednesdays, strength training on Tuesdays and Thursdays, and flexibility exercises on Fridays. Saturday can be dedicated to mind-body activities like yoga or tai chi to rejuvenate the mind and body.

Combining different types of activities not only provides a comprehensive approach to fitness but also prevents exercise monotony. By incorporating a mix of exercises, individuals can target multiple aspects of their health, such as endurance, strength, flexibility, and mental resilience.

Tips for Starting a Physical Activity Routine

For those new to physical activity or looking to revamp their routine, the following tips can help:

1. **Start Small and Progress Gradually**: Begin with shorter sessions, particularly if you're new to exercise, and gradually increase the duration and intensity over time.

2. **Listen to Your Body**: Pay attention to how your body responds to each type of exercise. If certain exercises cause discomfort, consider modifying the movements or focusing on other activities.

3. **Set Realistic Goals**: Setting achievable goals can provide motivation and a sense of accomplishment. For instance, aim to incorporate three types of activities each week and gradually increase to more sessions as fitness improves.

4. **Consider Professional Guidance**: If you're unsure where to start or have specific health conditions, consulting a fitness professional or physiotherapist can provide guidance tailored to your needs.

The Role of Physical Activity in Natural Wellness

Physical activity plays a significant role in natural wellness, complementing other health practices like herbal remedies, meditation, and mindful eating. By incorporating various types of physical activities, individuals can support holistic wellness goals, improve resilience, and enhance overall quality of life.

Consistent physical activity has far-reaching benefits that extend beyond physical health. It helps manage stress, supports healthy aging, and promotes mental clarity. For those interested in natural wellness, integrating physical activities into daily routines can provide a foundation for a healthier, more balanced life.

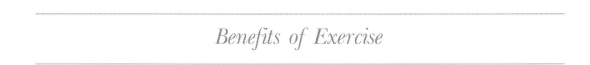

Benefits of Exercise

Exercise is a foundational component of holistic health, complementing natural remedies by enhancing overall physical and mental wellness. Integrating regular physical activity into daily life brings numerous health benefits, from improving cardiovascular health and metabolic function to enhancing mood and mental clarity. The benefits of exercise extend beyond physical fitness; they support immune function, reduce inflammation, and help stabilize emotional and mental health. This section explores these benefits in depth, offering insights into how regular exercise can improve well-being, amplify the effects of herbal remedies, and create a resilient foundation for health.

Physical Benefits of Exercise

1. **Enhanced Cardiovascular Health**: One of the primary benefits of regular exercise is its positive impact on heart health. Engaging in physical activities like brisk walking, running, swimming, or cycling strengthens the heart muscle, allowing it to pump blood more efficiently. This increased efficiency lowers blood pressure, improves circulation, and reduces the risk of cardiovascular diseases such as heart attacks, strokes, and hypertension. Regular cardiovascular exercise also helps maintain healthy cholesterol levels, which is essential for preventing arterial buildup and promoting long-term heart health.

2. **Improved Metabolic Function**: Exercise plays a crucial role in regulating metabolic processes, particularly in maintaining a healthy weight. Physical activity increases the rate at which calories are burned, supporting weight loss or weight maintenance, depending on individual goals. Additionally, exercise improves insulin sensitivity, meaning that the body can use blood glucose more effectively. This regulation helps prevent insulin resistance and lowers the risk of type 2 diabetes. A well-regulated metabolism also means that the body can efficiently convert nutrients into energy, which promotes vitality and reduces the risk of metabolic disorders.

3. **Enhanced Immune Function**: Physical activity has a significant impact on the immune system. Regular, moderate exercise stimulates the production of immune cells, particularly white blood cells, which are essential in identifying and eliminating pathogens. Exercise also promotes better circulation, allowing immune cells to travel more freely and efficiently throughout the body. This enhanced immune surveillance reduces the risk of infections and supports quicker recovery. While excessive, high-intensity exercise can temporarily weaken the immune response, moderate activity strengthens it, helping the body better resist illness and maintain resilience.

4. **Reduced Inflammation**: Inflammation is a natural response to injury or infection, but chronic inflammation can lead to a variety of health issues, including autoimmune disorders, cardiovascular disease, and cancer. Regular exercise helps regulate the inflammatory response by producing anti-inflammatory cytokines, which are proteins that counteract inflammation. Engaging in activities like yoga, walking, and

swimming helps reduce inflammatory markers, particularly in individuals who suffer from chronic conditions such as arthritis. This anti-inflammatory effect makes exercise a natural complement to herbal remedies that also target inflammation, such as turmeric and ginger.

5. **Increased Strength and Flexibility**: Strength and flexibility are important for maintaining an active, healthy lifestyle. Strength training exercises, such as weightlifting or resistance band workouts, build muscle mass, increase bone density, and improve posture. This is particularly beneficial for aging individuals, as it helps prevent osteoporosis and reduces the risk of falls and fractures. Flexibility exercises, such as stretching and yoga, improve the range of motion in joints and enhance balance. Together, strength and flexibility support functional movement, making daily activities easier and more enjoyable.

6. **Better Digestive Health**: Regular physical activity can improve digestive health by stimulating intestinal contractions, which helps move food through the digestive tract more efficiently. This can alleviate symptoms of constipation and bloating. Additionally, exercise reduces the risk of developing conditions like diverticulitis and colorectal cancer. Activities like walking, jogging, and yoga are particularly beneficial for promoting digestive health, especially when combined with a fiber-rich diet and herbal remedies that support digestion, such as fennel and peppermint.

Mental and Emotional Benefits of Exercise

1. **Reduced Symptoms of Depression and Anxiety**: Exercise is a powerful tool for managing symptoms of depression and anxiety. Physical activity triggers the release of endorphins, commonly known as "feel-good" hormones, which create a sense of happiness and well-being. Exercise also increases the levels of neurotransmitters like serotonin and dopamine, which play a crucial role in mood regulation. Engaging in regular exercise, particularly aerobic activities, can significantly reduce the symptoms of depression and anxiety, making it a natural and accessible remedy for mental health.

2. **Improved Cognitive Function and Memory**: Physical activity stimulates blood flow to the brain, which supports cognitive functions like memory, attention, and problem-solving skills. Exercise also promotes neurogenesis, the growth of new neurons, particularly in the hippocampus, a region of the brain associated with

memory. For older adults, regular exercise has been shown to slow cognitive decline and reduce the risk of neurodegenerative diseases like Alzheimer's. For individuals of all ages, exercise enhances mental clarity, helping them stay sharp and focused throughout the day.

3. **Stress Relief and Emotional Stability**: Physical activity serves as a natural stress reliever by lowering cortisol levels, a hormone associated with stress. Exercise helps stabilize the nervous system, allowing individuals to better manage their emotional responses to daily challenges. This stability is particularly beneficial for those who struggle with stress-related conditions, as it promotes a calm, balanced state of mind. Engaging in regular physical activity, whether through intense workouts or gentle practices like yoga, can significantly reduce stress and improve overall emotional resilience.

4. **Enhanced Sleep Quality**: Exercise has been shown to improve sleep quality by helping individuals fall asleep faster, stay asleep longer, and enjoy deeper sleep cycles. Physical activity reduces insomnia symptoms and promotes restorative sleep, which is crucial for mental and physical recovery. Exercise also helps regulate the body's circadian rhythm, the internal clock that dictates the sleep-wake cycle. A regular exercise routine, particularly in the morning or afternoon, can help individuals establish a healthy sleep pattern, leading to more restful nights and energized mornings.

Long-Term Health Benefits of Exercise

1. **Lower Risk of Chronic Diseases**: Regular physical activity reduces the risk of developing a range of chronic diseases, including heart disease, diabetes, and certain cancers. Exercise helps regulate blood pressure, improve cholesterol levels, and maintain a healthy weight, all of which contribute to disease prevention. Additionally, exercise has been shown to reduce the risk of osteoporosis by increasing bone density, particularly when combined with a diet rich in calcium and vitamin D.

2. **Increased Longevity**: Numerous studies have shown that regular exercise is associated with increased longevity. Physical activity reduces the risk of premature death from all causes, primarily by reducing the risk factors associated with chronic diseases. Exercise improves cardiovascular health, strengthens the immune system, and promotes mental resilience, all of which contribute to a longer, healthier life.

3. **Enhanced Quality of Life**: Exercise improves the overall quality of life by promoting physical, mental, and emotional well-being. Regular activity helps individuals feel more energetic, reduces pain and stiffness associated with aging, and enhances mental clarity. These benefits support a more active, fulfilling lifestyle, allowing individuals to participate fully in their daily activities and pursue their passions.

Practical Tips for Incorporating Exercise into Daily Life

1. **Start Small and Build Gradually**: For those new to exercise, starting with small, achievable goals is essential. Simple activities like walking, stretching, or light resistance training can be effective ways to begin. As fitness improves, individuals can gradually increase the duration and intensity of their workouts. This approach reduces the risk of injury and makes it easier to develop a consistent routine.

2. **Find Activities You Enjoy**: Enjoyment is a crucial factor in maintaining a long-term exercise routine. Experiment with different types of activities, such as swimming, dancing, hiking, or yoga, to find what resonates most. Engaging in enjoyable activities increases the likelihood of sticking with a routine, turning exercise into a pleasurable part of daily life.

3. **Set Realistic Goals**: Setting realistic, achievable goals helps maintain motivation and track progress. Goals can range from walking 10,000 steps daily to completing a certain number of workout sessions per week. Celebrating small victories along the way reinforces positive habits and encourages long-term commitment.

4. **Prioritize Consistency Over Intensity**: Consistency is key to reaping the long-term benefits of exercise. Rather than focusing on intense workouts, aim for regular, moderate activity. A consistent routine, even if it's a short walk each day, provides cumulative benefits over time.

5. **Integrate Exercise into Daily Routines**: Incorporating physical activity into daily tasks can make it easier to stay active. Simple actions like taking the stairs instead of the elevator, parking farther away from entrances, or doing household chores with added vigor can contribute to overall fitness. These small adjustments help increase daily movement without requiring a formal workout.

Complementing Exercise with Herbal Remedies

Exercise and herbal remedies work synergistically to enhance overall health and well-being. While exercise strengthens the body and mind, herbal remedies can provide additional support, particularly in areas like muscle recovery, energy enhancement, and mental clarity.

1. **Herbs for Muscle Recovery**: After exercise, herbs like turmeric and ginger can reduce inflammation and relieve muscle soreness. These anti-inflammatory herbs support faster recovery, allowing individuals to stay active without prolonged discomfort. Turmeric tea or ginger-infused water can be a refreshing post-workout drink that aids muscle recovery.

2. **Adaptogens for Energy and Stamina**: Adaptogenic herbs, such as ashwagandha and ginseng, are known for their ability to enhance endurance and energy levels. Incorporating these herbs into the diet can complement an active lifestyle by promoting sustained energy and reducing fatigue. Adaptogens can be taken in the form of teas, capsules, or powders added to smoothies.

3. **Mental Clarity and Focus**: Herbs like ginkgo biloba and gotu kola are associated with improved mental clarity and focus. For those engaging in activities that require concentration, such as yoga or Pilates, these herbs can enhance cognitive performance and make it easier to stay present during exercise.

Creating a Balanced Lifestyle with Exercise and Herbal Remedies

The combination of regular exercise and herbal remedies offers a comprehensive approach to wellness that addresses physical, mental, and emotional health. By establishing an active lifestyle supported by natural herbs, individuals can achieve a balanced, resilient foundation for overall well-being. Whether starting a new fitness routine or enhancing an existing one, incorporating these elements can make a profound impact on health and vitality.

Cardiovascular Health

Cardiovascular health is essential for overall well-being, impacting not only the heart and blood vessels but also contributing to the body's resilience, energy levels, and ability to combat chronic diseases. The cardiovascular system is responsible for circulating blood throughout the body, delivering oxygen, nutrients, and hormones to cells, and removing waste products like carbon dioxide. A healthy cardiovascular system supports nearly every function in the body, making it a cornerstone of good health. This section explores the key components of cardiovascular health, its significance, the risks of poor cardiovascular health, and actionable ways to maintain and improve it through natural means and lifestyle adjustments.

The Importance of Cardiovascular Health

Good cardiovascular health is crucial for longevity, quality of life, and the prevention of many diseases. When the heart, arteries, and veins function efficiently, blood flows freely, reducing the likelihood of blockages, clotting, or excessive strain on the heart. These conditions are essential because the cardiovascular system supports every cell, organ, and tissue in the body.

Cardiovascular health goes beyond just preventing heart disease. It influences cognitive health, mood stability, and physical endurance. Poor cardiovascular health can lead to fatigue, shortness of breath, and lower exercise tolerance, which affects daily life and overall productivity. Maintaining cardiovascular health enhances one's ability to cope with stress and recover from physical and emotional challenges.

Risks of Poor Cardiovascular Health

Poor cardiovascular health can result from a combination of genetic, lifestyle, and environmental factors. These risks are often compounded by unhealthy habits such as a poor diet, physical inactivity, smoking, and chronic stress. Over time, these factors can lead to plaque buildup in the arteries, high blood pressure, and high cholesterol levels, increasing the risk of heart disease, heart attacks, and strokes.

Chronic cardiovascular issues also increase the risk of conditions like peripheral artery disease, which restricts blood flow to the limbs, and can contribute to kidney disease and vision problems. Additionally, poor cardiovascular health can impair cognitive function, leading to memory loss, mood disorders, and reduced mental clarity.

Components of Cardiovascular Health

Achieving and maintaining cardiovascular health involves several key components:

1. **Heart Rate and Blood Pressure**: Maintaining a healthy heart rate and blood pressure is essential for reducing the strain on the heart. High blood pressure, or hypertension, increases the workload on the heart, leading to potential damage over time.

2. **Cholesterol Levels**: Keeping cholesterol levels balanced is vital to prevent plaque buildup in the arteries. High LDL (low-density lipoprotein) cholesterol can contribute to atherosclerosis, where arteries become narrow and hard due to plaque formation.

3. **Blood Sugar Control**: High blood sugar levels can damage blood vessels over time, making it essential for cardiovascular health to maintain balanced blood glucose. High blood sugar is particularly dangerous in individuals with diabetes, as it accelerates heart disease risk.

4. **Inflammation Levels**: Chronic inflammation in the body contributes to the development of cardiovascular disease. Addressing inflammation through diet, exercise, and stress management helps protect the cardiovascular system.

5. **Physical Fitness**: Regular exercise strengthens the heart muscle, improves circulation, and helps control blood pressure. Cardiovascular exercise, in particular, enhances heart and lung function, increasing endurance and overall fitness.

Natural Approaches to Support Cardiovascular Health

Several natural approaches can enhance cardiovascular health and reduce the risk of heart-related conditions. These include dietary changes, exercise, stress management, and the use of certain herbal remedies known for their heart-supportive properties.

Heart-Healthy Diet

A nutritious diet is one of the most effective ways to support cardiovascular health. The Mediterranean diet, rich in fruits, vegetables, whole grains, lean proteins, and healthy fats, has been shown to reduce cardiovascular disease risk. Omega-3 fatty acids, found in fatty fish like salmon and sardines, have anti-inflammatory effects and help reduce triglyceride levels, a type of fat in the blood that contributes to cardiovascular disease.

- **Example Foods for Cardiovascular Health**:
    - **Berries**: Rich in antioxidants like flavonoids, which reduce inflammation and improve blood vessel function.
    - **Leafy Greens**: High in nitrates, which help dilate blood vessels, improve blood flow, and lower blood pressure.
    - **Avocados**: Contain monounsaturated fats that support heart health by reducing bad cholesterol levels.

Physical Activity for a Strong Heart

Regular exercise is essential for cardiovascular health. Aerobic exercises like walking, running, cycling, and swimming are particularly beneficial because they elevate the heart rate, which strengthens the heart muscle and improves circulation. Aim for at least 150 minutes of moderate-intensity aerobic activity per week, as recommended by health experts. Strength training also supports cardiovascular health indirectly by enhancing muscle mass, which in turn boosts metabolism and improves insulin sensitivity, reducing the risk of high blood sugar levels. Flexibility and balance exercises, such as yoga, provide additional benefits by reducing stress and promoting overall physical resilience.

Herbal Remedies to Support Cardiovascular Health

Several herbal remedies are traditionally used to support heart health. While they are not substitutes for medical treatment, they can be beneficial as part of a heart-healthy lifestyle.

- **Hawthorn Berry**: Known for its potential to strengthen the heart muscle and improve blood flow. Hawthorn is rich in antioxidants, which combat oxidative stress, a contributor to cardiovascular disease.
- **Garlic**: Studies show that garlic can help reduce blood pressure and cholesterol levels. It contains a compound called allicin, which has been linked to improved heart health.
- **Ginger**: Possesses anti-inflammatory properties that benefit the cardiovascular system. Regular consumption of ginger may lower blood pressure and cholesterol levels.
- **Green Tea**: Contains polyphenols and catechins, which support cardiovascular health by reducing inflammation, lowering LDL cholesterol, and improving blood flow.

Managing Stress for Heart Health

Chronic stress negatively impacts cardiovascular health by increasing cortisol levels, which raises blood pressure and can lead to unhealthy behaviors such as overeating or smoking. Effective stress management techniques, like mindfulness meditation, deep breathing exercises, and yoga, can reduce stress and its harmful effects on the heart.

- **Example Practice**: Deep breathing exercises can lower blood pressure and slow the heart rate. Taking five minutes daily to practice deep breathing can make a significant difference in managing stress and supporting cardiovascular health.

Monitoring Cardiovascular Health

Regular check-ups and monitoring can help individuals maintain cardiovascular health. Blood pressure readings, cholesterol panels, and glucose tests provide insight into cardiovascular risk factors, enabling early intervention if needed. Many healthcare providers recommend yearly check-ups, but those with cardiovascular risk factors may benefit from more frequent monitoring.

Using wearable devices, such as fitness trackers, can also provide real-time insights into heart rate, activity levels, and sleep quality, helping individuals stay mindful of their cardiovascular health.

Lifestyle Habits to Support Cardiovascular Health

Developing a lifestyle that supports cardiovascular health involves making daily choices that benefit the heart and circulatory system. Avoiding smoking and limiting alcohol intake are two crucial steps, as both habits can harm cardiovascular health. Smoking damages blood vessels, increases blood pressure, and contributes to plaque buildup, while excessive alcohol intake can lead to high blood pressure, obesity, and heart disease.

Maintaining a healthy weight is another essential factor. Excess body weight puts additional strain on the heart and increases the risk of conditions like hypertension and type 2 diabetes, both of which contribute to cardiovascular disease.

The Role of Sleep in Cardiovascular Health

Adequate sleep is often overlooked but is essential for heart health. Poor sleep quality or insufficient sleep can increase the risk of hypertension, obesity, and diabetes, all of which strain the cardiovascular system. The American Heart Association recommends adults get 7–9 hours of sleep per night to promote cardiovascular health.

Sleep disorders, such as sleep apnea, are particularly harmful to heart health, as they cause repeated interruptions in breathing, which can lead to high blood pressure and other complications. Addressing sleep issues through lifestyle changes, sleep hygiene, or medical intervention, if needed, can make a significant difference in cardiovascular health.

Setting Realistic Goals for Cardiovascular Health

Improving cardiovascular health is a long-term commitment, but setting realistic, achievable goals can provide motivation. Start by identifying specific goals, such as reducing blood pressure or improving cholesterol levels, and then break these down into actionable steps.

For instance, if your goal is to lower cholesterol, you might aim to include heart-healthy foods, like oats and nuts, in your diet each day. If reducing blood pressure is a priority, regular physical activity, stress management, and cutting back on salt can be effective strategies.

By tracking progress and celebrating small victories along the way, individuals can stay motivated and maintain a heart-healthy lifestyle in the long term.

Building a Support System

Lastly, building a support system can enhance cardiovascular health efforts. Having friends, family members, or even a healthcare provider who encourages a heart-healthy lifestyle can make it easier to stick to dietary changes, stay active, and manage stress. Many people find that exercising with a friend, sharing recipes, or attending wellness classes creates a positive social experience that reinforces their commitment to heart health.

Support groups, both online and offline, provide a space for sharing challenges and tips, helping individuals feel less isolated in their journey toward better cardiovascular health.

Mental Clarity from Movement

Movement and exercise are powerful tools for enhancing mental clarity. Physical activity has a profound impact on cognitive functions, including memory, concentration, problem-solving, and overall mental sharpness. For centuries, humans have used physical movement not only to build physical strength but also to maintain mental acuity. Today, a growing body of scientific research supports the benefits of exercise for cognitive health, affirming its role in improving brain function, enhancing mood, and reducing stress. This section will explore how movement impacts mental clarity, the underlying mechanisms that make this possible, and practical strategies for leveraging exercise as a means to support cognitive health.

How Movement Improves Mental Clarity

1. **Enhanced Blood Flow to the Brain**: When we engage in physical activity, our heart rate increases, and blood flow is boosted throughout the body, including the brain. This increased circulation provides the brain with a steady supply of oxygen and nutrients that are essential for maintaining mental clarity. Enhanced blood flow to the brain is especially beneficial for areas like the prefrontal cortex and the hippocampus, regions associated with executive functions, memory, and emotional

regulation. This infusion of nutrients supports cellular health, promoting quicker thinking, sharper focus, and improved information processing.

2. **Release of Brain-Derived Neurotrophic Factor (BDNF)**: Exercise stimulates the production of brain-derived neurotrophic factor (BDNF), a protein that plays a critical role in brain function. BDNF is often referred to as "fertilizer for the brain" because it helps support the growth of new neurons and strengthens existing ones. This protein aids in neural plasticity, the brain's ability to reorganize and adapt by forming new neural connections. Neural plasticity is essential for learning and memory, and by boosting BDNF levels, exercise enables the brain to become more adaptable, which contributes to clearer, more flexible thinking.

3. **Reduction in Stress and Anxiety**: Movement serves as a natural stress reliever, helping to decrease levels of cortisol, the body's primary stress hormone. High levels of cortisol can impair cognitive functions, such as memory and concentration, making it difficult to think clearly. Physical activity helps to balance cortisol levels and promote the release of endorphins, which improve mood and increase a sense of well-being. Regular movement also decreases symptoms of anxiety, which can cloud judgment and reduce clarity. By stabilizing mood and lowering stress, movement paves the way for sharper focus and enhanced mental clarity.

4. **Improved Sleep Quality**: Quality sleep is essential for mental clarity, as it allows the brain to process information, consolidate memories, and clear out toxins. Regular physical activity has been shown to improve sleep quality by helping people fall asleep more quickly and experience deeper sleep cycles. As a result, those who engage in regular movement are more likely to wake up feeling refreshed and ready to tackle the day with a clear mind. Improved sleep also means better emotional regulation, which aids in decision-making and concentration.

5. **Enhanced Neurogenesis**: Neurogenesis, the process by which new neurons are formed in the brain, is particularly active in the hippocampus, a region involved in memory and learning. Exercise stimulates neurogenesis, which strengthens brain function and can slow the cognitive decline associated with aging. Regular movement helps the brain remain adaptable and resilient, allowing it to retain information more effectively, solve problems more creatively, and stay mentally sharp over the long term.

Practical Strategies for Using Movement to Boost Mental Clarity

1. **Aerobic Exercise**: Aerobic activities like running, walking, cycling, and swimming are some of the most effective ways to improve mental clarity. These exercises increase heart rate and oxygenate the blood, which supplies the brain with vital nutrients. Studies show that even moderate aerobic exercise can have immediate cognitive benefits, improving focus and mood. For individuals seeking to enhance mental clarity, incorporating at least 30 minutes of aerobic activity into their daily routine can make a noticeable difference.

2. **Mindful Movement Practices**: Mindful movement practices, such as yoga, tai chi, and qigong, combine physical activity with mindfulness, which enhances mental clarity by grounding the mind in the present moment. These practices improve focus, reduce mental clutter, and strengthen the mind-body connection. The rhythmic nature of mindful movement helps calm the nervous system, alleviating anxiety and promoting a state of relaxed alertness that allows for sharper thinking. Practicing mindful movement also helps develop concentration, as participants learn to stay present and attentive to each movement.

3. **High-Intensity Interval Training (HIIT)**: High-intensity interval training (HIIT) involves short bursts of intense exercise followed by brief rest periods. This form of exercise not only improves cardiovascular health but also boosts mental clarity by increasing BDNF production. HIIT workouts require focus and quick decision-making, training the brain to adapt to rapid changes. These workouts are particularly beneficial for individuals who struggle with focus, as the intensity requires concentration, making HIIT an excellent way to sharpen mental acuity.

4. **Outdoor Activities**: Engaging in outdoor activities, such as hiking, gardening, or simply walking in nature, can provide cognitive benefits that indoor workouts may not. Spending time in nature has been shown to reduce mental fatigue and restore attention, a phenomenon known as "attention restoration theory." Natural environments offer a break from urban stimuli and allow the mind to wander and recover from cognitive overload. Outdoor activities combine the benefits of movement with the rejuvenating effects of nature, promoting clearer thinking and a more relaxed state of mind.

5. **Balancing Physical and Mental Activity**: Alternating between physical and mental activities throughout the day can help sustain mental clarity. For example, taking a brisk walk after a period of focused work can clear the mind, reduce mental fatigue, and improve concentration when returning to the task. This approach, known as the "exercise snack," provides short breaks of movement that recharge the mind and prevent burnout. Integrating small bursts of activity throughout the day ensures that mental clarity remains consistent and that energy levels are sustained.

Real-World Examples of Movement for Mental Clarity

1. **Corporate Wellness Programs**: Many companies have implemented wellness programs that encourage employees to engage in physical activity during the workday. Activities like walking meetings, standing desks, and scheduled exercise breaks are becoming more common, as they have been shown to improve productivity, focus, and morale. These programs highlight the connection between physical activity and mental performance, and many employees report improved mental clarity and reduced stress as a result.

2. **Education and Movement**: Schools are beginning to incorporate movement into the classroom, recognizing the link between physical activity and cognitive function. Some schools use "brain breaks," short, structured movement activities, to help students regain focus and stay engaged. Physical education programs that prioritize active learning help students develop mental clarity, improving their ability to absorb and retain information.

3. **Using Movement as a Study Aid**: Students and individuals in cognitively demanding roles often use exercise as a study or work aid. Walking, cycling, or engaging in light physical activity during breaks from studying has been shown to improve retention and enhance focus. Even walking while reading or listening to recorded notes can enhance understanding and recall, making movement a valuable tool for students or professionals aiming to improve mental clarity.

4. **Movement for Aging Populations**: Older adults can also benefit from exercise to maintain cognitive health. Regular physical activity is known to reduce the risk of dementia and other cognitive impairments by promoting blood flow to the brain, reducing inflammation, and supporting neural plasticity. Movement programs

specifically designed for seniors, such as gentle yoga, water aerobics, or walking groups, offer a way to preserve mental clarity and enhance quality of life.

Combining Movement with Herbal Supplements for Optimal Mental Clarity

1. **Adaptogens for Focus and Stamina**: Adaptogenic herbs, such as ginseng, rhodiola, and ashwagandha, complement the mental clarity benefits of exercise by helping the body adapt to stress. These herbs support focus and stamina, particularly during physically demanding activities. Adaptogens are available as teas, capsules, or tinctures and can be taken before exercise to enhance endurance and reduce mental fatigue.

2. **Herbs for Circulation**: Improved circulation supports cognitive health by delivering oxygen and nutrients to the brain. Herbs like ginkgo biloba and gotu kola are known for their circulation-boosting properties, which enhance cognitive function and mental clarity. These herbs can be taken as supplements or brewed into teas, providing a natural boost to the cognitive benefits of physical activity.

3. **Calming Herbs for Mental Relaxation**: For individuals who experience anxiety or stress-related cognitive issues, calming herbs like chamomile, valerian, and passionflower can provide additional support. These herbs promote relaxation and reduce anxiety, making it easier to focus and think clearly. When used in combination with mindful movement practices like yoga or tai chi, calming herbs enhance the mental clarity gained from exercise by creating a sense of calm and balance.

Creating a Balanced Lifestyle for Mental Clarity

Achieving mental clarity through movement requires consistency, self-awareness, and a willingness to adapt routines to individual needs. Establishing a balanced lifestyle that incorporates physical activity, herbal support, and mindfulness practices can make a significant difference in cognitive health. Here are some guidelines for maintaining this balance:

1. **Prioritize Consistent Activity**: Regular movement, even if it's light activity, is more effective for mental clarity than sporadic intense workouts. Prioritizing activities that are enjoyable and sustainable will make it easier to maintain consistency.

2. **Listen to Your Body**: Different types of movement impact mental clarity in unique ways. Some people may find that high-intensity exercise boosts their focus, while

others benefit more from gentle, mindful practices. Experiment with various forms of movement to find what best supports your mental clarity.

3. **Integrate Herbal Support**: Herbal supplements can amplify the cognitive benefits of movement. For those seeking increased focus and stamina, adaptogens and circulation-boosting herbs can be valuable additions. Conversely, individuals looking for stress relief may find calming herbs beneficial.

4. **Practice Mindful Recovery**: Rest is essential for mental clarity. Ensuring that adequate sleep and recovery periods are incorporated into a movement routine allows the brain to process and recharge.

Chapter 2: Designing a Fitness Routine

A well-rounded workout is essential for physical fitness, overall health, and wellness. A balanced workout combines various elements that target different aspects of fitness, such as cardiovascular endurance, muscle strength, flexibility, balance, and coordination.

Components of a Balanced Workout

Incorporating these components into a workout routine ensures a holistic approach that improves physical capability, reduces the risk of injury, and enhances overall health. In this section, we will explore each component of a balanced workout, its importance, and practical tips for incorporating each aspect into a sustainable fitness routine.

The Importance of a Balanced Workout

A balanced workout program goes beyond merely achieving aesthetic goals; it fosters long-term health, resilience, and mental well-being. By including various fitness components, individuals can work towards achieving a high level of functional fitness, which helps in daily activities and increases resistance to injury. For instance, strong muscles support joints, flexible muscles prevent strains, and cardiovascular health ensures sustained energy. Regular, balanced workouts also improve posture, coordination, and mobility, and offer significant mental health benefits by reducing stress and enhancing mood.

Key Components of a Balanced Workout

1. **Cardiovascular   Endurance**

   Cardiovascular endurance is the body's ability to sustain prolonged physical activity, primarily affecting the heart, lungs, and circulatory system. Cardiovascular or aerobic exercises are activities that elevate the heart rate and increase respiration, thereby improving the body's ability to transport and utilize oxygen efficiently.

   o **Examples**: Running, cycling, swimming, and brisk walking are common forms of cardiovascular exercise. Engaging in activities like dancing or rowing also provides an enjoyable way to improve cardiovascular endurance.

- o **Benefits**: Cardiovascular exercise improves heart and lung function, lowers blood pressure, reduces cholesterol levels, and boosts overall energy. It is also effective for burning calories and managing weight, reducing the risk of heart disease and diabetes.
- o **Guidelines**: The American Heart Association recommends at least 150 minutes of moderate-intensity aerobic activity or 75 minutes of vigorous aerobic activity each week.

2. **Strength   Training**

Strength training involves exercises that improve muscle strength and endurance. Strengthening muscles enhances their ability to work without tiring, supports joints, and prevents injury. Muscle mass also contributes to a higher resting metabolic rate, aiding in weight management.

- o **Examples**: Weight lifting, bodyweight exercises like push-ups and squats, and resistance band exercises. Functional movements like deadlifts and lunges are also effective for strengthening multiple muscle groups.
- o **Benefits**: Increases muscle strength, bone density, and metabolism, helping to prevent conditions like osteoporosis and obesity. Strength training also improves posture, balance, and overall physical performance.
- o **Guidelines**: Aim for strength training exercises that target all major muscle groups at least twice a week, allowing adequate recovery between sessions.

3. **Flexibility**

Flexibility is the range of motion in the joints and muscles. Maintaining flexibility reduces stiffness and prevents injuries by allowing muscles and joints to move more freely. Regular stretching exercises are essential for preserving and improving flexibility, especially as people age.

- o **Examples**: Stretching exercises like dynamic stretches (e.g., leg swings) and static stretches (e.g., holding a hamstring stretch) are effective. Practices like yoga and Pilates also promote flexibility by working various muscle groups and improving the range of motion.
- o **Benefits**: Enhances mobility, reduces muscle soreness, and decreases the risk of injuries. Flexibility also supports proper alignment, balance, and posture, making everyday movements easier and more comfortable.

- o **Guidelines**: Incorporate flexibility exercises at least two to three times per week. Hold each stretch for 15-30 seconds, focusing on breathing deeply to relax the muscles.

4. **Balance and Coordination**

Balance and coordination exercises are crucial, especially for older adults, as they help prevent falls and improve stability. Good balance also enhances body control and reduces the risk of strains and sprains, which are common in both sports and daily activities.

- o **Examples**: Balance exercises include standing on one leg, heel-to-toe walking, and exercises that involve an unstable surface like a balance board. Tai Chi and yoga are also excellent for improving balance and coordination.
- o **Benefits**: Strengthens stabilizer muscles, improves posture, enhances athletic performance, and reduces the risk of falls and injuries. Good balance contributes to better movement efficiency in all types of activities.
- o **Guidelines**: Balance training can be practiced daily or incorporated into strength training routines. Start with simpler exercises and progress to more challenging moves as balance improves.

5. **Core Stability**

Core stability involves strengthening the muscles in the abdomen, lower back, and pelvis. A strong core is essential for almost every movement, from lifting objects to twisting and bending, as it stabilizes the spine and pelvis.

- o **Examples**: Exercises like planks, Russian twists, leg raises, and exercises involving an exercise ball strengthen the core muscles. Pilates also focuses on core strength and stability.
- o **Benefits**: Supports good posture, reduces lower back pain, and enhances athletic performance. Core stability improves balance and reduces the likelihood of injuries in the back and hips.
- o **Guidelines**: Incorporate core exercises into each workout session or dedicate specific days to core training. Avoid overexerting the lower back by practicing proper form during exercises.

Designing a Balanced Workout Routine

A balanced workout program involves combining these components in a structured and achievable way. By creating a weekly schedule that includes cardiovascular, strength, flexibility, and balance exercises, individuals can reap the full benefits of a balanced fitness routine.

Example Weekly Schedule

- **Day 1**: Cardio (e.g., 30 minutes of running or cycling)
- **Day 2**: Strength Training (upper body focus) + Core exercises
- **Day 3**: Flexibility and Balance (yoga or stretching session)
- **Day 4**: Cardio (e.g., swimming or brisk walking)
- **Day 5**: Strength Training (lower body focus) + Core exercises
- **Day 6**: Balance and Coordination exercises
- **Day 7**: Rest or light stretching

Integrating Natural Remedies for Muscle Recovery and Energy

For those seeking to enhance their workout experience naturally, certain herbs and supplements can support physical activity and recovery:

- **Turmeric**: Known for its anti-inflammatory properties, turmeric can help alleviate muscle soreness after a workout. It can be consumed as a supplement or added to meals.
- **Ginger**: Another anti-inflammatory herb, ginger helps reduce muscle pain and stiffness. Ginger tea or fresh ginger in smoothies can be beneficial post-workout.
- **Ashwagandha**: Often used to increase endurance and reduce stress, ashwagandha supports physical and mental performance. It's available in capsule or powder form.
- **Magnesium**: Essential for muscle function and relaxation, magnesium helps prevent muscle cramps and aids recovery. Magnesium-rich foods include spinach, almonds, and pumpkin seeds.

Practical Tips for a Balanced Workout Routine

1. **Progress Gradually**: When starting a balanced workout, begin with manageable exercises and durations. Gradually increase the intensity and complexity as fitness improves.
2. **Focus on Form**: Proper form is crucial, especially in strength training and flexibility exercises, to avoid injuries and ensure maximum benefit. Consider working with a trainer or using mirrors to monitor posture.

3. **Listen to Your Body**: Pay attention to how your body feels during and after each workout. Muscle soreness is normal, but sharp pain or excessive fatigue may indicate the need for rest or adjustments.

4. **Stay Consistent**: Consistency is key to seeing results. Aim to exercise regularly, even if some days are lighter than others. Consistent effort over time builds a strong foundation.

5. **Prioritize Recovery**: Allow muscles to rest and recover. Incorporating rest days and ensuring adequate sleep are essential for preventing burnout and muscle fatigue.

6. **Modify for Preferences and Goals**: Personalize the workout routine based on preferences, goals, and fitness level. Some individuals may enjoy strength training more than cardio, or vice versa. A balanced workout allows for flexibility to focus on areas of interest while covering all essential components.

The Role of Hydration and Nutrition

Proper hydration and nutrition are foundational to a successful workout program. Hydration supports endurance, reduces muscle fatigue, and aids recovery. Consuming a balanced diet rich in proteins, healthy fats, and carbohydrates fuels workouts and promotes muscle repair.

- **Hydration**: Aim to drink water before, during, and after workouts. Electrolyte drinks can be beneficial during intense or long-duration exercises.
- **Pre-Workout Nutrition**: Consuming a meal or snack with carbohydrates and a small amount of protein about an hour before exercise provides energy and supports muscle function.
- **Post-Workout Nutrition**: Protein-rich foods or shakes after a workout aid muscle repair and growth. Pairing protein with carbohydrates helps replenish energy stores.

Building a Support System

A support system can enhance consistency and motivation. Whether it's a workout buddy, a fitness class, or an online community, engaging with others who have similar goals encourages accountability and enjoyment.

Rest and Recovery Essentials

Rest and recovery are vital components of a healthy lifestyle and play an essential role in overall wellness. Just as physical activity is necessary for strengthening the body and enhancing mental clarity, adequate rest allows the body to rebuild, repair, and rejuvenate. Rest isn't merely about taking a break from physical exertion; it encompasses sleep quality, mental relaxation, and structured recovery practices that allow for holistic restoration. In this section, we'll explore the importance of rest, the physiological benefits of recovery, and effective strategies to incorporate these essentials into daily life.

The Importance of Rest and Recovery

1. **Muscle Repair and Growth**: Physical activity, especially activities that challenge the muscles, such as weightlifting, running, or high-intensity interval training, causes microscopic tears in muscle fibers. These small tears are necessary for muscle growth and strength but require time and proper nutrients to repair. During rest, the body heals these tears, reinforcing the muscle fibers to handle future stress more effectively. This repair process is what leads to stronger, more resilient muscles. Skipping rest periods can lead to overtraining, which often results in fatigue, muscle weakness, and even injury.

2. **Nervous System Restoration**: Exercise, particularly high-intensity activities, places stress on the nervous system, which is responsible for sending signals to and from the brain. The nervous system works tirelessly during exercise to maintain coordination, balance, and response time. However, just like muscles, the nervous system requires recovery to function optimally. Without adequate rest, individuals may experience decreased coordination, slower reflexes, and even mental fog. Rest periods allow the nervous system to regain strength, improving both physical and cognitive performance.

3. **Hormonal Balance**: Physical exertion, especially high-intensity or prolonged activities, triggers the release of various hormones, including cortisol, adrenaline, and growth hormone. While these hormones support physical activity by providing energy and increasing alertness, chronic overexertion without adequate recovery can disrupt their balance. Elevated cortisol levels, for instance, can lead to chronic stress, anxiety, and even suppressed immune function. Rest and relaxation help bring hormone levels back to baseline, supporting mental stability and physical health.

4. **Immune System Support**: Regular exercise supports the immune system by promoting circulation and reducing inflammation. However, intense or prolonged exertion without proper rest can weaken immune function, making the body more susceptible to infections and illnesses. Rest days give the immune system time to repair any inflammation that might arise from physical exertion, enhancing the body's natural defenses and preventing the negative impacts of overtraining on immunity.

5. **Mental Health Benefits**: Recovery isn't only about physical repair; it's essential for mental well-being. Constant physical strain and lack of adequate rest can lead to feelings of burnout, mental fatigue, and decreased motivation. Incorporating rest days allows the brain to reset and recover, improving focus, mood, and overall mental clarity. The restorative effects of rest support long-term commitment to physical health and prevent burnout.

Effective Rest and Recovery Practices

1. **Quality Sleep**: Sleep is the cornerstone of rest and recovery. During deep sleep, the body releases growth hormone, which is essential for muscle repair, tissue growth, and immune function. Sleep also provides a mental reset, allowing the brain to process emotions, memories, and new information. Prioritizing 7-9 hours of quality sleep each night is one of the best ways to support overall recovery. To enhance sleep quality, maintain a regular sleep schedule, create a relaxing bedtime routine, and keep the sleep environment comfortable and free of distractions.

2. **Active Recovery**: Not all rest needs to be passive. Active recovery involves engaging in low-intensity activities, such as walking, stretching, or gentle yoga, which increase circulation and promote muscle recovery without placing undue stress on the body. Active recovery encourages blood flow to the muscles, which aids in the removal of metabolic waste products, such as lactic acid, and delivers fresh oxygen and nutrients to speed up healing. Integrating active recovery days into a fitness routine allows for gentle movement while supporting the recovery process.

3. **Hydration and Nutrition**: Proper hydration and balanced nutrition are essential for effective recovery. Water aids in nutrient transport, temperature regulation, and waste elimination, all of which support recovery. Additionally, nutrients like protein,

carbohydrates, and essential fats are vital for muscle repair, energy replenishment, and reducing inflammation. After exercise, consuming a balanced meal that includes protein for muscle repair and carbohydrates for energy replenishment is key to accelerating recovery.

4. **Stretching and Flexibility Exercises**: Stretching and flexibility exercises enhance muscle elasticity, reduce stiffness, and support joint health. Gentle stretching after workouts helps reduce muscle tightness and can prevent soreness. Yoga and other flexibility-based practices help to restore muscle length, which may shorten slightly from intense exercise. Incorporating stretching into a recovery routine promotes flexibility, reduces muscle tension, and aids in mental relaxation.

5. **Massage Therapy**: Massage therapy is a recovery method that helps reduce muscle soreness, increase blood flow, and decrease muscle tightness. Massage not only provides physical benefits but also promotes relaxation by reducing stress levels. Self-massage using foam rollers or massage balls is a convenient and affordable way to target tight muscles and alleviate tension. Professional massage therapy, such as Swedish or sports massage, can also accelerate recovery by reducing inflammation and promoting lymphatic drainage.

6. **Herbal Remedies for Recovery**: Certain herbs and natural supplements support the recovery process by reducing inflammation, soothing sore muscles, and promoting relaxation. Herbs like turmeric, ginger, and arnica are known for their anti-inflammatory properties, making them beneficial for recovery. Turmeric, which contains curcumin, is particularly effective at reducing exercise-induced inflammation. Arnica, available in cream form, is widely used to relieve muscle soreness. Chamomile and valerian root are beneficial for promoting relaxation, aiding sleep, and reducing stress, all of which support holistic recovery.

Real-World Application of Recovery Practices

1. **Athletes and Recovery Days**: Many athletes incorporate scheduled rest days into their training to allow for adequate recovery. For instance, professional runners often take one to two rest days per week and schedule "easy" days with light running or cross-training to promote active recovery. By balancing intense workouts with rest and lighter activity, athletes are able to maintain peak performance, prevent injury, and avoid burnout.

2. **Workplace Wellness**: Recovery is essential not only for athletes but also for individuals in demanding work environments. Long hours, especially those involving physical labor or high stress, require adequate recovery. Companies that prioritize workplace wellness may encourage breaks, offer relaxation spaces, or even sponsor recovery programs like yoga or stretching sessions. These initiatives help employees recharge, reduce stress, and improve productivity, highlighting the importance of recovery in diverse settings.

3. **Mindfulness and Meditation for Recovery**: Meditation and mindfulness practices are powerful tools for mental recovery. These practices allow the mind to rest, reducing stress and promoting a state of calm. Mindfulness meditation involves focusing on the present moment, which can alleviate mental fatigue and provide a sense of relaxation. Incorporating mindfulness practices into a rest day can support mental recovery, reduce cortisol levels, and improve overall well-being.

4. **Sleep Hygiene Practices**: Individuals who struggle with sleep may find it helpful to implement sleep hygiene practices that support restful sleep. Techniques such as avoiding caffeine in the evening, dimming lights before bedtime, and engaging in a calming pre-sleep routine, such as reading or gentle stretching, prepare the body for quality sleep. By optimizing sleep hygiene, individuals can enhance their natural recovery processes, leading to better physical and mental performance.

Creating a Balanced Recovery Routine

To maximize the benefits of rest and recovery, it's essential to develop a balanced routine that supports both physical and mental rejuvenation. Here are some guidelines to create an effective recovery routine:

1. **Schedule Regular Rest Days**: Designate at least one day each week for complete rest, especially after high-intensity workouts or physically demanding tasks. These rest days allow the body to recover fully, helping prevent injury and fatigue.

2. **Incorporate Active Recovery**: On non-intensive days, incorporate active recovery to promote circulation without straining the body. Light walks, stretching, and mobility exercises are excellent ways to keep moving while supporting recovery.

3. **Focus on Nutrition and Hydration**: Proper nutrition and hydration are the foundation of effective recovery. Consuming a post-exercise meal with protein and carbohydrates helps repair muscles and restore glycogen levels. Staying hydrated

before, during, and after physical activity supports cellular recovery and reduces the likelihood of cramps or soreness.

4. **Utilize Herbal Support**: Herbal remedies can be effective for enhancing recovery. Consuming turmeric tea or incorporating ginger into meals can help manage inflammation. Valerian root tea or chamomile can be particularly useful for promoting relaxation and enhancing sleep quality.

5. **Practice Mindful Relaxation**: Engaging in relaxation techniques, such as deep breathing exercises, meditation, or progressive muscle relaxation, supports mental clarity and reduces stress levels. These practices provide a mental reset, complementing physical rest and contributing to overall well-being.

6. **Set a Consistent Sleep Schedule**: Prioritizing consistent sleep patterns optimizes the body's natural recovery process. Going to bed and waking up at the same time each day reinforces the body's internal clock, improving sleep quality and enhancing both mental and physical restoration.

7. **Evaluate and Adjust**: Recovery needs may vary depending on factors such as age, physical activity level, and stress. Evaluate your recovery routine regularly and make adjustments as needed. Pay attention to signals from your body, such as fatigue, soreness, or mood changes, and prioritize rest if needed.

Stretching Techniques

Stretching is a fundamental component of physical fitness and wellness, supporting flexibility, muscle recovery, and overall range of motion. When done correctly, stretching can prevent injuries, enhance athletic performance, and promote a sense of relaxation and well-being. However, not all stretching techniques serve the same purpose. Each type of stretch affects muscles and joints differently and should be applied appropriately depending on one's goals, activity level, and physical condition. In this section, we'll explore the various stretching techniques, their benefits, and practical ways to incorporate them into daily routines for optimal physical and mental health.

The Benefits of Stretching

Stretching is often an underestimated part of fitness but offers numerous health advantages. Regular stretching helps improve flexibility by lengthening muscles and soft tissues, thus enhancing joint range of motion. By reducing muscle stiffness, stretching also decreases the risk of strains and injuries. Furthermore, flexibility plays a significant role in functional fitness, as it enables ease of movement and agility, which are crucial in everyday activities.

Beyond physical benefits, stretching has a positive impact on mental well-being. Slow, mindful stretching activates the parasympathetic nervous system, promoting relaxation and reducing stress levels. Incorporating stretching techniques into daily routines can improve posture, circulation, and recovery, especially after intense workouts. Improved blood flow to the muscles also accelerates recovery by delivering nutrients and oxygen that aid in the healing process.

Types of Stretching Techniques

1. **Static Stretching**

Static stretching involves elongating a muscle and holding the position for a set period, typically between 15 and 60 seconds. This form of stretching is most beneficial after a workout, as it helps relax muscles and alleviate tension.

- o **Examples**: Hamstring stretch (sitting and reaching for toes), quadriceps stretch (pulling one foot towards the glutes), shoulder stretch (reaching one arm across the body).

- o **Benefits**: Static stretching increases flexibility and promotes muscle relaxation. Holding a stretch for an extended time helps the muscle lengthen and relax, making it less susceptible to injury.

- o **When to Use**: Static stretching is ideal for a cool-down after exercise, helping to reduce muscle soreness and aiding in recovery. It's also suitable as a stand-alone activity for relaxation and flexibility improvement.

2. **Dynamic Stretching**

Dynamic stretching involves moving parts of your body through a full range of motion in a controlled, smooth, and deliberate manner. Unlike static stretching, dynamic stretching is active and warms up the muscles by increasing blood flow and activating the nervous system.

- o **Examples**: Arm circles, leg swings, walking lunges, high knees, and torso twists.

- o **Benefits**: Dynamic stretching improves flexibility, coordination, and circulation. It's particularly effective for preparing the muscles for more intense activity, as it activates the muscles without overstretching them.

- **When to Use**: This technique is ideal for a warm-up before physical activities such as running, sports, or strength training. Dynamic stretching primes the muscles and joints for movement, which can enhance performance and reduce the risk of injury.

3. **Ballistic Stretching**

Ballistic stretching uses momentum to force a muscle beyond its normal range of motion by making quick, bouncing movements. It aims to increase flexibility rapidly but can be risky if not performed correctly, as it can lead to overstretching or muscle tears.

- **Examples**: Bouncing down repeatedly to touch your toes, swinging legs forward forcefully.
- **Benefits**: When done cautiously and with proper guidance, ballistic stretching can improve flexibility and range of motion. However, it's best suited for experienced athletes or individuals in specific sports that require explosive movements.
- **When to Use**: Ballistic stretching should be limited to advanced athletes who have the strength and control to manage rapid movements safely. It's not recommended for beginners or as a general fitness warm-up.

4. **Proprioceptive Neuromuscular Facilitation (PNF) Stretching**

PNF stretching involves alternating between contracting and relaxing muscles to increase flexibility. Typically done with a partner or using resistance, this method requires the muscle to be stretched, then contracted, then stretched again.

- **Examples**: Hamstring stretch with a partner providing resistance, stretching a muscle to the limit, holding it, then contracting it against resistance before stretching again.
- **Benefits**: PNF stretching is one of the most effective techniques for improving flexibility. The contract-relax method enables muscles to stretch beyond their usual range.
- **When to Use**: PNF is ideal for athletes or those looking to achieve greater flexibility. It requires caution and proper technique, preferably with the assistance of a trainer or partner, to ensure that muscles aren't overstretched.

5. **Active Stretching**

Active stretching involves holding a position using only the muscles of the opposing group. This technique engages certain muscles to hold a stretch without any external force, making it effective for building both flexibility and strength.

- o **Examples**: Lifting a leg in front and holding it in the air using only the opposing leg muscles, rather than with hands or a support.
- o **Benefits**: Active stretching helps improve strength in addition to flexibility, as the muscles work to hold the position. It also promotes muscle control and stability.
- o **When to Use**: Active stretching can be done as part of a warm-up, cool-down, or standalone flexibility routine. It's particularly useful for those looking to build strength and control while improving flexibility.

6. **Passive Stretching**

Passive stretching, also known as relaxed stretching, involves holding a stretch with the assistance of gravity, a partner, or an object. It's a gentle form of stretching that requires minimal muscle engagement.

- o **Examples**: Leaning against a wall to stretch the calves, using a strap to pull a leg into a stretch while lying on your back.
- o **Benefits**: Passive stretching is excellent for relaxation, flexibility, and muscle recovery. By minimizing muscle engagement, it helps release tension and promote relaxation.
- o **When to Use**: Passive stretching is ideal for cooldowns, yoga sessions, or before bed to release tension and stress. It's also helpful in rehabilitation settings, as it minimizes strain on the muscles.

Practical Tips for Incorporating Stretching into a Routine

1. **Choose the Right Technique**: Tailor your stretching technique to the specific goals of your workout. For instance, use dynamic stretches to warm up before a high-intensity workout, and static or passive stretching to cool down afterward.
2. **Hold and Control**: When performing static or PNF stretches, hold each position steadily without bouncing. Aim to hold each stretch for at least 15-30 seconds, allowing the muscles time to lengthen and relax.

3. **Breathe Deeply**: Breathing is essential during stretching, as it helps relax muscles and increase the effectiveness of each stretch. Focus on taking deep, controlled breaths, especially during static and passive stretching.

4. **Avoid Overstretching**: Stretch only until you feel a gentle pull, not pain. Pushing beyond comfort can cause muscle strain or injury. Over time, your flexibility will improve naturally with consistent practice.

5. **Make Stretching a Habit**: Regular stretching is key to reaping its benefits. Aim to incorporate some form of stretching every day, even if it's just a few minutes in the morning or before bed.

6. **Use Props as Needed**: For passive stretches, use straps, yoga blocks, or cushions to support and deepen stretches without adding strain. This approach is particularly helpful in stretching exercises for beginners.

Enhancing Stretching with Natural Remedies

Stretching is even more beneficial when combined with natural methods to support muscle recovery and relaxation:

- **Aromatherapy**: Using essential oils like lavender or eucalyptus during stretching promotes relaxation. Lavender reduces muscle tension, while eucalyptus invigorates and improves focus. Add a few drops to a diffuser in your stretching space or use a diluted oil directly on sore muscles.

- **Warm Compresses**: Applying a warm compress or heating pad to tight muscles before stretching can enhance flexibility. The warmth increases blood flow to the muscles, reducing stiffness and easing movement.

- **Herbal Teas**: Consuming chamomile or ginger tea post-stretching helps reduce inflammation and promotes relaxation. Chamomile has soothing properties, while ginger aids in muscle recovery due to its anti-inflammatory benefits.

Sample Stretching Routine for a Balanced Program

Here's a sample routine to incorporate different stretching techniques effectively:

- **Warm-Up**: Start with 5-10 minutes of dynamic stretching, such as leg swings, arm circles, and torso twists, to prepare muscles for movement.

- **Workout-Specific Stretches**: Incorporate ballistic stretching carefully if you're doing high-energy activities. Otherwise, stick to dynamic and active stretching for balance and control.

- **Cooldown**: Use static and passive stretches to relax the muscles, focusing on areas worked during the session. Hold each stretch for at least 20-30 seconds.
- **Dedicated Flexibility Session**: Once a week, spend 20-30 minutes focusing on flexibility through a combination of PNF, passive, and active stretching.

The Importance of Hydration

Hydration is a fundamental aspect of health that influences nearly every system in the body. Water is often described as the "essence of life," and it's easy to see why: it accounts for about 60% of the adult human body and is involved in vital functions, including temperature regulation, joint lubrication, nutrient transport, and waste elimination. Adequate hydration supports physical performance, cognitive function, skin health, digestion, and detoxification, making it essential to well-being. Despite its importance, hydration is often overlooked, with many people living in a state of mild dehydration without realizing it. This section delves into why hydration matters, the risks of inadequate hydration, and practical tips to stay properly hydrated for optimal health.

The Role of Water in the Body

1. **Cellular Health and Function**: Water is essential for cellular processes. It acts as a medium where biochemical reactions occur, facilitates the transport of nutrients and oxygen into cells, and helps remove waste products. Cells rely on water to maintain their shape, structure, and function, and when hydration is insufficient, these processes are compromised, leading to fatigue, dizziness, and decreased cellular efficiency.

2. **Temperature Regulation**: One of the primary functions of water in the body is to regulate temperature. Through the process of sweating, the body releases heat, which is then evaporated to cool down the skin's surface. This cooling mechanism is critical during physical activity or exposure to high temperatures. Dehydration reduces the body's ability to sweat effectively, leading to an increased risk of overheating and, in severe cases, heat exhaustion or heatstroke.

3. **Joint Lubrication and Muscle Function**: Water is a key component of synovial fluid, which lubricates joints, reducing friction and enabling smooth movement. Proper hydration is essential for cushioning joints, which is especially important for

those with physically demanding lifestyles or activities. Additionally, muscles require water to contract effectively; even a small decrease in hydration can lead to muscle cramps, stiffness, and diminished physical performance.

4. **Digestive Health and Waste Elimination**: Water plays a crucial role in digestion, from saliva production in the mouth to moving waste through the intestines. It helps dissolve nutrients for absorption in the intestines and softens stools, facilitating regular bowel movements and preventing constipation. When hydration is inadequate, the body may struggle with waste elimination, leading to digestive issues such as constipation, bloating, and an increased risk of developing kidney stones.

5. **Nutrient Transport and Absorption**: Water is a primary component of blood, which transports nutrients, oxygen, and waste products throughout the body. Proper hydration maintains blood volume and promotes efficient circulation, ensuring that nutrients and oxygen reach cells efficiently. Inadequate hydration can lead to reduced blood volume, impacting nutrient delivery and causing cells to function less effectively.

6. **Cognitive Function and Mood Regulation**: Dehydration, even in mild forms, can have a significant impact on cognitive function. Studies have shown that hydration levels influence mood, memory, concentration, and reaction time. Dehydration can lead to irritability, fatigue, and a decrease in alertness. The brain requires adequate hydration to perform at its best, and a lack of water may contribute to feelings of stress and anxiety, impairing overall mental well-being.

Signs of Dehydration

Dehydration occurs when the body loses more water than it takes in. While severe dehydration has obvious symptoms, such as extreme thirst, rapid heartbeat, and confusion, mild dehydration often goes unnoticed. Common signs of dehydration include:

- Thirst: Thirst is the body's way of signaling a need for hydration, but it often only appears when mild dehydration is already present.

- Dark yellow urine: Urine color is a useful indicator of hydration. Pale, clear urine indicates adequate hydration, while dark yellow or amber-colored urine suggests dehydration.
- Dry skin and lips: Skin elasticity depends on hydration, and dry, flaky skin or chapped lips may indicate inadequate water intake.
- Fatigue: Dehydration causes the body to conserve energy, leading to feelings of tiredness and lethargy.
- Headaches: Dehydration can lead to decreased blood flow to the brain, causing headaches or migraines.
- Dizziness or light-headedness: Low hydration levels can lead to a drop in blood pressure, causing dizziness.

Being aware of these signs allows individuals to address dehydration early, preventing it from escalating into a more severe condition.

Hydration Needs and Factors That Influence Them

While the "8 cups of water a day" guideline is commonly cited, hydration needs vary based on individual factors, including age, weight, physical activity, climate, and health conditions.

1. **Physical Activity**: Those who engage in regular physical activity, especially high-intensity workouts or outdoor sports, require more water to compensate for fluid lost through sweat. Athletes often require additional hydration to replace not only water but also electrolytes lost during extended exercise sessions.

2. **Climate and Environment**: People living in hot or humid climates, or at high altitudes, lose more water through sweat and require additional hydration. Cold climates can also influence hydration needs, as cold air tends to be dry, leading to water loss through respiration.

3. **Health Conditions**: Certain health conditions, such as kidney disease, diabetes, or digestive disorders, can influence hydration needs. For example, individuals with diabetes may need more water to manage blood sugar levels, while those with kidney issues need to be mindful of their hydration to avoid strain on the kidneys.

4. **Age**: Children and older adults are at higher risk of dehydration. Children may not recognize or communicate thirst as effectively, while older adults may experience a diminished sense of thirst, requiring conscious efforts to stay hydrated.

5. **Pregnancy and Breastfeeding**: Pregnant and breastfeeding women have increased hydration needs to support fetal development and milk production. Proper hydration is essential for maternal and infant health during these periods.

Practical Tips for Staying Hydrated

1. **Drink Water Regularly Throughout the Day**: Rather than waiting until you feel thirsty, make it a habit to drink water consistently throughout the day. Carry a reusable water bottle as a reminder to stay hydrated.

2. **Infuse Water with Natural Flavors**: If plain water feels monotonous, try infusing it with fruits, herbs, or vegetables. Lemon, cucumber, mint, and berries can add a refreshing twist to water, making it more enjoyable to drink without added sugars or artificial flavors.

3. **Set Hydration Goals**: Set a daily water intake goal based on your activity level and environment. Tracking water intake using a journal or an app can help ensure you meet your hydration needs.

4. **Consume Hydrating Foods**: Fruits and vegetables with high water content, such as watermelon, cucumber, oranges, and strawberries, contribute to daily hydration needs. Soups and broths are also excellent choices for maintaining hydration.

5. **Monitor Urine Color**: Checking the color of your urine throughout the day provides immediate feedback on your hydration status. Aim for a pale yellow color, indicating adequate hydration.

6. **Avoid Excessive Caffeine and Alcohol**: Caffeinated and alcoholic beverages have a diuretic effect, leading to increased water loss. If consumed, balance these beverages with an equal amount of water to minimize dehydration.

7. **Hydrate Before, During, and After Exercise**: Hydrating before, during, and after physical activity helps replenish fluids lost through sweat and supports physical performance. During exercise, particularly intense or prolonged sessions, consider adding an electrolyte solution to maintain electrolyte balance.

8. **Listen to Your Body**: Trust your body's signals and respond to thirst. If you're feeling thirsty, don't ignore it; take it as a cue to hydrate.

Herbal Infusions for Hydration and Electrolyte Support

Herbal infusions can be a refreshing alternative to plain water and offer additional benefits. Some herbs provide not only hydration but also a source of natural electrolytes and antioxidants:

1. **Coconut Water**: Known as "nature's sports drink," coconut water is rich in potassium, magnesium, and other electrolytes, making it an excellent hydrating beverage. It is particularly beneficial after exercise or during warm weather, as it helps replenish electrolyte levels naturally.

2. **Lemon Balm and Mint Tea**: Lemon balm and mint are hydrating herbs with soothing properties. They can be brewed into a cooling infusion that hydrates while also aiding digestion and calming the mind.

3. **Hibiscus Tea**: Hibiscus is not only hydrating but also packed with antioxidants. Its tart flavor is refreshing and can be enjoyed cold, making it a great option for hot days. Hibiscus tea also supports cardiovascular health and helps regulate blood pressure.

4. **Ginger and Lemon Water**: Ginger provides warmth, while lemon offers vitamin C and antioxidants. This combination helps boost the immune system and supports digestion, all while keeping you hydrated.

5. **Aloe Vera Juice**: Aloe vera is hydrating and soothing, and it is particularly beneficial for digestive health. Adding a small amount of aloe vera juice to water or an herbal tea creates a hydrating, gut-friendly beverage.

Hydration Myths and Misconceptions

1. **Myth: Only Water Counts for Hydration**: While water is the most efficient hydrator, other beverages, such as herbal teas, milk, and even coffee in moderate amounts, can contribute to daily hydration. Foods high in water content, like fruits and vegetables, also play a role in keeping the body hydrated.

2. **Myth: Thirst Is the Best Indicator of Hydration**: Thirst is an indication of hydration needs, but it is not always reliable. Mild dehydration can occur before thirst is perceived, especially in older adults or those with high physical demands. Regular water intake throughout the day is a more effective strategy for staying hydrated.

3. **Myth: Clear Urine Indicates Perfect Hydration**: While pale yellow urine is ideal

Chapter 3: Nutrition for Fitness and Recovery

When it comes to optimizing physical performance and recovery, nutrition plays a pivotal role. Pre- and post-workout meals are essential in fueling the body, enhancing performance, and aiding in recovery.

Pre- and Post-Workout Nutrition

The right foods, consumed at the right times, can significantly affect energy levels, muscle repair, and overall endurance. This section explores the ideal foods, timing, and nutritional balance for pre- and post-workout nourishment, highlighting how simple yet strategic choices can lead to improved fitness outcomes.

The Importance of Pre-Workout Nutrition

Pre-workout nutrition serves the fundamental purpose of preparing the body for physical exertion by ensuring that there is adequate fuel for sustained energy and focus. When exercising, the body draws on glycogen reserves in the muscles for energy. A well-balanced pre-workout meal can help maximize glycogen stores, thereby supporting endurance and delaying fatigue.

Beyond glycogen, amino acids from protein sources are essential as they help maintain muscle integrity, reduce the risk of breakdown, and support muscle endurance. Proper hydration also comes into play here, as even mild dehydration can lead to fatigue and decreased performance.

Timing Pre-Workout Nutrition

When it comes to the timing of pre-workout meals, a common recommendation is to consume food approximately 2-3 hours before exercising. This allows ample time for digestion and ensures that nutrients are readily available for energy. For those who prefer a smaller snack closer to their workout, something light yet nutrient-dense 30-60 minutes prior can provide an energy boost without the discomfort of a full stomach.

If planning a substantial meal, aim for the following composition:

- **Carbohydrates**: Complex carbohydrates provide slow-releasing energy and maintain blood sugar stability.
- **Proteins**: A moderate amount of lean protein supports muscle protection.
- **Fats**: Include a small amount of healthy fats, as they provide a slow, steady energy source when digested along with carbohydrates.

For closer-to-workout snacks, opt for easy-to-digest items with a higher carbohydrate and protein content to deliver immediate energy and muscle protection.

Ideal Pre-Workout Foods

The foods selected before a workout should provide a balanced source of energy, aiding both performance and endurance. Here are some practical and effective pre-workout meal and snack options:

1. **Oatmeal with Fresh Fruit and Nuts**
   o Oatmeal is a rich source of complex carbohydrates and provides a steady release of energy. Add fresh fruit for natural sugars and vitamins, while nuts contribute a touch of healthy fat and protein.

2. **Banana with Almond Butter**
   o Bananas are an excellent source of fast-digesting carbohydrates and potassium, which supports muscle function. A small serving of almond butter adds protein and fat, creating a balanced snack that's easy on the stomach.

3. **Greek Yogurt with Berries and Honey**
   o Greek yogurt is high in protein, while berries offer antioxidants that help reduce exercise-induced inflammation. Honey adds natural sugars for an energy boost.

4. **Whole-Grain Toast with Avocado and a Boiled Egg**
   o Whole-grain toast provides complex carbohydrates, while avocado and a boiled egg offer healthy fats and protein. This combination sustains energy levels and reduces muscle breakdown.

5. **Smoothie with Spinach, Banana, and Protein Powder**
   o Blending spinach, banana, and protein powder creates a nutrient-rich, easy-to-digest option that provides essential carbohydrates, proteins, and minerals for sustained energy and hydration.

The Role of Hydration in Pre-Workout Nutrition

Hydration is crucial, as it supports muscle function, joint lubrication, and temperature regulation. Dehydration can lead to early fatigue, cramping, and impaired coordination, which are counterproductive to any workout goals. As a general guideline, drink around 16-20 ounces of water at least 2-3 hours before exercising, and another 8 ounces about 20-30 minutes before the workout.

Post-Workout Nutrition: Refueling and Recovery

Post-workout nutrition is essential to the recovery process, as it helps restore depleted glycogen, repairs muscle tissues, and reduces inflammation. This meal or snack should ideally be consumed within 30-60 minutes after exercise, as this is when muscles are most receptive to nutrient absorption, maximizing repair and growth.

The primary goals of post-workout nutrition are:

1. **Glycogen Replenishment**: Carbohydrates help replenish glycogen stores used during exercise.

2. **Muscle Repair and Growth**: Proteins provide essential amino acids necessary for muscle recovery and growth.

3. **Reducing Inflammation**: Foods with antioxidants and anti-inflammatory properties aid in reducing exercise-induced muscle damage.

Ideal Post-Workout Foods

A well-balanced post-workout meal includes a blend of carbohydrates and proteins, and potentially some healthy fats, which can further assist in reducing inflammation. Below are some effective options:

1. **Grilled Chicken with Quinoa and Steamed Vegetables**
   - Chicken offers a lean protein source, while quinoa provides complex carbs and essential amino acids. Steamed vegetables add fiber, vitamins, and minerals, supporting overall recovery.

2. **Protein Smoothie with Berries, Spinach, and Chia Seeds**
   - A smoothie is a convenient option that's easy to digest post-workout. The protein powder helps repair muscles, berries offer antioxidants, and chia seeds add fiber, omega-3 fatty acids, and protein.

3. **Scrambled Eggs with Whole-Grain Toast and Avocado**

o Eggs are a complete protein, containing all essential amino acids. Whole-grain toast provides slow-release carbohydrates, while avocado contributes healthy fats to support muscle recovery.

4. **Brown Rice with Black Beans and Vegetables**
   o Brown rice and black beans make a complete protein and carbohydrate meal that's rich in fiber, vitamins, and minerals, making it an excellent post-workout recovery option for sustained energy.

5. **Cottage Cheese with Pineapple and Walnuts**
   o Cottage cheese is high in casein protein, which is slowly digested and supports prolonged muscle recovery. Pineapple contains bromelain, an enzyme with anti-inflammatory effects, and walnuts add omega-3 fats.

Additional Natural Remedies for Enhanced Recovery

Incorporating certain natural remedies alongside post-workout nutrition can further aid in reducing soreness and inflammation, supporting faster recovery. Here are some options to consider:

- **Ginger Tea**: Ginger has anti-inflammatory properties that reduce muscle soreness. A cup of ginger tea post-exercise can help alleviate discomfort.
- **Turmeric Smoothie**: Adding turmeric to a post-workout smoothie provides curcumin, a compound that helps reduce inflammation and speeds up muscle recovery.
- **Tart Cherry Juice**: Tart cherry juice is known for its antioxidant properties and has been shown to reduce muscle pain and improve recovery time.
- **Herbal Muscle Rubs**: Applying a natural rub with arnica or peppermint oil can help ease muscle soreness, particularly after intense physical activity.

Practical Tips for Pre- and Post-Workout Nutrition

1. **Balance Macronutrients**: Both pre- and post-workout meals should balance carbohydrates and proteins, with small amounts of healthy fats to sustain energy without causing digestive issues.

2. **Incorporate Antioxidant-Rich Foods**: Foods high in antioxidants, such as berries, dark leafy greens, and nuts, can reduce oxidative stress caused by exercise and improve recovery.

3. **Hydrate Before and After**: Hydration is just as essential as food for muscle function and recovery. Aim to drink water before, during, and after a workout to maintain fluid balance.

4. **Avoid High-Fat Foods Before Exercise**: While fats are an important part of a balanced diet, consuming heavy, high-fat meals before exercise can slow digestion and lead to discomfort.

5. **Listen to Your Body**: Nutritional needs can vary based on the intensity of the workout and individual tolerance. Experiment with different foods and timings to find what best supports your energy levels and recovery.

Sample Pre- and Post-Workout Meal Plan

Pre-Workout (2-3 hours before)

- Oatmeal with banana, a handful of berries, and a sprinkle of almonds
- Hydrate with water or herbal tea

Pre-Workout Snack (30 minutes before)

- A small smoothie with spinach, a half-banana, and a scoop of protein powder
- 8 ounces of water

Post-Workout (within 30-60 minutes after)

- Grilled chicken with quinoa and a side of steamed vegetables
- Water with a slice of lemon or a glass of coconut water for added electrolytes

Evening Recovery Snack (if needed)

- Cottage cheese with pineapple and a few walnuts
- Herbal tea with ginger or chamomile for relaxation

Hydration and Electrolytes

Hydration is an essential component of health, impacting everything from energy levels to cognitive function and physical performance. While drinking enough water is a primary focus for hydration, maintaining the balance of electrolytes is equally important.

Electrolytes, such as sodium, potassium, calcium, and magnesium, play a crucial role in keeping the body's fluids balanced, supporting nerve function, and enabling muscles to contract effectively. In this section, we'll explore the relationship between hydration and electrolytes, how the two work together to support overall wellness, and practical tips for ensuring adequate electrolyte balance in your daily hydration routine.

The Role of Electrolytes in Hydration

1. **Sodium**: Sodium is one of the primary electrolytes responsible for fluid balance in the body. It works with potassium to regulate the amount of water inside and outside of cells, enabling cells to function optimally. Sodium is essential for maintaining blood pressure and ensuring that nerves and muscles work correctly. Without enough sodium, dehydration symptoms such as confusion, fatigue, and muscle weakness can develop, even if water intake is sufficient.

2. **Potassium**: Potassium is crucial for maintaining cellular fluid balance, particularly in collaboration with sodium. It helps control nerve signals and muscle contractions, including the regulation of the heartbeat. Potassium plays a role in maintaining the body's pH balance and blood pressure. Without enough potassium, individuals may experience muscle cramps, weakness, and irregular heart rhythms, often exacerbated by physical activity.

3. **Calcium**: While often associated with bone health, calcium also functions as an electrolyte. It is involved in muscle contractions and nerve transmission, working to ensure that muscles contract and relax smoothly. Calcium is vital in preventing muscle spasms, particularly during exercise when calcium loss can be higher due to sweating.

4. **Magnesium**: Magnesium is known for its role in over 300 biochemical reactions in the body, including the regulation of muscle and nerve function, blood sugar levels, and blood pressure. Magnesium acts as a stabilizer for many enzymatic activities, promoting muscle relaxation and preventing cramps. Low levels of magnesium can lead to fatigue, muscle cramps, and irritability, especially under stress.

The Importance of Electrolyte Balance in Daily Hydration

The balance of electrolytes is essential for hydration to be effective. Simply drinking water without adequate electrolyte intake can lead to an imbalance, particularly if large amounts of water are consumed over a short period. Electrolytes help maintain the right osmotic balance, preventing the cells from becoming overly diluted with water or, conversely, too concentrated with electrolytes.

1. **Preventing Hyponatremia**: Hyponatremia occurs when sodium levels in the blood become dangerously low, often due to drinking excessive amounts of water without adequate sodium intake. This condition causes water to move into cells, leading to swelling. For brain cells, in particular, this can result in confusion, nausea, and, in severe cases, seizures. Consuming beverages that contain a balanced amount of electrolytes, especially in hot weather or during intense physical activities, can prevent this condition.

2. **Regulating Blood Pressure and Fluid Balance**: Sodium and potassium work together to manage blood pressure. When sodium levels are high, they retain water, which increases blood volume and, consequently, blood pressure. Potassium balances sodium's effect by helping to remove excess water through urination. Proper hydration with electrolyte balance supports stable blood pressure levels.

3. **Enhancing Physical Performance**: Electrolytes are particularly important for those who are physically active. During exercise, the body loses water and electrolytes through sweat. Without replenishing electrolytes, muscle function can diminish, leading to cramping and fatigue. Proper electrolyte balance during and after physical activity can help maintain performance and reduce muscle soreness.

4. **Supporting Cognitive and Mood Stability**: Dehydration and electrolyte imbalance can impact cognitive function, leading to confusion, irritability, and reduced concentration. Potassium and magnesium, in particular, support the nervous system, stabilizing mood and aiding in clear thinking. Proper electrolyte intake can help sustain mental clarity and emotional well-being.

Recognizing Electrolyte Imbalance Symptoms

Electrolyte imbalances can occur due to inadequate intake, excessive sweating, illness, or prolonged physical activity without proper hydration. Recognizing the symptoms of imbalance can help individuals address the issue before it worsens:

- **Muscle cramps and spasms**: Low levels of potassium, calcium, or magnesium often lead to muscle cramps, particularly in the legs.

- **Fatigue and weakness**: Electrolyte imbalances can lead to overall fatigue, even if hydration seems adequate.
- **Dizziness and headaches**: Low sodium or potassium can result in light-headedness and headaches, especially when standing up.
- **Heart palpitations or irregular heartbeat**: Electrolytes play a role in maintaining a stable heart rhythm; imbalances may result in an irregular heartbeat.
- **Confusion or irritability**: Electrolyte depletion, particularly of sodium and magnesium, can affect mental clarity and mood, leading to confusion, irritability, or difficulty focusing.

Sources of Electrolytes in Food and Beverages

Electrolytes are naturally found in many foods and beverages, and a well-rounded diet can typically meet daily needs. For those with increased needs due to physical activity or heat exposure, specific foods and drinks can help replenish electrolytes.

1. **Bananas**: Known for their potassium content, bananas are a great source of this electrolyte, making them ideal for post-workout snacks to prevent cramps.
2. **Coconut Water**: Often called "nature's sports drink," coconut water provides potassium, magnesium, and calcium, making it a refreshing option for rehydration after exercise.
3. **Leafy Greens**: Spinach, kale, and other leafy greens contain magnesium and potassium, supporting hydration and muscle relaxation.
4. **Avocados**: Avocados are rich in potassium and magnesium, supporting heart health, hydration, and muscle recovery.
5. **Dairy Products**: Milk, yogurt, and cheese are high in calcium and can be beneficial for hydration, especially after exercise, helping to prevent muscle cramps.
6. **Salted Nuts and Seeds**: Nuts and seeds provide magnesium and potassium, while adding a small amount of salt can ensure a balanced sodium intake.
7. **Watermelon and Cantaloupe**: These fruits are hydrating due to their high water content and also contain potassium and magnesium.
8. **Broths and Soups**: Bone broths and soups are hydrating options rich in sodium, potassium, and other electrolytes, making them excellent for post-exercise recovery.

Hydration Strategies for Maintaining Electrolyte Balance

1. **Drink Electrolyte-Enhanced Water During Physical Activity**: For those engaging in prolonged or intense physical activities, drinking electrolyte-enhanced water can prevent depletion. Choose beverages with natural electrolytes, avoiding those high in added sugars.

2. **Include a Variety of Electrolyte-Rich Foods in Your Diet**: Relying on food sources to meet electrolyte needs can be effective. Incorporate fruits, vegetables, nuts, and dairy products to ensure balanced intake.

3. **Use Electrolyte Tablets or Powders When Needed**: Electrolyte tablets or powders can be added to water to boost electrolyte levels, especially for those in high-heat environments or engaging in long-duration exercise. Ensure that these supplements are free of artificial additives and excessive sugars.

4. **Listen to Your Body's Cues**: Pay attention to signs of electrolyte imbalance, such as muscle cramps or light-headedness. Adjust hydration practices based on physical activity level, climate, and personal needs.

5. **Balance Water Intake with Electrolytes**: Drinking large amounts of plain water without electrolytes can dilute sodium levels in the blood, leading to hyponatremia. This is particularly important for athletes or those exposed to hot climates. In such cases, drinking water with a balanced electrolyte content is essential.

6. **Monitor Salt Intake Carefully**: While sodium is essential, it's easy to consume too much in modern diets. Balance sodium intake by choosing natural sources and minimizing processed foods, which are often high in added salt.

Electrolyte Myths and Misunderstandings

1. **Myth: All Electrolyte Drinks Are Healthy**: Many commercial electrolyte drinks are loaded with sugars and artificial ingredients. Opt for natural options like coconut water, or use unsweetened electrolyte tablets, especially if consuming these drinks regularly.

2. **Myth: You Only Need Electrolytes After Intense Exercise**: While exercise increases electrolyte needs, factors like high temperatures, illness, or dietary imbalances can also necessitate additional electrolytes. Staying mindful of electrolyte intake during any period of increased physical or environmental stress is beneficial.

3. **Myth: Salt Alone Can Restore Electrolyte Balance**: While salt provides sodium, electrolyte balance requires other minerals, such as potassium, magnesium,

and calcium. Focusing solely on sodium can lead to an imbalance and exacerbate hydration issues.

4. **Myth: Drinking Lots of Water is the Best Hydration Strategy**: Over-hydration without electrolytes can lead to diluted blood sodium levels. Effective hydration combines both water and electrolyte intake, especially under conditions where sweating or water loss is high.

The Role of Herbal Infusions in Electrolyte Support

Certain herbal infusions can provide natural electrolyte support while also offering other health benefits. These infusions are easy to prepare and can be a valuable addition to your hydration routine:

1. **Nettle Tea**: Nettle is rich in minerals like potassium and magnesium, making it a beneficial tea for maintaining electrolyte balance. It also supports kidney function, which helps in the elimination of waste while maintaining fluid levels.

2. **Hibiscus and Lemon Balm Tea**: Hibiscus provides natural antioxidants, while lemon balm offers mild hydration support and can help with relaxation. Together, they make a refreshing, mildly hydrating infusion.

3. **Lemon and Ginger Water**: Lemon offers vitamin C and potassium, while ginger provides a gentle warming effect, making this infusion beneficial for cold environments. Ginger can also help with digestion, enhancing the overall benefit of hydration.

4. **Aloe Vera Juice**: Small amounts of aloe vera juice in water can aid hydration, as it is naturally rich in minerals. Be cautious with dosage, as too much aloe can have a laxative effect.

Incorporating a mix of electrolyte-rich foods, balanced hydration practices, and herbal infusions can help maintain optimal hydration and electrolyte levels, supporting energy, cognitive function, and physical health. Proper electrolyte balance is crucial for anyone looking to enhance their overall health and well-being, and focusing on natural, whole food sources can provide sustained support throughout the day.

Foods Rich in Electrolytes

Electrolytes are essential minerals that carry an electric charge, enabling vital physiological processes such as muscle contraction, fluid balance, and nerve function. The body loses electrolytes through sweat and other metabolic processes, particularly during physical activity, hot weather, or illness. This makes it essential to replenish these minerals through diet to prevent dehydration, muscle cramps, and overall fatigue. Understanding foods rich in electrolytes can empower you to maintain optimal health and energy levels naturally.

Understanding Electrolytes and Their Functions

The key electrolytes in the body include sodium, potassium, calcium, magnesium, chloride, bicarbonate, and phosphate. Each plays a unique role in maintaining cellular functions and fluid balance. Here's a closer look at these primary electrolytes and their physiological functions:

1. **Sodium**: Maintains fluid balance and aids in nerve and muscle function. Found abundantly in extracellular fluids, sodium is crucial for hydration and cellular function.

2. **Potassium**: Works closely with sodium to support cellular fluid balance and is vital for muscle contraction and nerve transmission.

3. **Calcium**: Known for its role in bone health, calcium also plays a role in muscle contraction, nerve signaling, and blood clotting.

4. **Magnesium**: Supports over 300 enzymatic reactions, including muscle function, nerve function, and protein synthesis. It also helps regulate blood pressure.

5. **Chloride**: Often paired with sodium in salt, chloride aids in maintaining a proper fluid balance and is essential for digestion.

6. **Phosphate**: Crucial for cellular energy production and bone health. Phosphate is a component of ATP, the energy molecule in cells.

7. **Bicarbonate**: Maintains the body's pH balance, which is critical for normal cellular function.

A diet rich in electrolyte-containing foods helps replenish these essential minerals and supports overall health and vitality. Below are various foods categorized by their dominant electrolyte to guide you in making well-rounded, electrolyte-rich dietary choices.

Sodium-Rich Foods

Sodium is commonly associated with table salt, but many whole foods provide this electrolyte naturally. The key is to consume sodium in balanced amounts, as excessive sodium intake can lead to high blood pressure and other health issues.

- **Celery**: This crunchy vegetable provides a mild source of sodium and is also rich in water content, aiding hydration.
- **Beets**: Not only are beets a good source of sodium, but they also contain nitrates, which help improve blood flow.
- **Carrots**: While primarily recognized for their vitamin A content, carrots also contribute a small but beneficial amount of sodium.
- **Spinach**: This leafy green provides sodium alongside potassium and magnesium, making it an excellent choice for electrolyte replenishment.

Adding a pinch of sea salt to homemade dishes can also boost sodium intake in moderation while adding trace minerals like iodine.

Potassium-Rich Foods

Potassium is essential for muscle health, blood pressure regulation, and heart health. It counteracts sodium and helps prevent muscle cramps, especially in active individuals.

- **Bananas**: Known as a top source of potassium, bananas are convenient and easy to incorporate into various meals.
- **Avocados**: Avocados offer high potassium content and healthy fats, making them a great addition to meals and snacks.
- **Sweet Potatoes**: These tubers are packed with potassium, vitamins A and C, and fiber, which support energy and digestive health.
- **Tomatoes**: Fresh tomatoes and tomato products provide potassium and antioxidants like lycopene, beneficial for heart health.
- **Oranges**: These citrus fruits provide potassium, vitamin C, and natural sugars, making them ideal for hydration and energy.
- **Spinach and Swiss Chard**: Both leafy greens are potassium-dense and contain magnesium, supporting muscle and heart health.

Calcium-Rich Foods

Calcium is known for its role in maintaining bone density, but it also plays a role in heart rhythm regulation, muscle function, and neurotransmission. Here are foods high in calcium:

- **Dairy Products**: Milk, cheese, and yogurt are primary sources of calcium, offering easily absorbable forms of this mineral.
- **Leafy Greens**: Kale, bok choy, and collard greens are high in calcium and provide additional fiber and vitamins.
- **Broccoli and Brussels Sprouts**: These cruciferous vegetables contain a moderate amount of calcium and are beneficial for overall health.
- **Sardines and Canned Salmon**: These fish contain bones that are rich in calcium and are also high in omega-3 fatty acids.
- **Almonds**: A handful of almonds provides calcium along with healthy fats and magnesium, supporting heart health and energy.

Magnesium-Rich Foods

Magnesium plays a crucial role in muscle and nerve function, energy production, and blood pressure regulation. It's often referred to as the "relaxation mineral" due to its calming effect on muscles and nerves.

- **Pumpkin Seeds**: One of the richest sources of magnesium, pumpkin seeds also provide zinc, which supports immune function.
- **Dark Chocolate**: Besides its high magnesium content, dark chocolate contains antioxidants that benefit heart health.
- **Legumes**: Beans, lentils, and chickpeas are high in magnesium and fiber, making them excellent for heart and digestive health.
- **Whole Grains**: Quinoa, brown rice, and oats are rich in magnesium, which supports muscle relaxation and overall energy.
- **Leafy Greens**: Spinach, Swiss chard, and kale are high in magnesium and other essential nutrients, ideal for overall wellness.

Chloride-Rich Foods

Chloride helps maintain fluid balance and is often consumed alongside sodium as part of table salt. However, certain whole foods also provide this essential electrolyte.

- **Seaweed**: Besides being high in iodine, seaweed provides chloride and other minerals beneficial for thyroid and cellular health.
- **Celery and Olives**: These are natural sources of chloride that can help support electrolyte balance in a healthy diet.

- **Rye Bread**: This type of bread provides chloride and other minerals, adding diversity to grain choices.

Phosphate-Rich Foods

Phosphate is critical for energy production and bone health. Many foods rich in protein are also good sources of phosphate.

- **Meat and Poultry**: Chicken, turkey, and pork contain high levels of phosphate essential for cellular energy.
- **Eggs**: Not only are eggs a source of complete protein, but they also provide phosphorus needed for bone and cellular health.
- **Whole Grains**: Barley, oats, and brown rice are rich in phosphorus and fiber, supporting digestive and cardiovascular health.
- **Nuts and Seeds**: Almonds, chia seeds, and sunflower seeds provide phosphorus alongside magnesium and healthy fats.

Bicarbonate and pH-Balancing Foods

Bicarbonate is naturally produced by the body to maintain pH balance, but certain foods help maintain this balance, promoting better metabolic function.

- **Green Leafy Vegetables**: Spinach, kale, and other greens help promote alkalinity in the body, aiding in pH balance.
- **Lemons and Limes**: Despite their acidic nature, they have an alkalizing effect once metabolized, supporting overall pH balance.
- **Apples and Pears**: These fruits contain natural bicarbonate precursors, which help balance the body's pH levels.

Natural Sources of Electrolyte-Rich Beverages

For those who prefer beverages, certain natural drinks provide electrolytes while hydrating the body:

1. **Coconut Water**: Known as nature's sports drink, coconut water is rich in potassium, sodium, and magnesium, making it ideal for hydration.
2. **Herbal Teas**: Teas made from nettle, dandelion, and chamomile offer trace electrolytes and have mild diuretic properties, supporting fluid balance.
3. **Lemon Water with a Pinch of Salt**: Adding lemon and a pinch of salt to water provides a simple, homemade electrolyte drink that helps with rehydration and electrolyte replenishment.

Practical Tips for Incorporating Electrolyte-Rich Foods

1. **Include a Variety of Vegetables**: Opt for a colorful range of vegetables, such as leafy greens, carrots, tomatoes, and beets, which collectively provide a balance of electrolytes.

2. **Add Fruits High in Potassium**: Bananas, oranges, and melons are easy to incorporate into smoothies, salads, or as standalone snacks for potassium and fluid balance.

3. **Snack on Nuts and Seeds**: Almonds, sunflower seeds, and pumpkin seeds provide magnesium, calcium, and phosphorus, making them an ideal snack for electrolyte balance.

4. **Use Dairy or Alternatives**: Milk, yogurt, and cheese are excellent sources of calcium and phosphorus. For those who prefer dairy-free options, fortified plant-based milks offer similar benefits.

5. **Opt for Whole Grains**: Whole grains like quinoa, brown rice, and oats provide magnesium, potassium, and phosphorus, which aid in energy and fluid regulation.

Sample Meal Plan for Electrolyte Balance

Breakfast: Greek yogurt with fresh berries, chia seeds, and a sprinkle of almonds
- **Electrolytes**: Potassium, calcium, and magnesium

Lunch: Spinach and kale salad with tomatoes, carrots, avocado, and a sprinkle of pumpkin seeds
- **Electrolytes**: Potassium, magnesium, and sodium

Snack: Smoothie with banana, spinach, coconut water, and a touch of honey
- **Electrolytes**: Potassium, magnesium, and natural sugars for energy

Dinner: Grilled salmon with quinoa, steamed broccoli, and a side of roasted sweet potatoes
- **Electrolytes**: Potassium, calcium, phosphorus, and magnesium

By incorporating a variety of these electrolyte-rich foods into your diet, you can maintain optimal hydration, energy, and overall health naturally.

Chapter 4: Fitness Recovery Herbal Recipes

A rnica, derived from the flowering plant *Arnica montana*, has been a staple in natural medicine for centuries, renowned for its ability to relieve pain, reduce inflammation, and expedite the healing process for bruises and sprains.

Arnica Muscle Rub

An arnica muscle rub, when applied topically, can help alleviate muscle soreness, stiffness, and minor injuries, making it a valuable remedy for athletes, those recovering from physical strain, and anyone experiencing muscular discomfort. In this section, we'll explore the benefits, uses, and methods of creating an effective arnica muscle rub, as well as the science behind its powerful effects.

Understanding Arnica: The Basics

Arnica belongs to the daisy family (*Asteraceae*) and is primarily grown in Europe and Siberia, thriving in mountain regions. Its bright yellow flowers are harvested for medicinal use, and the compounds within arnica are known to contain numerous beneficial properties for pain relief and healing. The active ingredients in arnica include sesquiterpene lactones, helenalin, flavonoids, and essential oils, each playing a role in reducing inflammation and improving circulation in affected areas.

1. **Helenalin**: Helenalin is the primary anti-inflammatory compound in arnica. It inhibits inflammatory enzymes, which helps reduce swelling and pain in muscle tissue. While powerful, helenalin can also be toxic if ingested, which is why arnica is strictly for topical use.

2. **Flavonoids**: These antioxidants combat oxidative stress within muscle tissues, promoting cell repair and helping muscles recover after exercise or injury. The presence of flavonoids in arnica enhances its ability to soothe and repair muscle tissue.

3. **Essential Oils**: Arnica contains a variety of essential oils that provide its distinctive scent and contribute to its soothing effects. These oils help in reducing discomfort and promoting relaxation when massaged into the skin.

The Benefits of Using Arnica Muscle Rub

Arnica muscle rubs offer a range of benefits for muscle recovery and pain management. Whether dealing with sore muscles from a workout, a minor injury, or general aches and pains, arnica's anti-inflammatory and analgesic properties can provide relief naturally and effectively.

1. **Pain Relief**: Arnica's ability to reduce inflammation directly affects the perception of pain in muscles and joints. When applied as a muscle rub, arnica's compounds work to numb the pain, offering natural relief without the need for pharmaceuticals.

2. **Reduced Inflammation**: Inflammation is the body's response to injury, and while it is part of the healing process, excessive inflammation can lead to prolonged pain and stiffness. Arnica inhibits inflammatory markers, helping the body control the inflammation process for faster recovery.

3. **Improved Circulation**: Arnica promotes blood flow to the affected area, which is crucial for healing. Improved circulation ensures that nutrients and oxygen reach damaged tissues more efficiently, aiding in quicker recovery and reducing the buildup of lactic acid, which can cause muscle soreness.

4. **Alleviates Bruising and Swelling**: Arnica's compounds are particularly effective at reducing bruising by speeding up the reabsorption of blood in bruised tissues. This is especially beneficial for individuals who experience frequent bruising or minor muscle injuries.

5. **Prevention of Muscle Stiffness**: For those who engage in regular physical activity, arnica muscle rub can help prevent stiffness by relaxing muscles and reducing the tension that leads to soreness. Using arnica rub as a post-workout treatment can help muscles recover faster and stay flexible.

Preparing Your Own Arnica Muscle Rub

Creating a homemade arnica muscle rub allows you to control the ingredients and customize the blend according to your needs. Here's a step-by-step guide on how to prepare a simple, effective arnica rub at home.

Ingredients

1. **Arnica Oil**: The primary ingredient, arnica oil, can be made by infusing dried arnica flowers in a carrier oil. Alternatively, pre-made arnica oil is available in most health stores.

2. **Carrier Oil**: A neutral oil like olive oil, coconut oil, or jojoba oil works well as a base for the rub. Coconut oil, in particular, has anti-inflammatory properties and solidifies at room temperature, making it ideal for a muscle rub.

3. **Beeswax**: Beeswax adds thickness to the rub, creating a balm-like consistency that is easy to apply.

4. **Essential Oils**: Essential oils like peppermint, eucalyptus, and lavender add cooling and soothing effects, enhancing the muscle rub's pain-relieving properties.

5. **Vitamin E Oil**: Adding a few drops of vitamin E oil helps extend the shelf life of the muscle rub while providing additional skin benefits.

Instructions

1. **Prepare the Arnica Infusion**: If making your own arnica oil, place dried arnica flowers in a clean jar and cover them with your chosen carrier oil. Let this mixture infuse for two weeks, shaking it occasionally to help release the active compounds from the flowers.

2. **Strain the Oil**: Once infused, strain the oil through a cheesecloth or fine strainer to remove the arnica flowers.

3. **Melt the Beeswax**: In a double boiler, melt the beeswax until it becomes liquid. Beeswax provides the thick consistency and stability to the rub, ensuring it stays solid at room temperature.

4. **Combine Ingredients**: Add the arnica-infused oil to the melted beeswax, stirring well. Add a few drops of essential oils and vitamin E oil, then mix until fully incorporated.

5. **Pour into Containers**: Transfer the mixture into clean, airtight containers and let it cool. Once solidified, your arnica muscle rub is ready for use.

Application Techniques and Tips

1. **Massage Gently**: Apply a small amount of arnica rub to the affected area and massage it gently. Allow the rub to absorb fully into the skin, which may take a few minutes. Massaging helps improve circulation and enhances the absorption of arnica's active compounds.

2. **Frequency of Use**: For best results, apply the arnica muscle rub two to three times per day. After intense physical activity or if dealing with muscle soreness, apply the rub immediately after a warm bath or shower to maximize absorption.

3. **Avoid Broken Skin**: Arnica should not be applied to broken or irritated skin, as it can cause further irritation. Ensure that the application area is free of cuts or abrasions.

4. **Store Properly**: To maintain the potency of your arnica rub, store it in a cool, dark place. Proper storage ensures that the oils and active ingredients remain effective for several months.

Practical Scenarios for Using Arnica Muscle Rub

1. **After Workouts or Physical Activity**: If you regularly engage in high-intensity workouts or endurance activities, applying arnica rub post-exercise can reduce the likelihood of delayed onset muscle soreness (DOMS). For example, marathon runners often experience soreness and inflammation that arnica can help alleviate, enabling them to recover faster.

2. **For Desk Workers**: Muscle stiffness and discomfort aren't limited to athletes. Those who spend long hours at a desk can also benefit from arnica rub, particularly for neck, shoulder, and back tension. Apply a small amount of arnica rub to these areas after a workday to relieve tightness.

3. **For Minor Injuries and Bruises**: Arnica rub is ideal for minor muscle strains, sprains, and bruises that result from everyday activities. For instance, if you accidentally bump your leg and develop a bruise, applying arnica rub can help reduce the discoloration and speed up healing.

4. **Pre-Bed Relaxation Routine**: For individuals who struggle with muscle tightness that disrupts sleep, a pre-bed arnica rub routine can relax muscles and promote better rest. By massaging sore areas before bedtime, you can create a soothing ritual that helps you unwind and prepare for a restful night.

Safety Considerations

While arnica is effective when used correctly, it's important to be mindful of the following safety considerations:

1. **External Use Only**: Arnica is not safe for internal use due to the risk of toxicity. Ingesting arnica can cause severe side effects, including nausea and irregular heart rhythms. Always use arnica externally and keep it out of reach of children.

2. **Allergic Reactions**: People with allergies to plants in the Asteraceae family, such as daisies, chrysanthemums, or marigolds, may also be sensitive to arnica. Conduct a patch test before using the rub extensively. Apply a small amount on the forearm and wait 24 hours to check for any adverse reactions.

3. **Avoid Prolonged Use on Large Areas**: Arnica should be used sparingly and not applied over large areas for extended periods. While it is effective for targeted pain relief, excessive use may cause skin irritation or other side effects.

4. **Pregnancy and Breastfeeding**: Consult a healthcare provider before using arnica during pregnancy or breastfeeding, as the effects on these groups have not been extensively studied.

Additional Ingredients to Enhance the Arnica Rub

For those looking to customize their arnica rub, here are some additional ingredients that can provide added benefits:

1. **Comfrey**: Known for its cell-regenerative properties, comfrey root or leaf can be infused with arnica for a stronger muscle recovery rub. Comfrey helps repair tissues and reduce inflammation, making it an excellent addition for muscle and joint pain.

2. **Menthol Crystals**: Adding a small amount of menthol crystals can create a cooling effect, which provides immediate relief for sore muscles. Menthol also helps improve blood flow and can make the arnica rub feel refreshing.

3. **Turmeric Powder**: Turmeric's anti-inflammatory properties make it a powerful addition to muscle rubs. Its active compound, curcumin, enhances the pain-relieving effects of arnica while providing a warm sensation.

4. **Ginger Oil**: Ginger oil warms muscles and encourages relaxation, pairing well with arnica's properties for a deeper sense of relief. Ginger is especially beneficial for sore joints and muscles that feel cold and tense.

Creating an arnica muscle rub at home offers a personalized and natural solution for managing muscle soreness, stiffness, and minor injuries.

Nettle, known scientifically as *Urtica dioica*, has a long-standing history as a valuable medicinal herb in various traditional healing practices, particularly for its revitalizing effects on health. A nettle infusion, which involves steeping dried nettle leaves in hot water over an extended period, unlocks a range of benefits, providing the body with a concentrated dose of vitamins, minerals, and other beneficial compounds.

Understanding the Nutritional Value of Nettle

Nettle leaves are incredibly nutrient-dense, and when prepared as an infusion, they deliver essential minerals and vitamins that support various body systems:

1. **Vitamins**: Nettle is rich in vitamins A, C, K, and several B vitamins. Vitamin C enhances immune function and aids iron absorption, while vitamin K plays a role in blood clotting and bone health. The B vitamins support energy production and stress management.

2. **Minerals**: Nettle is especially high in minerals like iron, calcium, magnesium, potassium, and silica. Iron is essential for red blood cell production, while calcium and magnesium are critical for bone health and muscle relaxation. Potassium contributes to proper fluid balance, and silica strengthens connective tissues, including skin, hair, and nails.

3. **Phytonutrients**: Nettle leaves contain chlorophyll, which is known for its detoxifying properties, and flavonoids that provide antioxidant support. This helps reduce oxidative stress in the body, which contributes to cellular aging and disease.

Preparing a Nettle Infusion

Making a nettle infusion is a straightforward process, but it requires time to allow the nutrients to fully release into the water. Here's a simple method to prepare it:

1. **Ingredients**:
   o 1 ounce (about 28 grams) of dried nettle leaves
   o 1 quart (4 cups) of boiling water

2. **Instructions**:
   o Place the dried nettle leaves into a quart-sized jar.
   o Pour the boiling water over the leaves, filling the jar to the top.

- Cover the jar with a lid and let it steep for 4 to 8 hours or overnight.
- Strain the liquid into another container, pressing out as much liquid as possible from the nettle leaves.
- Store the infusion in the refrigerator and drink 1 to 2 cups daily.

The extended steeping time allows the nettle leaves to release a significant amount of minerals and other beneficial compounds, resulting in a deeply nourishing infusion.

Health Benefits of Nettle Infusion

1. Supports Iron Levels and Blood Health

Nettle is an excellent plant-based source of iron, which is essential for the production of hemoglobin—a protein in red blood cells responsible for carrying oxygen throughout the body. Low iron levels can lead to fatigue, weakness, and anemia. Nettle also contains vitamin C, which enhances the absorption of non-heme iron (the type found in plants), making it especially beneficial for those looking to increase their iron levels naturally.

For individuals who experience heavy menstruation, nettle infusion can help replenish iron levels lost during the menstrual cycle. It may also be beneficial for vegetarians and vegans, who might find it challenging to consume sufficient iron from their diet alone.

2. Bone Health and Mineral Density

The high calcium and magnesium content in nettle makes it a supportive ally for bone health. Calcium is critical for bone density, while magnesium aids in the proper absorption of calcium into the bones. Additionally, the presence of vitamin K in nettle contributes to bone health, as it plays a role in bone mineralization and the maintenance of bone structure.

Regular consumption of nettle infusion can help maintain healthy bones, particularly for individuals at risk of osteoporosis or those seeking to support their musculoskeletal health naturally.

3. Anti-Inflammatory and Joint Health

Nettle has been used in herbal medicine to reduce inflammation, particularly for those suffering from arthritis or other joint-related issues. The plant contains anti-inflammatory compounds, such as flavonoids and quercetin, which help reduce the production of inflammatory cytokines in the body.

Some people with arthritis report relief from joint pain and swelling after incorporating nettle into their diet, especially when combined with other lifestyle practices, like a nutrient-dense diet and regular physical activity. The calcium and magnesium in nettle also aid in reducing muscle cramps and promoting overall relaxation.

4. Promotes Kidney and Urinary Health

Nettle is a natural diuretic, which means it helps the body eliminate excess water and flush out toxins through urine. This makes nettle infusion an excellent choice for supporting kidney function and urinary tract health. Regular consumption can aid in preventing urinary tract infections (UTIs) by promoting regular urination and flushing out bacteria.

Its mild diuretic effect is beneficial for individuals who experience bloating or water retention, as it encourages the excretion of excess fluids. Additionally, nettle's anti-inflammatory properties may help reduce discomfort associated with urinary tract inflammation.

5. Skin Health and Radiance

Rich in antioxidants and chlorophyll, nettle infusion can support skin health by reducing oxidative stress and providing nutrients that promote collagen production. Chlorophyll has detoxifying properties, which help cleanse the body from the inside, promoting clearer and more radiant skin.

Silica, another component found in nettle, is essential for maintaining the elasticity and strength of the skin. Regular consumption of nettle infusion may also benefit individuals with eczema, acne, or other skin conditions, as it helps reduce inflammation and redness.

6. Enhanced Hair Growth and Strength

Nettle has been traditionally used to support hair growth and prevent hair loss. The minerals in nettle, particularly iron and silica, strengthen hair follicles, which can lead to improved hair texture and reduced hair fall. Silica contributes to hair shine and resilience, while iron helps prevent hair thinning associated with iron deficiency.

In addition to drinking nettle infusion, some individuals use nettle-infused water as a hair rinse to promote scalp health and nourish the hair shaft directly.

7. Immune System Support

Nettle infusion provides several nutrients, such as vitamin C, which enhances immune function and helps the body defend itself against infections. Vitamin C also supports the production of white blood cells, which play a crucial role in the immune response.

The flavonoids in nettle also provide antioxidant protection, helping to shield the immune system from oxidative damage caused by environmental factors and stress. Consistent consumption of nettle infusion can contribute to a more resilient immune system, particularly during colder months or periods of increased stress.

Practical Tips for Incorporating Nettle Infusion

To maximize the benefits of nettle infusion, consider the following practical tips:

- **Begin with Small Amounts**: If you are new to nettle infusion, start with a small amount and gradually increase your intake to allow your body to adjust.
- **Combine with Other Herbal Infusions**: Nettle pairs well with other nutrient-rich herbs like red raspberry leaf and oat straw, which also support overall wellness.
- **Use Nettle Infusion as a Base for Smoothies**: Instead of plain water, use nettle infusion in your morning smoothie for an added nutritional boost.
- **Flavoring the Infusion**: Nettle has an earthy flavor, which some people find strong. Adding a splash of lemon juice or a bit of honey can improve the taste and make it more enjoyable.

Precautions and Considerations

Although nettle infusion is generally safe, certain precautions should be kept in mind:

1. **Pregnancy and Breastfeeding**: While nettle infusion is often considered safe during pregnancy and lactation, it's best to consult with a healthcare provider to determine the appropriate amount and frequency.
2. **Kidney Issues**: Since nettle is a diuretic, those with kidney conditions or fluid restrictions should consult a healthcare professional before consuming it regularly.
3. **Medication Interactions**: Nettle can interact with medications like blood thinners, diuretics, and blood pressure medications. If you are taking any of these, discuss nettle infusion with your healthcare provider.

Sourcing Quality Nettle for Infusion

To ensure you're getting the most from your nettle infusion, it's essential to use high-quality dried nettle leaves:

- **Look for Organic**: Choose organic dried nettle leaves to avoid pesticide residues and ensure the highest nutrient quality.
- **Purchase from Reputable Sources**: Purchase dried nettle leaves from trusted herbal suppliers who test their products for contaminants.

- **Harvesting Your Own**: If you have access to fresh nettles, you can harvest them yourself. Be sure to wear gloves, as the tiny hairs on fresh nettle leaves can sting. Once dried or infused, however, the stinging property is neutralized.

Incorporating nettle infusion into your daily routine can be a powerful way to enhance overall well-being, supporting energy, skin, immunity, and even hair health. The ritual of preparing and drinking nettle infusion also promotes mindfulness, as it connects you to the natural world and the healing properties of plants.

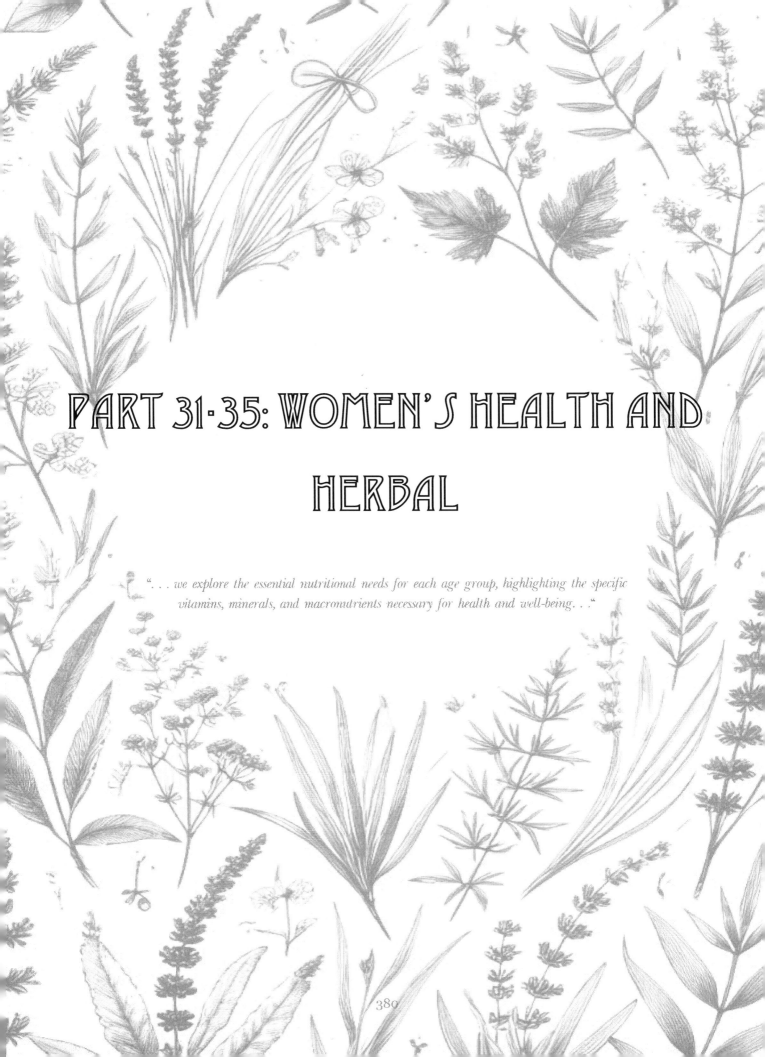

PART 31-35: WOMEN'S HEALTH AND HERBAL

". . . we explore the essential nutritional needs for each age group, highlighting the specific vitamins, minerals, and macronutrients necessary for health and well-being. . ."

Chapter 1: Women's Health Across Life Stages

Nutritional needs change as we move through life, influenced by factors like growth, activity level, hormonal shifts, and metabolism. A well-balanced diet, adapted to each stage of life, can ensure we meet our body's requirements for growth, maintenance, and energy. Here, we explore the essential nutritional needs for each age group, highlighting the specific vitamins, minerals, and macronutrients necessary for health and well-being.

Nutritional Needs at Different Ages

Nutritional Needs in Infancy (0-1 Year)

Infants undergo rapid growth and development, which means their nutritional requirements are significantly higher relative to their size. For the first six months, breast milk or formula provides all essential nutrients, with breast milk being the gold standard. Rich in antibodies, healthy fats, and proteins, breast milk is essential for immune support and growth. Formula, designed to mimic breast milk, is also a suitable source, especially in cases where breastfeeding isn't an option.

- **Protein**: Needed for growth and cellular repair, infants get sufficient protein from breast milk or formula.
- **Fats**: Essential fatty acids like DHA and ARA are crucial for brain and vision development.
- **Iron**: Around six months, iron stores in infants begin to deplete, making iron-fortified cereals or pureed meats a beneficial introduction to prevent iron deficiency.
- **Vitamin D**: For infants, particularly those who are breastfed, a vitamin D supplement is often recommended to support bone health, as breast milk contains limited amounts.

As infants reach 6 months and beyond, introducing solids provides a chance to support their growing needs for energy, iron, and vitamins. Soft, nutrient-dense foods, such as pureed vegetables, fruits, and iron-rich cereals, become essential building blocks for developing a varied and nutritious diet.

Nutritional Needs in Early Childhood (1-5 Years)

Toddlers and young children are active explorers, requiring energy-dense foods to fuel their high activity levels and rapid growth. While their appetites can be unpredictable, creating a well-rounded diet rich in vitamins, minerals, and macronutrients is key.

- **Calcium and Vitamin D**: Essential for bone growth, calcium is needed in larger amounts during early childhood. Milk, cheese, and fortified plant milks are great sources, with vitamin D aiding calcium absorption.
- **Iron**: An essential mineral, iron supports energy levels and brain development. Foods like lean meats, eggs, beans, and fortified cereals can prevent iron deficiency, which is common in young children.
- **Healthy Fats**: While adults are often advised to limit fats, young children benefit from healthy fats found in avocados, nuts (if allergy-safe), and fatty fish. These fats support brain development, a crucial aspect at this stage.

Balanced meals should include a variety of food groups, with emphasis on whole grains, lean proteins, vegetables, and fruits. Encouraging healthy eating habits early on can set the foundation for a lifetime of balanced nutrition.

Nutritional Needs in Childhood and Pre-Adolescence (6-12 Years)

As children grow, their bodies continue to require higher amounts of essential nutrients to support cognitive development, immune function, and physical activity. This age group benefits from a diet rich in nutrients that sustain their energy levels and promote growth.

- **Protein**: Adequate protein intake supports muscle development and the maintenance of tissues. Sources include poultry, eggs, dairy, and legumes.
- **Fiber**: Found in whole grains, fruits, and vegetables, fiber supports digestive health and can prevent childhood constipation, a common issue at this age.

- **Calcium and Vitamin D**: Bone development continues to be a priority, and this age group requires calcium and vitamin D to build a strong skeletal foundation. Including dairy or fortified alternatives ensures these needs are met.
- **B Vitamins**: B vitamins, such as B6 and B12, are necessary for energy production and red blood cell formation. Whole grains, meats, and leafy greens are good sources.

Maintaining variety is critical at this stage. To keep meals appealing and nutritionally balanced, encourage a rainbow of colors on the plate, aiming for vegetables, lean proteins, and whole grains.

Nutritional Needs in Adolescence (13-18 Years)

Adolescence brings about intense physical changes and increased nutritional needs due to growth spurts and hormonal shifts. This age group often requires more calories, protein, and specific vitamins and minerals to support their rapid development.

- **Protein**: Protein intake is essential for muscle growth and overall body repair, especially for teens involved in sports. Lean meats, fish, dairy, and plant-based proteins like beans and tofu provide adequate protein.
- **Iron**: Iron needs increase due to growth and, in girls, menstrual blood loss. Iron-rich foods like red meat, beans, and dark leafy greens are beneficial. Pairing iron with vitamin C-rich foods can improve absorption.
- **Calcium and Vitamin D**: Since adolescence is a crucial period for bone development, adequate calcium and vitamin D are essential to prevent future osteoporosis. Milk, cheese, yogurt, and fortified foods are helpful sources.
- **Folic Acid**: For both boys and girls, folic acid is important for DNA synthesis and cell growth. Green vegetables, legumes, and fortified grains are recommended.

Adolescents often develop their own food preferences, so it's beneficial to educate them about healthy choices. Emphasizing balanced meals and the benefits of whole foods can help teens make informed dietary decisions.

Nutritional Needs in Early Adulthood (19-40 Years)

Young adults generally reach their peak physical condition, but nutritional needs remain critical to sustain energy, muscle health, and cognitive function. The primary focus for this age group is maintaining a well-balanced diet that supports a busy lifestyle.

- **Protein**: Protein remains essential for muscle maintenance and cellular repair. Incorporate lean meats, fish, dairy, and plant-based options like lentils and quinoa to meet daily requirements.
- **Antioxidants**: Antioxidants, including vitamins C and E, help reduce oxidative stress, which is especially important as young adults often lead high-stress lives. Berries, nuts, and leafy greens provide these protective compounds.
- **Healthy Fats**: Omega-3 fatty acids support heart health and cognitive function, essential during the working years. Fish, flaxseeds, and walnuts are great sources.
- **Fiber**: Fiber helps with digestion and can support weight management. Whole grains, fruits, and vegetables are key to a diet rich in fiber.

Balancing macronutrients, minimizing processed foods, and staying hydrated are essential components for overall health during early adulthood.

Nutritional Needs in Middle Age (41-60 Years)

During middle age, the focus shifts to preventing chronic diseases, maintaining muscle mass, and supporting heart and brain health. Hormonal changes, such as menopause, can also influence nutritional requirements.

- **Calcium and Vitamin D**: With a natural decline in bone density, calcium and vitamin D become more critical to prevent osteoporosis. Dairy products, leafy greens, and fortified foods can help maintain bone strength.
- **Fiber**: Higher fiber intake helps regulate blood sugar and supports heart health, which is particularly important in middle age. Beans, whole grains, and vegetables are excellent sources.
- **Antioxidants**: Antioxidants like vitamins C, E, and beta-carotene help reduce inflammation and protect against age-related diseases. Colorful fruits and vegetables like carrots, bell peppers, and citrus are highly beneficial.
- **Magnesium**: Magnesium aids in muscle function and energy production. It's also beneficial for reducing blood pressure. Nuts, seeds, and whole grains provide magnesium naturally.

Middle age is also a time when many become more aware of weight management. Balanced portions, regular physical activity, and reducing added sugars and processed foods are effective strategies for this life stage.

Nutritional Needs in Older Adulthood (60+ Years)

As we age, our metabolism slows, and our body becomes less efficient at absorbing nutrients, making nutrient-dense food choices critical. Older adults should focus on maintaining muscle mass, bone health, and cognitive function.

- **Protein**: Maintaining muscle mass is essential to prevent frailty and improve recovery from illness or injury. Protein sources like lean meat, fish, dairy, eggs, and plant-based proteins are ideal.
- **Calcium and Vitamin D**: Aging bones require additional calcium and vitamin D to prevent fractures and osteoporosis. Consider dairy products, fortified plant milks, and supplements if necessary.
- **Fiber**: Fiber is essential for digestive health and can reduce the risk of heart disease. Whole grains, fruits, vegetables, and legumes are excellent choices.
- **Vitamin B12**: Older adults are at a higher risk of B12 deficiency, as the body's ability to absorb this vitamin decreases with age. Meat, fish, dairy, and fortified cereals are good sources.
- **Hydration**: Older adults are more susceptible to dehydration, so maintaining proper fluid intake is essential for kidney health and cognitive clarity.

Nutritional habits in older adulthood should prioritize easy-to-digest foods, often consumed in smaller portions, to ensure sufficient nutrient intake without causing digestive discomfort.

Herbal and Natural Supplements for Different Life Stages

Herbal remedies and natural supplements can complement a balanced diet and provide additional support throughout the various stages of life.

1. **Infancy and Childhood**: Herbs like chamomile and ginger can be safe in very small doses to support digestion and relieve colic in infants. Always consult a pediatrician before introducing any herbs.
2. **Adolescence**: Herbs like peppermint and green tea can support digestive health, while adaptogens such as ashwagandha may assist with stress management, particularly during exams.

3. **Adulthood and Middle Age**: Ashwagandha and turmeric are popular adaptogens that support stress relief and reduce inflammation. Omega-3 supplements can support heart and brain health.

4. **Older Adulthood**: Turmeric, ginger, and ginkgo biloba are beneficial for reducing inflammation, aiding cognitive health, and maintaining mobility.

By understanding and adapting to the nutritional needs unique to each age group, we can better support health, prevent disease, and ensure a vibrant and balanced life across all stages.

Supporting Reproductive Health

Reproductive health is a crucial component of overall wellness, impacting both physical and emotional well-being. In both men and women, reproductive health is influenced by a range of factors including hormones, nutrition, lifestyle choices, and stress. Herbs and natural remedies have been used throughout history to support reproductive function, balance hormones, and address specific concerns such as fertility, menstrual health, and libido. This section delves into natural strategies to nurture reproductive health holistically, with an emphasis on herbal remedies that promote balance and resilience in the body.

Understanding the Foundations of Reproductive Health

Reproductive health is complex, involving numerous systems working together. Hormones play a central role, as they regulate the menstrual cycle, sperm production, libido, and pregnancy. Nutrition is another key factor, providing the body with essential vitamins and minerals required for fertility and hormone production. Stress management and lifestyle choices also affect reproductive health, as chronic stress and unhealthy habits can lead to hormone imbalances, reduced libido, and challenges with conception.

Hormonal Balance and Its Importance

Balanced hormones are fundamental for reproductive health in both men and women. Hormones such as estrogen, progesterone, and testosterone influence sexual function, mood, and reproductive capacity. Imbalances can lead to issues such as irregular menstrual cycles, polycystic ovarian syndrome (PCOS), endometriosis, low libido, and infertility. Supporting the endocrine system—the system responsible for hormone production—through herbs and lifestyle practices can help restore hormonal balance and support reproductive health.

Herbs for Female Reproductive Health

For women, reproductive health encompasses menstruation, ovulation, and potential pregnancy. Herbal remedies can offer support for menstrual regularity, fertility, and relief from discomfort related to hormonal fluctuations.

1. Red Raspberry Leaf

Red raspberry leaf is known as the "woman's herb" for its toning effects on the uterus and support for menstrual health. This herb contains essential nutrients such as calcium, magnesium, and iron, which promote strong uterine muscles and regular menstruation. Red raspberry leaf is often consumed as a tea and can help reduce cramps and heavy bleeding.

- **How to Use**: Brew red raspberry leaf tea daily, particularly in the luteal phase (second half) of the menstrual cycle, to prepare the body for menstruation and ease cramps.

2. Vitex (Chaste Tree Berry)

Vitex, also known as chaste tree berry, is a powerful herb for regulating the menstrual cycle and balancing estrogen and progesterone levels. It stimulates the pituitary gland, which in turn encourages the production of luteinizing hormone (LH) to balance the menstrual cycle. Vitex is especially useful for conditions like PMS, PCOS, and luteal phase defects, which can impact fertility.

- **How to Use**: Vitex is commonly taken as a tincture or capsule, with a typical dose being 500–1000 mg per day. Consistency is key, as vitex works gradually to bring balance over a period of several months.

3. Maca Root

Maca root is a well-known adaptogen native to Peru, used for enhancing fertility and balancing hormones. It supports the hypothalamus and pituitary glands, which regulate hormone production in both men and women. Maca also increases libido and energy levels, making it beneficial for reproductive health and general vitality.

- **How to Use**: Maca powder can be added to smoothies or taken in capsule form. Begin with a small amount (around 1/2 teaspoon of powder) and gradually increase, as maca can be energizing.

4. Dong Quai

Dong quai is an herb commonly used in Traditional Chinese Medicine for its ability to regulate menstruation, relieve cramps, and support blood flow to the pelvic region. Known as a "female ginseng," dong quai nourishes the blood, making it especially helpful for women with light or irregular periods. It also has mild estrogenic properties, which can balance low estrogen levels.

- **How to Use**: Dong quai is available in capsule, tea, and tincture forms. Many women take it during the follicular phase (first half) of their cycle to support estrogen and blood flow.

Herbs for Male Reproductive Health

Male reproductive health relies on factors such as testosterone levels, sperm production, and prostate health. Certain herbs have been traditionally used to support male fertility, libido, and reproductive function.

1. Ashwagandha

Ashwagandha, a well-known adaptogen, is valued for its ability to reduce stress and increase energy. For men, it is especially beneficial because it supports testosterone production, enhances libido, and promotes sperm health. By reducing cortisol levels, ashwagandha may also improve hormonal balance and overall vitality.

- **How to Use**: Ashwagandha can be taken in powder or capsule form, with a typical dose of 500–1000 mg daily. Adding ashwagandha powder to smoothies or taking it with warm milk is a popular approach.

2. Saw Palmetto

Saw palmetto is frequently used to support prostate health and regulate testosterone levels in men. It reduces the conversion of testosterone to dihydrotestosterone (DHT), a hormone associated with prostate enlargement and hair loss. Additionally, saw palmetto can help enhance libido and sperm health.

- **How to Use**: Saw palmetto is available as capsules, soft gels, and tinctures. Men typically take around 160–320 mg daily for reproductive support.

3. Tribulus Terrestris

Tribulus is an herb that has been traditionally used to boost testosterone levels, increase libido, and improve sperm health. It is often included in fertility blends for men due to its aphrodisiac effects and ability to support erectile function.

- **How to Use**: Tribulus is available in capsules, powders, and tinctures. A typical dose is around 500–750 mg daily.

4. Panax Ginseng

Panax ginseng, also known as Korean ginseng, is another adaptogen known for enhancing male reproductive health. It has been shown to improve sperm quality, boost libido, and enhance stamina. Ginseng can help balance hormones and improve erectile function by enhancing nitric oxide production, which improves blood flow.

- **How to Use**: Panax ginseng is available in capsules, powders, and teas. Men can take 200–400 mg daily for reproductive benefits.

Nutritional Support for Reproductive Health

Alongside herbal remedies, a nutrient-dense diet is fundamental for reproductive wellness. Certain vitamins and minerals are especially crucial for reproductive health:

- **Folic Acid**: Essential for women of childbearing age, folic acid reduces the risk of birth defects and supports healthy cellular function.
- **Zinc**: Zinc is vital for hormone balance and sperm production. It also supports ovulation and progesterone production in women.
- **Omega-3 Fatty Acids**: Found in fish, flaxseeds, and walnuts, omega-3s are anti-inflammatory and support hormone production.
- **Vitamin E**: Known as the "fertility vitamin," vitamin E supports egg health and protects sperm from oxidative damage.

Lifestyle Practices to Support Reproductive Health

1. **Stress Management**: Chronic stress can interfere with hormone production, making stress management practices essential. Techniques like meditation, deep breathing exercises, and yoga can help reduce cortisol levels, creating a more favorable environment for reproductive health.

2. **Regular Exercise**: Moderate exercise improves circulation, supports weight management, and reduces stress. However, it's essential to avoid excessive high-intensity exercise, which can increase cortisol levels and negatively impact fertility.

3. **Adequate Sleep**: Quality sleep is crucial for hormone regulation. Aim for 7–9 hours of restful sleep each night to support the body's reproductive processes and overall health.

4. **Limit Exposure to Endocrine Disruptors**: Chemicals found in plastics, pesticides, and certain personal care products can disrupt hormone balance. Opt for organic foods, use glass or stainless-steel containers, and choose natural personal care products to reduce exposure to endocrine disruptors.

Using Herbal Remedies Safely

While herbal remedies offer valuable support for reproductive health, they should be used responsibly:

- **Consult a Healthcare Provider**: Before starting any new herbal regimen, it's wise to consult a healthcare provider, especially if you have pre-existing health conditions or are taking medications.

- **Understand the Timing**: Certain herbs are best taken during specific phases of the menstrual cycle. For example, red raspberry leaf is often used during the luteal phase, while dong quai is generally taken during the follicular phase.

- **Listen to Your Body**: Herbs can have varying effects based on individual constitution. If you notice any adverse effects, discontinue use and consult a professional.

Integrating Herbs and Nutrition for Optimal Reproductive Health

Combining herbal remedies with a nutrient-rich diet, stress management practices, and adequate rest provides a holistic approach to supporting reproductive health. Regularly incorporating herbs such as red raspberry leaf, ashwagandha, and saw palmetto, alongside lifestyle practices, creates a supportive foundation for reproductive vitality.

Whether you are looking to address specific reproductive concerns, enhance fertility, or simply support long-term hormonal balance, natural remedies offer a range of safe and effective options. By understanding the role of herbs and nutrition in reproductive health, individuals can make empowered choices that nurture their bodies and support their overall well-being.

Balancing Hormones Naturally

Hormones act as messengers in the body, regulating processes from metabolism to mood, energy, and reproductive health. When these hormones fall out of balance, it can lead to issues such as weight gain, fatigue, mood swings, and digestive problems. Natural remedies, lifestyle choices, and dietary changes can support a balanced hormonal state, providing a pathway to improved health without the side effects often associated with synthetic hormone treatments.

Understanding Hormone Imbalance

Hormones can become imbalanced for many reasons, including stress, poor diet, lack of sleep, exposure to toxins, and natural aging. Key hormones like estrogen, progesterone, testosterone, cortisol, and thyroid hormones are all sensitive to these influences, and any fluctuation can impact overall health.

- **Estrogen and Progesterone**: These are primarily female hormones but also play essential roles in male health. An imbalance can lead to symptoms like irregular menstrual cycles, mood changes, and weight gain.
- **Testosterone**: This hormone is crucial for muscle mass, energy, and libido in both men and women. Low levels can cause fatigue and depression.
- **Cortisol**: Known as the "stress hormone," cortisol helps manage our response to stress. Chronic stress can cause cortisol levels to stay elevated, leading to weight gain and reduced immunity.
- **Thyroid Hormones**: These hormones regulate metabolism, energy, and mood. Imbalances can lead to symptoms such as weight changes, fatigue, and mood instability.

Restoring balance often requires a holistic approach that includes dietary adjustments, herbal remedies, and lifestyle modifications. Let's explore some natural ways to address hormone imbalances.

1. Dietary Changes for Hormone Balance

A nutrient-rich diet is foundational for hormonal health. Food influences hormone production, metabolism, and cellular health, so a balanced diet can support hormonal balance naturally.

- **Healthy Fats**: Hormones are made from fat and cholesterol, so consuming healthy fats is vital for hormone production. Avocado, coconut oil, olive oil, and nuts provide essential fatty acids that help maintain hormone production.
- **Fiber**: Dietary fiber supports hormone health by helping the body eliminate excess hormones, particularly estrogen. Fiber-rich foods like vegetables, fruits, and whole grains can assist in detoxification and help prevent hormone build-up.
- **Protein**: Protein is essential for hormone production. Lean meats, fish, eggs, beans, and lentils are excellent sources of protein that can help regulate hunger hormones like ghrelin and maintain muscle mass.
- **Cruciferous Vegetables**: Vegetables such as broccoli, cauliflower, and Brussels sprouts contain compounds that help the body metabolize and excrete excess estrogen, helping to balance this hormone naturally.
- **Omega-3 Fatty Acids**: Found in fish, flaxseed, and walnuts, omega-3s reduce inflammation, which can positively impact hormone health. They also support the production of hormone-regulating neurotransmitters.

Incorporating these foods into daily meals can lay the foundation for balanced hormones and provide essential nutrients that keep the body functioning optimally.

2. Herbal Remedies for Hormone Balance

Herbs have long been used in traditional medicine to support hormonal health. Several herbs contain phytoestrogens, adaptogens, and other compounds that can stabilize hormone levels.

- **Ashwagandha**: This adaptogen helps the body manage stress by regulating cortisol levels. Ashwagandha has been shown to improve energy, mood, and sleep, which can be beneficial in managing overall hormone health.
- **Maca Root**: Known as a "hormone balancer," maca root supports the endocrine system and can alleviate symptoms of menopause, such as hot flashes and mood swings. It is also beneficial for men, as it may improve libido and energy levels.
- **Chasteberry (Vitex)**: Often used to treat PMS and menstrual irregularities, chasteberry supports progesterone production. This can be particularly helpful for women who experience symptoms associated with low progesterone, like mood swings or irregular cycles.
- **Red Clover**: High in phytoestrogens, red clover can help balance estrogen levels, especially during menopause. These phytoestrogens mimic estrogen in the body, potentially reducing symptoms like hot flashes and night sweats.
- **Holy Basil**: This adaptogenic herb supports adrenal health, making it beneficial for managing cortisol levels. Holy basil can also improve mental clarity and reduce anxiety, both of which positively impact hormonal balance.

Adding these herbs as teas, tinctures, or supplements can help the body adjust naturally to changes in hormone levels.

3. Managing Stress for Hormonal Balance

Stress is one of the biggest disruptors of hormonal balance, leading to elevated cortisol levels, which can affect other hormones, such as thyroid and sex hormones. Finding effective ways to manage stress is essential for maintaining hormonal health.

- **Meditation and Mindfulness**: Regular meditation can help reduce stress, lower cortisol levels, and improve mood. Practicing mindfulness, even for just 10 minutes a day, can make a significant difference in managing stress.
- **Exercise**: Physical activity, especially low-impact exercises like yoga and walking, reduces stress levels by promoting endorphin release. Yoga, in particular, is beneficial for hormone health, as it can reduce cortisol and improve adrenal function.
- **Deep Breathing Exercises**: Practicing deep breathing can activate the parasympathetic nervous system, helping to reduce stress and cortisol levels. Techniques such as 4-7-8 breathing or alternate nostril breathing can be effective for calming the nervous system.

Consistent stress management practices can help the body maintain a more balanced hormonal state by reducing the impact of cortisol on other hormones.

4. Sleep and Hormonal Health

Quality sleep is a crucial factor in maintaining hormonal health. Poor sleep disrupts the body's natural circadian rhythms, leading to imbalances in cortisol, insulin, and growth hormone. Aim for 7-9 hours of quality sleep each night.

- **Establish a Routine**: Going to bed and waking up at the same time each day can regulate your circadian rhythm, which supports balanced hormone production.
- **Create a Relaxing Environment**: Reducing screen time before bed and keeping the bedroom cool and dark can promote better sleep. Avoid caffeine and large meals close to bedtime.
- **Consider Magnesium Supplements**: Magnesium can help relax muscles and promote sleep. Magnesium glycinate or citrate taken before bed can improve sleep quality, supporting hormone balance indirectly.

A well-rested body is better equipped to regulate hormones and support overall health, making sleep hygiene a key component of any hormone-balancing regimen.

5. Physical Activity and Hormones

Exercise plays a role in balancing hormones by improving insulin sensitivity, reducing stress, and promoting the release of endorphins, the "feel-good" hormones.

- **Strength Training**: Strength training increases testosterone levels, which can benefit both men and women by enhancing muscle mass, energy, and mood.
- **Cardiovascular Exercise**: Aerobic activities like walking, jogging, and cycling improve cardiovascular health and increase endorphins, which reduce stress and support a balanced hormonal profile.
- **Yoga and Pilates**: These low-impact exercises reduce cortisol levels and promote relaxation. Yoga, in particular, includes poses that stimulate the endocrine system and support hormonal balance.

Regular exercise, tailored to your body's needs, can serve as a powerful tool in the quest for hormone health.

6. Detoxifying for Hormonal Balance

Toxins from the environment, food, and even household products can disrupt hormone balance. Many of these toxins, known as endocrine disruptors, mimic or interfere with the body's natural hormones, leading to imbalances.

- **Avoid Processed Foods**: Processed foods often contain additives, preservatives, and chemicals that may disrupt hormone function. Opt for whole, organic foods to reduce exposure to toxins.
- **Use Natural Personal Care Products**: Many conventional personal care products contain parabens and phthalates, which can disrupt hormones. Natural alternatives can reduce the body's toxin load.
- **Stay Hydrated**: Drinking plenty of water helps flush toxins from the body. Adding lemon to water can improve hydration and aid liver detoxification.

By reducing exposure to toxins and supporting the body's natural detox processes, you can create a healthier environment for your hormones.

7. Supplementation for Hormone Support

In addition to dietary changes and lifestyle modifications, certain supplements can help maintain hormonal balance.

- **Vitamin D**: Essential for hormone health, vitamin D acts as a hormone in the body and can support thyroid and sex hormone balance. Sunlight is a natural source, but supplements may be necessary for those with limited sun exposure.
- **Magnesium**: This mineral supports over 300 enzyme processes in the body, including those involved in hormone production. It can be found in leafy greens, nuts, and seeds or taken as a supplement.
- **Zinc**: Zinc supports the immune system and hormone production, particularly testosterone. Foods rich in zinc, such as pumpkin seeds and shellfish, can help maintain adequate levels.
- **Probiotics**: A healthy gut microbiome aids in hormone balance by improving digestion and nutrient absorption. Probiotics from foods like yogurt, sauerkraut, or supplements can support a balanced microbiome.

These supplements should be taken based on individual needs and, if possible, under the guidance of a healthcare professional.

8. Hydration and Hormones

Staying hydrated is essential for cellular function and hormone transportation. Dehydration can stress the body, elevating cortisol levels and impacting other hormones.

- **Drink Adequate Water**: Aim for at least 8 cups of water daily. Herbal teas can also contribute to hydration, and some, like chamomile, provide additional stress-relief benefits.

- **Electrolyte Balance**: Electrolytes like potassium, magnesium, and sodium are crucial for maintaining fluid balance. They can be replen

Chapter 2: Nutrition for Women's Health

Maintaining strong and healthy bones is fundamental for overall physical well-being and longevity. Bones provide structure to the body, protect vital organs, and enable mobility, while also serving as a reservoir for essential minerals.

Essential Nutrients for Bone Health

Bone health is particularly important because bones naturally lose density and strength with age, increasing the risk of fractures and conditions such as osteoporosis. Ensuring that the body receives essential nutrients to support bone density and integrity can play a crucial role in promoting long-term skeletal health and reducing the likelihood of bone-related issues. In this section, we will explore the key nutrients necessary for maintaining strong bones and delve into the ways in which these nutrients contribute to bone health. We'll also examine how incorporating these nutrients into a daily diet can help build and maintain bone density across the lifespan.

Understanding Bone Health and Density

Bone density peaks in early adulthood, generally around the age of 30. After this peak, bone density begins to decline gradually, with more rapid losses typically occurring in postmenopausal women and older adults. This natural process of bone remodeling involves both bone formation by osteoblasts and bone resorption by osteoclasts. Maintaining a balance between these two processes is critical for preserving bone mass. Essential nutrients provide the building blocks needed for bone formation, mineralization, and repair, supporting bone density and helping prevent structural weakness.

Calcium: The Foundation of Bone Health

Calcium is one of the most well-known nutrients essential for bone health. It plays a foundational role in bone structure, as around 99% of the body's calcium is stored in bones and teeth. Calcium is required for the mineralization process, where calcium phosphate crystals are laid down in the bone matrix to create a rigid structure. Insufficient calcium intake leads to the body withdrawing calcium from bones to support other vital functions, such as muscle contraction and blood clotting, which weakens bones over time.

- **Sources of Calcium**: Dairy products like milk, yogurt, and cheese are rich sources of calcium. However, for those who are lactose intolerant or vegan, calcium-fortified plant-based milk (such as almond, soy, or oat milk), leafy greens like kale and broccoli, and nuts like almonds can provide an alternative source.
- **Daily Recommended Intake**: Adults typically require around 1,000 mg of calcium per day, with increased needs for postmenopausal women and older adults at about 1,200 mg daily to support bone density and reduce the risk of osteoporosis.

Vitamin D: Facilitating Calcium Absorption

Vitamin D is vital for bone health as it facilitates calcium absorption in the intestines. Without adequate vitamin D, the body cannot absorb sufficient calcium from dietary sources, even if intake is adequate. Vitamin D also plays a role in bone remodeling by supporting osteoclast and osteoblast activity, which helps maintain bone density. Deficiency in vitamin D is associated with bone loss, fractures, and conditions such as rickets in children and osteomalacia in adults.

- **Sources of Vitamin D**: Sunlight exposure is one of the most effective ways to get vitamin D, as the skin synthesizes it when exposed to UV rays. Dietary sources include fatty fish like salmon, trout, and sardines, as well as egg yolks and fortified foods such as milk and cereals.
- **Daily Recommended Intake**: Most adults require at least 600-800 IU of vitamin D daily. For individuals with limited sun exposure, a vitamin D supplement may be necessary, especially during winter months or in areas with less sunlight.

Magnesium: Supporting Bone Structure and Calcium Metabolism

Magnesium is a crucial mineral that contributes to bone density and strength. About 60% of the body's magnesium is stored in bones, where it aids in bone formation and supports calcium metabolism. Magnesium deficiency can lead to impaired bone growth and an increased risk of osteoporosis, as it affects the activity of osteoblasts and osteoclasts, as well as the function of parathyroid hormone (PTH), which regulates calcium levels in the blood.

- **Sources of Magnesium**: Leafy green vegetables, nuts (such as almonds and cashews), seeds, whole grains, and legumes are excellent sources of magnesium. Dark chocolate is also a rich source of magnesium, making it a nutritious treat for supporting bone health.
- **Daily Recommended Intake**: The recommended daily intake for magnesium is around 310-420 mg for adults. Incorporating a variety of magnesium-rich foods into daily meals can support bone health and provide additional benefits for muscle and nerve function.

Vitamin K: Activating Bone-Building Proteins

Vitamin K is essential for bone health due to its role in activating proteins that bind calcium to the bone matrix. One of these proteins, osteocalcin, relies on vitamin K for its activity. Without adequate vitamin K, bones may become weaker and more prone to fractures. Vitamin K also helps regulate calcium deposition, preventing calcium from accumulating in soft tissues and supporting overall bone mineralization.

- **Sources of Vitamin K**: Leafy greens such as kale, spinach, and collard greens are rich in vitamin K. Other sources include broccoli, Brussels sprouts, and fermented foods like natto (fermented soybeans).
- **Daily Recommended Intake**: Adults generally need about 90-120 mcg of vitamin K daily. Those on blood-thinning medications should consult with healthcare providers before increasing vitamin K intake, as it may interact with certain medications.

Phosphorus: Partnering with Calcium for Bone Formation

Phosphorus, alongside calcium, is a primary component of bone mineral density. Phosphorus contributes to the formation of hydroxyapatite, the mineralized form of calcium phosphate that gives bones and teeth their structure. Adequate phosphorus intake is essential for maintaining bone health, but excessive phosphorus can disrupt calcium balance, leading to weakened bones.

- **Sources of Phosphorus**: Phosphorus is found in dairy products, meat, fish, poultry, nuts, seeds, and legumes. Many processed foods also contain phosphorus in the form of additives, though naturally occurring phosphorus from whole foods is preferable.

- **Daily Recommended Intake**: Adults generally require about 700 mg of phosphorus daily. Since phosphorus is present in many foods, most people achieve adequate intake through a balanced diet.

Protein: Building the Bone Matrix

Protein is a fundamental component of bone health because it forms the collagen matrix, a scaffold that provides flexibility and strength to bones. Collagen supports bone resilience and the ability to absorb impact, reducing the likelihood of fractures. Protein deficiency can lead to decreased bone density, as bones lose essential structural proteins, particularly in older adults.

- **Sources of Protein**: Lean meats, poultry, fish, eggs, dairy products, legumes, nuts, and seeds are excellent sources of protein. For vegetarians and vegans, plant-based proteins such as beans, tofu, tempeh, and quinoa offer sufficient protein to support bone health.
- **Daily Recommended Intake**: Adults generally require about 50-70 grams of protein daily, though individual needs vary based on factors such as age, activity level, and overall health.

Vitamin C: Supporting Collagen Synthesis

Vitamin C is vital for bone health as it supports the synthesis of collagen, a protein that forms the foundation of bone structure. Vitamin C acts as a cofactor in collagen production, helping to strengthen the bone matrix and enhancing the flexibility of bones. Vitamin C deficiency is associated with weaker bones and an increased risk of fractures due to reduced collagen production.

- **Sources of Vitamin C**: Citrus fruits, strawberries, bell peppers, broccoli, and Brussels sprouts are rich in vitamin C. Including a variety of fruits and vegetables in daily meals helps maintain adequate vitamin C levels.
- **Daily Recommended Intake**: Adults typically need around 65-90 mg of vitamin C daily. Consuming foods rich in vitamin C alongside iron-rich foods also improves iron absorption, which is beneficial for overall health.

Boron: A Trace Mineral for Bone Health

Boron is a lesser-known mineral that plays a role in bone health by supporting the metabolism of calcium, magnesium, and vitamin D. Boron helps improve bone mineral density and may reduce the risk of bone loss, especially in postmenopausal women.

- **Sources of Boron**: Boron is found in foods such as apples, grapes, raisins, nuts, legumes, and leafy greens. Although boron is required in small amounts, it contributes to bone health by enhancing the body's use of other bone-supportive nutrients.
- **Daily Recommended Intake**: There is no established daily requirement for boron, but an intake of 1-3 mg per day is generally considered beneficial for bone health.

Omega-3 Fatty Acids: Reducing Bone Inflammation

Omega-3 fatty acids are known for their anti-inflammatory properties, which can support bone health by reducing inflammation associated with bone loss. Omega-3s also promote osteoblast activity, contributing to bone formation and density.

- **Sources of Omega-3s**: Fatty fish such as salmon, mackerel, and sardines are excellent sources of omega-3s. Flaxseeds, chia seeds, and walnuts also provide plant-based omega-3s for those following a vegetarian or vegan diet.
- **Daily Recommended Intake**: It's recommended to consume at least two servings of fatty fish per week or supplement with fish oil for adequate omega-3 intake. For those following a plant-based diet, incorporating flaxseed oil or chia seeds can provide necessary omega-3s.

Lifestyle and Dietary Tips for Stronger Bones

1. **Regular Weight-Bearing Exercise**: Activities such as walking, running, weightlifting, and yoga stimulate bone growth and improve bone density. Exercise encourages osteoblast activity, which is essential for bone formation.
2. **Maintain a Balanced Diet**: A diet rich in vegetables, fruits, whole grains, lean protein, and dairy products or fortified alternatives provides a range of nutrients that support bone health.

3. **Limit Caffeine and Alcohol**: Excessive caffeine and alcohol consumption can interfere with calcium absorption and increase the risk of bone loss. Limiting intake of these substances can help preserve bone density.

4. **Get Sufficient Sun Exposure**: Sunlight is a primary source of vitamin D, essential for calcium absorption. Aim for about 10-30 minutes of sun exposure a few times a week, depending on skin type and climate.

Integrating these essential nutrients and lifestyle practices into daily routines fosters an environment for robust bone health, supporting the body's skeletal structure and resilience throughout life.

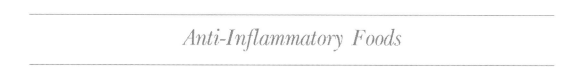

Anti-Inflammatory Foods

Inflammation is a natural response by the immune system to infection, injury, or stress. However, chronic inflammation can lead to numerous health issues, including heart disease, diabetes, arthritis, and even certain cancers. One of the most effective ways to combat chronic inflammation is through diet. Certain foods possess powerful anti-inflammatory properties, helping to reduce inflammation naturally and improve overall health. Let's explore these foods, why they're effective, and how they can be incorporated into a balanced, inflammation-fighting diet.

Understanding Chronic Inflammation

Before diving into specific foods, it's important to understand what chronic inflammation is and why it occurs. Unlike acute inflammation, which is a short-term response to immediate injury or infection, chronic inflammation is a prolonged and often low-grade response that persists over time. It may be caused by factors such as poor diet, high levels of stress, lack of exercise, exposure to environmental toxins, or autoimmune disorders. Over time, this chronic inflammation can damage tissues and organs, setting the stage for disease.

1. Leafy Green Vegetables

Leafy greens, such as spinach, kale, and Swiss chard, are loaded with antioxidants and nutrients that help reduce inflammation. These vegetables are high in vitamins A, C, and K, as well as minerals like magnesium, which is known for its anti-inflammatory effects. The antioxidants in leafy greens help neutralize free radicals—unstable molecules that contribute to inflammation and cell damage.

- **Spinach**: Rich in vitamins C and E, as well as beta-carotene, spinach helps lower levels of inflammation. Vitamin E, in particular, has been shown to protect the body from pro-inflammatory molecules known as cytokines.
- **Kale**: Kale contains quercetin, an antioxidant that helps lower inflammation and is associated with a reduced risk of chronic diseases.
- **Swiss Chard**: Packed with magnesium, Swiss chard is excellent for people with chronic inflammation. Low levels of magnesium have been linked to higher levels of inflammatory markers in the body.

Incorporating leafy greens into daily meals is easy—add them to salads, smoothies, or as a side to your main dish. These vegetables offer a nutrient-dense, low-calorie way to combat inflammation naturally.

2. Berries

Berries, including strawberries, blueberries, raspberries, and blackberries, are rich in antioxidants and polyphenols that combat inflammation. They are also high in fiber, which promotes a healthy gut—a key component in managing inflammation.

- **Blueberries**: Blueberries contain anthocyanins, a type of antioxidant that reduces inflammation and oxidative stress. Studies have shown that eating blueberries regularly can lower markers of inflammation in at-risk populations.
- **Strawberries**: High in vitamin C and ellagic acid, strawberries help protect cells from inflammatory damage. They are also linked to lower levels of CRP (C-reactive protein), a marker of inflammation in the body.
- **Raspberries**: These berries are rich in antioxidants like quercetin and catechins, which help reduce inflammation in the body.

Berries can be added to yogurt, smoothies, or eaten as a snack. They provide a sweet, nutritious boost that helps keep inflammation at bay.

3. Fatty Fish

Fatty fish, such as salmon, mackerel, sardines, and trout, are among the best sources of omega-3 fatty acids, which are renowned for their anti-inflammatory effects. Omega-3 fatty acids reduce inflammation by decreasing the production of pro-inflammatory molecules in the body.

- **Salmon**: High in both EPA and DHA, the two main types of omega-3 fatty acids, salmon is highly effective at reducing inflammation, especially in people with inflammatory conditions like arthritis.
- **Mackerel**: This fish is not only rich in omega-3s but also contains selenium, an antioxidant mineral that helps reduce inflammation and support immune health.
- **Sardines**: Sardines are a great choice for reducing inflammation as they contain both EPA and DHA, as well as vitamin D, which has anti-inflammatory properties.

Consuming fatty fish at least twice a week can significantly reduce chronic inflammation. For those who don't eat fish, fish oil supplements may be an alternative to obtain similar anti-inflammatory benefits.

4. Turmeric

Turmeric, a bright yellow spice commonly used in curry dishes, has been used for centuries in traditional medicine for its anti-inflammatory properties. The active compound in turmeric, curcumin, has powerful anti-inflammatory effects and is often compared to over-the-counter anti-inflammatory drugs.

Curcumin works by blocking NF-kB, a molecule that travels into the nuclei of cells and turns on genes related to inflammation. Studies have shown that curcumin can help alleviate symptoms of arthritis, inflammatory bowel disease, and other inflammatory conditions.

To improve curcumin absorption, consume turmeric with black pepper, which contains piperine—a compound that boosts curcumin absorption by up to 2,000%. Add turmeric to soups, stews, or try it as a tea with a dash of black pepper and honey.

5. Ginger

Ginger is another powerful anti-inflammatory food that has been used for centuries to relieve inflammation and pain. Ginger contains bioactive compounds like gingerol and shogaol, which have been shown to reduce inflammation in conditions such as arthritis and gastrointestinal issues.

Ginger works by inhibiting the production of pro-inflammatory cytokines and reducing oxidative stress. It is particularly effective for reducing pain and inflammation associated with osteoarthritis.

Ginger can be added to meals, made into a tea, or taken as a supplement for its anti-inflammatory effects. Consuming ginger regularly can offer relief from chronic inflammation and improve overall health.

6. Extra Virgin Olive Oil

Extra virgin olive oil is a staple in the Mediterranean diet, which is known for its anti-inflammatory benefits. It is rich in monounsaturated fats and contains oleocanthal, a compound with anti-inflammatory properties similar to ibuprofen.

Studies have shown that people who consume extra virgin olive oil regularly have lower levels of inflammation and are less likely to develop heart disease. The oleocanthal in olive oil works by inhibiting enzymes involved in the inflammatory process, offering a natural way to reduce inflammation without side effects.

Use extra virgin olive oil as a base for salad dressings, drizzle it over cooked vegetables, or add it to sauces. Its mild flavor and health benefits make it an excellent choice for reducing inflammation.

7. Green Tea

Green tea is loaded with antioxidants, particularly epigallocatechin gallate (EGCG), which has strong anti-inflammatory effects. EGCG inhibits the production of pro-inflammatory molecules and helps reduce the risk of chronic diseases associated with inflammation.

Research has shown that regular consumption of green tea can lower levels of inflammation and decrease the risk of conditions like heart disease, arthritis, and Alzheimer's. Additionally, green tea supports healthy weight management, which is essential for reducing inflammation.

Enjoy green tea as a warm beverage, or try it iced for a refreshing anti-inflammatory drink. Drinking a few cups of green tea daily can significantly contribute to lowering inflammation in the body.

8. Nuts and Seeds

Nuts and seeds, including almonds, walnuts, flaxseeds, and chia seeds, are excellent sources of anti-inflammatory nutrients like fiber, omega-3 fatty acids, and antioxidants.

- **Almonds**: High in vitamin E, an antioxidant that fights inflammation and supports immune health, almonds are a great snack for those looking to reduce inflammation.
- **Walnuts**: Walnuts are rich in omega-3 fatty acids and polyphenols, both of which have been shown to reduce markers of inflammation.
- **Flaxseeds and Chia Seeds**: These seeds are packed with alpha-linolenic acid (ALA), a type of omega-3 that helps reduce inflammation. They are also high in fiber, which supports gut health.

Add nuts and seeds to your diet by sprinkling them on salads, yogurt, or oatmeal. Their combination of healthy fats, fiber, and antioxidants makes them a valuable addition to an anti-inflammatory diet.

9. Tomatoes

Tomatoes are high in lycopene, an antioxidant with potent anti-inflammatory properties. Lycopene is particularly effective at reducing inflammation associated with heart disease, as well as lowering oxidative stress in the body.

Cooking tomatoes increases the bioavailability of lycopene, making cooked tomato products like tomato sauce or roasted tomatoes especially beneficial. Include tomatoes in salads, sauces, or as a side dish to enjoy their anti-inflammatory benefits.

10. Garlic

Garlic contains sulfur compounds that stimulate the immune system and reduce inflammation. Allicin, one of the main active compounds in garlic, has been shown to reduce inflammation in conditions like arthritis and support cardiovascular health.

Consuming raw garlic provides the most anti-inflammatory benefits, though it can also be cooked or taken as a supplement. Adding garlic to meals can enhance flavor while providing powerful anti-inflammatory support.

Incorporating Anti-Inflammatory Foods into Your Diet

To maximize the benefits of these anti-inflammatory foods, aim for a balanced diet rich in a variety of whole foods. Avoid processed foods, sugary snacks, and refined oils, which can contribute to inflammation. By focusing on nutrient-dense options, you can support your body's natural ability to manage and reduce inflammation, leading to better health and overall well-being.

Chapter 3: Herbal Remedies for Women's Health

Menstrual discomfort is a common experience for many people, manifesting in symptoms like cramps, bloating, mood swings, headaches, and fatigue. While pharmaceutical options like over-the-counter pain relievers are widely used, there is a growing interest in herbal solutions that provide natural, effective relief with fewer side effects.

Herbal Solutions for Menstrual Relief

Herbs can offer gentle support by reducing inflammation, balancing hormones, easing muscle spasms, and addressing emotional symptoms, making them an appealing choice for holistic menstrual care.

In this section, we'll explore various herbs known for their benefits in alleviating menstrual symptoms, their mechanisms of action, and how they can be safely incorporated into a menstrual care routine.

Understanding Menstrual Discomfort and Herbal Relief

Menstrual pain, or dysmenorrhea, is often caused by the release of prostaglandins, hormone-like substances that trigger uterine contractions to expel the uterine lining. High levels of prostaglandins are associated with more severe cramps, as they increase the intensity and frequency of these contractions. Other factors, like hormonal imbalances and lifestyle stressors, can also contribute to premenstrual syndrome (PMS) symptoms, which can vary widely from physical pain to mood-related challenges.

Herbs can work in a variety of ways to help manage these symptoms. Some herbs act as anti-inflammatories to reduce the intensity of cramps, while others support hormone balance or calm the nervous system. These plant-based remedies can often be used together, providing a comprehensive approach to menstrual relief.

1. Ginger (Zingiber officinale)

Ginger has a long history of use in traditional medicine for its anti-inflammatory and analgesic properties, making it an excellent choice for menstrual cramps. Studies suggest that ginger can reduce the production of prostaglandins, which may alleviate cramping. Additionally, ginger is known to help reduce bloating, nausea, and fatigue, common symptoms associated with menstruation.

- **How to Use Ginger**: Ginger tea is a popular and soothing way to consume ginger for menstrual relief. Boil a small piece of fresh ginger root in water for 10-15 minutes, then strain and drink. For those who prefer a stronger dose, ginger supplements are available in capsule form.
- **Safety Note**: Ginger is generally safe when consumed in moderate amounts. However, excessive intake can cause digestive discomfort in some individuals. Consult with a healthcare provider if you are pregnant or have a medical condition.

2. Chamomile (Matricaria chamomilla)

Chamomile is widely known for its calming effects on the nervous system, making it a go-to remedy for emotional symptoms like irritability and anxiety associated with PMS. It also contains anti-inflammatory compounds that help reduce cramping by relaxing the uterine muscles. Chamomile can aid with insomnia, a common issue for those experiencing PMS or menstrual pain, providing a more restful sleep and better overall mood.

- **How to Use Chamomile**: Chamomile tea is the most common way to enjoy this herb's benefits. Steep dried chamomile flowers in hot water for 5-10 minutes. For convenience, chamomile is also available in capsule form or as an essential oil for aromatherapy.
- **Safety Note**: Chamomile is generally considered safe for most people. However, individuals with allergies to plants in the daisy family should avoid it. Also, it may interact with blood-thinning medications.

3. Cramp Bark (Viburnum opulus)

As its name suggests, cramp bark is specifically known for relieving menstrual cramps. The herb works as a muscle relaxant, helping to ease uterine spasms and reduce pain. Cramp bark also has sedative properties that may help alleviate stress and tension often experienced during menstruation.

- **How to Use Cramp Bark**: Cramp bark can be taken as a tea, tincture, or in capsule form. A tincture may be particularly effective due to its concentrated form. To make cramp bark tea, steep one teaspoon of dried cramp bark in a cup of hot water for 15 minutes.

- **Safety Note**: Cramp bark is generally safe when used as directed. However, pregnant women should avoid it as it may stimulate the uterus.

4. Red Raspberry Leaf (Rubus idaeus)

Red raspberry leaf is rich in fragarine, a compound known to tone and relax the uterine muscles, which can reduce menstrual cramps. It is also packed with vitamins and minerals, including vitamin C, magnesium, and iron, which are beneficial for those experiencing fatigue and low energy during menstruation. This herb is often used to support overall reproductive health, making it a valuable addition to menstrual care.

- **How to Use Red Raspberry Leaf**: Red raspberry leaf is commonly consumed as a tea. Simply steep one to two teaspoons of dried leaves in hot water for 10-15 minutes. Drinking this tea regularly throughout the menstrual cycle may help prepare the body and reduce cramps.
- **Safety Note**: Red raspberry leaf is safe for most individuals, though it's recommended to consult a healthcare provider if you are pregnant.

5. Dong Quai (Angelica sinensis)

Dong Quai, also known as "female ginseng," is a powerful herb in traditional Chinese medicine for balancing hormones and relieving menstrual cramps. It promotes blood flow, which can reduce stagnation and alleviate cramping. Dong Quai also has mild sedative properties, making it beneficial for mood swings and anxiety.

- **How to Use Dong Quai**: Dong Quai can be taken as a tea, tincture, or capsule. Due to its slightly bitter taste, many prefer the capsule form.
- **Safety Note**: Avoid Dong Quai if you are pregnant, breastfeeding, or taking blood-thinning medications, as it may interact with these conditions.

6. Vitex (Vitex agnus-castus)

Vitex, or chaste tree berry, is commonly used to balance hormones by supporting the pituitary gland, which regulates hormone production. Vitex has been shown to reduce symptoms of PMS, including mood swings, breast tenderness, and cramps, making it an ideal herb for those seeking relief from hormonal fluctuations during the menstrual cycle.

- **How to Use Vitex**: Vitex is typically taken as a tincture or capsule. It works best when taken consistently over a period of time, often several months, to gradually help balance hormones.
- **Safety Note**: Vitex is generally safe for most individuals but may take several weeks or months to produce noticeable effects. Consult a healthcare provider if taking hormonal medications or if pregnant.

7. Fennel (Foeniculum vulgare)

Fennel is known for its antispasmodic and anti-inflammatory properties, which can help reduce the intensity of menstrual cramps. Additionally, fennel can alleviate bloating and digestive discomfort that often accompany menstruation. Its mild estrogenic effects make it a gentle choice for balancing hormones.

- **How to Use Fennel**: Fennel tea is an effective and convenient way to consume this herb. Crush a teaspoon of fennel seeds and steep in hot water for 10 minutes. Fennel can also be added to meals or chewed after meals for digestive support.
- **Safety Note**: Fennel is safe for most people when used in moderate amounts. Pregnant individuals should consult a healthcare provider before using fennel.

Practical Tips for Incorporating Herbal Remedies into a Menstrual Care Routine

1. **Start Early**: To maximize the benefits of herbal remedies, consider starting them a few days before your period begins. Many herbs work preventively, helping to reduce the buildup of prostaglandins and alleviate cramps before they become severe.
2. **Combine Herbs for Synergistic Effects**: Some herbs work well together to create a more comprehensive effect. For example, combining ginger, chamomile, and fennel can provide a soothing tea that addresses cramps, digestive issues, and emotional symptoms.
3. **Consistency is Key**: For herbs like Vitex, which work to balance hormones over time, consistency is essential. Consider incorporating these herbs daily for a few months to see optimal results.
4. **Practice Self-Care Alongside Herbal Remedies**: Herbs can be a powerful addition to menstrual care, but they work best when combined with other supportive practices. Regular exercise, a balanced diet rich in nutrients like magnesium and

omega-3 fatty acids, and adequate rest can complement herbal remedies and promote a more comfortable menstrual experience.

5. **Monitor Your Body's Response**: Everyone's body responds differently to herbs, so it's important to pay attention to how you feel. If a particular herb doesn't seem effective or causes unwanted side effects, consider trying a different option.

Herbal solutions provide a gentle, natural approach to managing menstrual discomfort. By understanding the properties and effects of each herb, individuals can create a personalized menstrual care plan that suits their unique needs and preferences. Whether used individually or in combination, these herbs offer effective ways to alleviate cramps, balance hormones, and support emotional well-being, empowering people to navigate their menstrual cycles with greater comfort and confidence.

Natural Remedies for Menopause

Menopause marks a significant transition in a woman's life, characterized by a natural decline in reproductive hormones, particularly estrogen and progesterone. This hormonal shift often leads to various symptoms such as hot flashes, mood swings, sleep disturbances, and fatigue, which can impact a woman's quality of life. While menopause is a normal biological process, managing its symptoms with natural remedies can provide relief and enhance well-being without the potential side effects of pharmaceutical treatments. Let's explore effective, natural solutions for alleviating menopause symptoms, grounded in holistic practices and herbal medicine.

Understanding Menopause and Its Symptoms

Menopause generally occurs between the ages of 45 and 55, signaling the end of a woman's menstrual cycles. The transition usually unfolds in three stages: perimenopause, menopause, and postmenopause. Perimenopause, the period leading up to menopause, is often when symptoms first arise. During menopause itself, symptoms can become more intense, eventually subsiding in postmenopause.

Common symptoms include:

- **Hot flashes**: Sudden feelings of warmth, usually in the face and chest, that can last for seconds to minutes.
- **Night sweats**: Similar to hot flashes but occurring during sleep, often disturbing rest.
- **Mood swings**: Emotional fluctuations due to hormonal changes.
- **Vaginal dryness**: Reduced estrogen levels can lead to dryness, impacting comfort and intimacy.
- **Weight gain and metabolism changes**: Hormonal shifts can lead to slower metabolism and weight gain.

While these symptoms are typical, their intensity and duration vary among women, making personalized approaches to symptom relief beneficial.

1. Phytoestrogens: Nature's Hormone Balancers

Phytoestrogens are plant compounds that mimic estrogen in the body. By interacting with estrogen receptors, phytoestrogens can help balance hormone levels, reducing menopause symptoms like hot flashes and mood swings. Phytoestrogens are particularly useful during perimenopause and early menopause, when estrogen fluctuations are most pronounced.

- **Soy**: Soy is one of the richest sources of phytoestrogens, specifically isoflavones, which have been shown to alleviate hot flashes and improve mood. Incorporate soy-based foods such as tofu, tempeh, and soy milk into your diet for added benefits.
- **Flaxseeds**: Rich in lignans, another type of phytoestrogen, flaxseeds help balance hormones and are also high in fiber, which supports digestive health. Ground flaxseeds can be added to smoothies, yogurt, or oatmeal.
- **Red Clover**: Known for its high concentration of isoflavones, red clover has been studied for its effects on reducing hot flashes and improving bone health. Red clover is available as an herbal tea or supplement.

While phytoestrogens are generally safe, they should be consumed in moderation, especially for women with a history of hormone-sensitive conditions.

2. Black Cohosh for Hot Flashes and Mood

Black cohosh, a herb native to North America, has a long history of use in alleviating menopausal symptoms, particularly hot flashes and mood disturbances. It contains compounds that interact with serotonin receptors, which can help regulate body temperature and mood. Black cohosh does not contain phytoestrogens, making it a suitable choice for women who prefer a non-estrogenic remedy.

Black cohosh is commonly available in capsule or tincture form, and studies have shown its effectiveness in reducing the frequency and intensity of hot flashes. While generally safe, it is recommended to use black cohosh under the guidance of a healthcare provider, especially if taken for extended periods.

3. Adaptogenic Herbs: Managing Stress and Hormonal Balance

Adaptogens are a category of herbs that help the body adapt to stress and restore balance, making them ideal for addressing the hormonal fluctuations and emotional challenges of menopause. Some of the most effective adaptogens for menopause include:

- **Ashwagandha**: Known for its stress-relieving properties, ashwagandha helps regulate cortisol levels and supports restful sleep. This can be particularly beneficial for women experiencing night sweats and insomnia.
- **Maca Root**: A Peruvian root with hormone-balancing properties, maca helps alleviate mood swings and increase energy levels. Maca powder can be added to smoothies or taken as a supplement.
- **Rhodiola Rosea**: This adaptogen is known for its ability to reduce fatigue and improve focus, both of which can be affected during menopause.

Incorporating adaptogens into a daily routine can enhance resilience to stress and stabilize mood, helping to create a more balanced emotional state during menopause.

4. Herbal Teas for Relaxation and Symptom Relief

Herbal teas provide a gentle, soothing way to relieve menopause symptoms. Certain herbs, when brewed as teas, can have calming effects, relieve hot flashes, and support digestion.

- **Chamomile Tea**: Known for its calming properties, chamomile tea can help with sleep disturbances and reduce anxiety. Its anti-inflammatory properties also benefit digestion.
- **Peppermint Tea**: Peppermint has a cooling effect, making it an excellent remedy for hot flashes. It can also ease digestive issues, which are common during menopause.
- **Lemon Balm Tea**: This herb has been shown to reduce mood swings and anxiety, providing a sense of calm and aiding sleep.

Herbal teas are easy to incorporate and can be enjoyed throughout the day. Drinking a calming tea before bed can help relax the body and prepare for a restful night's sleep.

5. Essential Oils for Symptom Management

Aromatherapy, using essential oils, can provide menopause relief by alleviating anxiety, promoting relaxation, and even reducing hot flashes. Essential oils can be used in a diffuser, added to a carrier oil for massage, or applied to pulse points.

- **Clary Sage Oil**: Known for balancing hormones, clary sage oil helps alleviate hot flashes and improve mood. Studies have shown that inhaling clary sage oil can reduce cortisol levels, helping to manage stress.
- **Lavender Oil**: With its calming properties, lavender oil promotes relaxation and improves sleep quality, making it ideal for night sweats and sleep disturbances.
- **Peppermint Oil**: Applied topically (with a carrier oil) to the neck or wrists, peppermint oil has a cooling effect, which can help reduce the intensity of hot flashes.

Using essential oils is a simple, non-invasive way to enhance relaxation and reduce menopause symptoms. However, always dilute essential oils before applying them to the skin.

6. Nutritional Support for Bone Health

Menopause increases the risk of osteoporosis due to declining estrogen levels, which affects bone density. Supporting bone health with nutrition is essential to prevent bone loss and maintain strength.

- **Calcium**: Calcium is the building block of bones. Good sources include dairy products, leafy greens, almonds, and fortified plant milks. Aim for about 1,200 mg of calcium per day.
- **Vitamin D**: Vitamin D helps the body absorb calcium, making it essential for bone health. Sun exposure is the best source, but supplements or foods like fatty fish, eggs, and fortified cereals can help.
- **Magnesium**: This mineral supports bone health and aids calcium absorption. It can be found in foods like spinach, pumpkin seeds, and dark chocolate.

A well-rounded diet rich in these nutrients can support bone health, reduce the risk of fractures, and help prevent osteoporosis.

7. Regular Exercise to Enhance Mood and Physical Health

Exercise is one of the most effective natural remedies for managing menopause symptoms. Regular physical activity can reduce hot flashes, improve mood, support weight management, and enhance sleep quality.

- **Aerobic Exercise**: Activities like walking, jogging, and swimming can improve cardiovascular health, which is important as the risk of heart disease increases after menopause.
- **Strength Training**: Weight-bearing exercises help maintain bone density and muscle mass, which tend to decline with age.
- **Yoga and Stretching**: Yoga can help reduce stress, improve flexibility, and enhance mental clarity. Certain poses also aid in balancing hormones and alleviating hot flashes.

Incorporating 30 minutes of moderate exercise most days of the week provides numerous benefits, from improved mood to enhanced physical health.

8. Sleep Hygiene for Better Rest

Sleep disturbances are common during menopause due to factors like night sweats, anxiety, and hormonal changes. Adopting good sleep hygiene practices can help improve sleep quality:

- **Establish a Routine**: Go to bed and wake up at the same time each day to regulate your internal clock.
- **Create a Relaxing Environment**: Keep the bedroom cool, dark, and quiet. Consider using a fan to help manage night sweats.
- **Limit Caffeine and Alcohol**: Both can interfere with sleep, especially if consumed in the evening.

Improving sleep quality supports overall well-being and helps reduce other menopause symptoms, making it a vital part of any natural approach to menopause management.

9. Mindfulness and Meditation for Stress Reduction

Mindfulness and meditation practices are powerful tools for managing stress, which can exacerbate menopause symptoms. Techniques like deep breathing, guided meditation, and mindfulness exercises help reduce anxiety, improve emotional balance, and foster a sense of calm.

Spending just 10-15 minutes daily on mindfulness can make a difference in mood and stress management. Apps like Headspace or Calm offer guided meditations tailored to different needs, including stress reduction and sleep suppor

Chapter 4: Women's Health Recipes

Red clover (Trifolium pratense) has been valued for centuries as a natural remedy for various ailments, particularly in women's health. This perennial flowering plant, often found in fields and meadows, boasts numerous beneficial properties, making it a popular choice in herbal medicine.

Red Clover Infusion

Its therapeutic uses span from supporting hormonal balance to offering relief for respiratory and skin conditions. Among its most accessible and beneficial preparations is the red clover infusion, a gentle herbal tea that harnesses the plant's potent phytochemicals and nutrients. Red clover is particularly known for its high isoflavone content—compounds with estrogen-like effects that can provide hormonal support, especially during perimenopause and menopause. Beyond hormonal health, red clover is packed with vitamins, minerals, and antioxidants that support immunity, skin health, and bone strength. This infusion offers a mild, earthy flavor, making it easy to incorporate into a daily routine for those seeking natural wellness support.

Nutritional Profile of Red Clover

The efficacy of red clover as an herbal remedy is rooted in its rich nutrient profile. The flowers, which are primarily used in infusions, contain various beneficial compounds, including:

- **Isoflavones**: These are phytoestrogens, which mimic estrogen in the body. Isoflavones like biochanin A, formononetin, and genistein are known to balance hormones and have been studied for their potential in reducing menopausal symptoms.

- **Vitamins**: Red clover is a source of vitamin C, vitamin E, and several B vitamins, including niacin (B3) and thiamine (B1), all of which support skin health, energy levels, and immune function.

- **Minerals**: Rich in calcium, magnesium, potassium, and phosphorus, red clover infusion provides essential minerals for bone health and muscle function.
- **Antioxidants**: In addition to isoflavones, red clover contains other antioxidants, such as flavonoids and coumarins, that protect the body from oxidative stress.
- **Tannins**: These compounds have astringent properties, which can aid in toning tissues and supporting skin health.

Health Benefits of Red Clover Infusion

Red clover infusion is known for offering a range of health benefits, many of which are supported by both traditional use and modern studies. These benefits primarily address hormonal health, respiratory wellness, and skin care, making it a versatile addition to a natural health routine.

1. Hormonal Balance and Menopause Support

Red clover is perhaps best known for its role in balancing hormones, particularly in women experiencing menopause. The isoflavones in red clover mimic estrogen, which can help alleviate symptoms related to estrogen deficiency, such as hot flashes, night sweats, and mood swings. Studies have shown that red clover extract and infusions can reduce the frequency and intensity of hot flashes, providing a natural alternative to hormone replacement therapy (HRT).

For women in perimenopause, when hormone levels begin to fluctuate, red clover infusion can provide gentle support by smoothing out these fluctuations. This makes it particularly useful for those looking for non-pharmaceutical solutions to manage the transition into menopause.

2. Bone Health

Isoflavones in red clover not only impact hormonal balance but also play a role in bone health. Estrogen is essential for maintaining bone density, and as estrogen levels decrease during menopause, the risk of osteoporosis and fractures increases. Red clover's estrogenic compounds may help slow bone loss and improve bone density. Additionally, its mineral content, including calcium, magnesium, and potassium, supports bone strength and overall skeletal health.

Red clover infusion, taken regularly, can be an effective addition to a bone health regimen, especially for those who prefer natural alternatives to synthetic supplements. The minerals and isoflavones work together to reinforce bone density and reduce the risk of osteoporosis.

3. Skin Health and Detoxification

The antioxidants and anti-inflammatory compounds in red clover make it beneficial for skin health. Traditionally, red clover has been used to support skin conditions such as eczema, psoriasis, and acne due to its ability to reduce inflammation and promote healing. The infusion works internally by flushing out toxins and supporting liver health, which in turn can lead to clearer skin.

The infusion's detoxifying properties stem from its mild diuretic effect, which encourages the body to eliminate waste and reduce water retention. A healthy liver and efficient elimination process are essential for maintaining clear skin, making red clover infusion a valuable component of a skin-care routine.

4. Respiratory Health

In traditional medicine, red clover has been used as an expectorant, helping to clear the respiratory tract of mucus and ease coughs. Its mild antispasmodic effects can relieve symptoms of bronchitis and asthma, making it a useful remedy for supporting lung health. Drinking red clover infusion during cold and flu season may help soothe the respiratory system and provide relief from congestion.

The infusion's ability to support respiratory health can be particularly helpful for individuals with chronic respiratory conditions. While it should not replace medical treatment, it can offer a complementary approach to managing symptoms.

5. Cardiovascular Health

Red clover's isoflavones have also been studied for their potential benefits in supporting heart health. By mimicking estrogen, these compounds can positively impact cholesterol levels, helping to reduce LDL (bad cholesterol) while increasing HDL (good cholesterol). Regular consumption of red clover infusion may contribute to better cardiovascular health by supporting balanced cholesterol levels and improving circulation.

Additionally, red clover's antioxidant properties help protect blood vessels from oxidative stress, which can reduce the risk of atherosclerosis and other cardiovascular issues.

Preparing Red Clover Infusion

Making a red clover infusion is simple and requires only dried red clover flowers, which can be sourced from reputable herbal suppliers or health food stores.

1. **Ingredients**:
   o 1 tablespoon of dried red clover flowers
   o 1 cup of boiling water
2. **Instructions**:
   o Place the dried red clover flowers in a teapot or mug.
   o Pour the boiling water over the flowers and cover.
   o Allow the infusion to steep for 10-15 minutes for a milder infusion, or up to 30 minutes for a stronger, more therapeutic effect.
   o Strain the flowers and enjoy the infusion warm or cool.

For therapeutic use, it's recommended to drink one to three cups of red clover infusion daily. Regular consumption over time may be necessary to experience the full benefits, especially for hormonal support.

Incorporating Red Clover Infusion into Daily Wellness

Red clover infusion can be easily incorporated into a daily wellness routine, offering a gentle but effective way to support overall health. For those interested in holistic approaches, the infusion can be combined with other herbal teas to create a personalized herbal regimen. Here are some practical tips for making red clover infusion a regular part of your day:

- **Morning Start**: Begin your day with a warm cup of red clover infusion to support detoxification and boost your body's natural healing processes.
- **Afternoon Support**: Drinking red clover in the afternoon can help manage mid-day hormonal fluctuations and provide a gentle energy lift.
- **Evening Relaxation**: Red clover's mild sedative properties make it a soothing drink in the evening, supporting relaxation and restful sleep.

Safety and Precautions

While red clover is generally considered safe for most individuals, certain precautions should be taken to avoid potential interactions or side effects:

- **Pregnancy and Breastfeeding**: Due to its estrogenic effects, red clover should be avoided by pregnant or breastfeeding women unless advised otherwise by a healthcare provider.

- **Blood-Thinning Medications**: Red clover contains natural blood-thinning compounds, so individuals taking anticoagulant medications should consult with a healthcare provider before using red clover.
- **Hormone-Sensitive Conditions**: People with hormone-sensitive conditions, such as breast or uterine cancer, should exercise caution with red clover, as its estrogen-like compounds may affect hormone balance.

Combining Red Clover with Other Herbs

To enhance the effects of red clover, it can be combined with other complementary herbs for a more targeted approach. Some popular combinations include:

- **Red Clover and Nettle**: For an infusion that supports both hormonal and bone health, nettle provides additional minerals like iron and calcium.
- **Red Clover and Lemon Balm**: Lemon balm can add a calming effect, making this combination ideal for easing tension and promoting relaxation.
- **Red Clover and Peppermint**: Peppermint adds a refreshing flavor and can support digestion, making it an excellent choice for those with digestive discomfort related to hormonal changes.

Each of these combinations can be prepared by mixing the dried herbs in equal parts and brewing them in a similar manner to red clover infusion alone.

Red clover infusion offers a rich source of natural compounds that can support various aspects of health, especially for women seeking hormonal balance, bone health, and cardiovascular support. As a safe, versatile, and enjoyable herbal remedy, red clover has earned its place in traditional medicine and modern wellness practices alike.

Dong Quai Tincture

Dong Quai (Angelica sinensis), often referred to as "female ginseng," has been a cornerstone of Traditional Chinese Medicine (TCM) for centuries. Known for its ability to support women's health, Dong Quai is particularly celebrated for its effects on reproductive health and hormonal balance. From menstrual cramps to menopausal symptoms, Dong Quai is highly valued for its broad range of therapeutic properties. In the United States, as more individuals turn to natural and herbal remedies for health issues, Dong Quai tincture has gained popularity as a holistic approach to managing various women's health concerns.

In this section, we'll explore the potential benefits of Dong Quai tincture, how to use it, its preparation, safety considerations, and its therapeutic role within the broader context of natural health and wellness.

Understanding Dong Quai and Its Properties

Dong Quai is a perennial herb native to the high-altitude regions of China, Japan, and Korea. The root of the plant is the primary component used in herbal medicine and is known for its warm, sweet, and slightly bitter properties. According to TCM, Dong Quai is believed to invigorate and nourish the blood, promote energy flow, and regulate menstruation, making it highly regarded as a female tonic.

Key bioactive compounds in Dong Quai include:

- **Ferulic Acid**: A compound with antioxidant, anti-inflammatory, and vasodilatory effects, which helps reduce oxidative stress and inflammation.
- **Ligustilide**: Known for its antispasmodic properties, ligustilide helps alleviate muscle cramps and can relieve menstrual pain.
- **Polysaccharides**: These compounds support immune function and have potential adaptogenic effects, helping the body cope with physical and emotional stress.
- **Coumarins**: These compounds help improve blood circulation, support cardiovascular health, and can be mildly sedative.

These compounds work synergistically to provide a range of health benefits, particularly for women's health. Dong Quai's role in supporting hormonal balance, reducing pain, and enhancing blood flow makes it a versatile herb for addressing menstrual and menopausal discomforts.

Benefits of Dong Quai Tincture

Dong Quai tincture, a concentrated liquid form of the herb, is a convenient way to harness the plant's medicinal properties. Below are some of the key benefits that Dong Quai tincture can offer, especially for women seeking natural remedies for reproductive health:

1. **Hormonal Balance and Menstrual Health**

Dong Quai is often recommended for its effects on hormonal balance, particularly in cases of irregular menstrual cycles. The herb helps regulate estrogen levels, which can aid in alleviating symptoms associated with premenstrual syndrome (PMS) and menopause. By improving the blood flow and relieving stagnation, Dong Quai also helps in reducing menstrual cramps, which makes it a valuable natural solution for dysmenorrhea (painful periods). Many women find relief from PMS symptoms such as mood swings, bloating, and breast tenderness when using Dong Quai regularly.

2. Menopausal Symptom Relief

For women going through menopause, Dong Quai offers an alternative to hormone replacement therapy (HRT) for alleviating symptoms such as hot flashes, night sweats, and mood swings. The phytoestrogenic compounds in Dong Quai interact with estrogen receptors in the body, offering a mild estrogenic effect that helps stabilize fluctuating hormone levels. This can provide significant relief from symptoms without the side effects associated with synthetic hormone treatments.

3. Improved Circulation and Cardiovascular Health

Dong Quai's coumarin content helps to thin the blood, supporting better circulation and reducing the risk of clot formation. This property not only helps improve overall cardiovascular health but also supports efficient nutrient delivery throughout the body, which is essential for physical and mental vitality. For individuals experiencing fatigue or reduced stamina, Dong Quai can help improve energy levels by enhancing blood flow and oxygenation.

4. Enhanced Immune Function

The polysaccharides in Dong Quai have immune-boosting properties, helping the body fight infections and recover from illnesses. This makes Dong Quai tincture a valuable remedy during periods of stress or seasonal changes when the immune system may be compromised. Regular use can provide the body with the additional support it needs to maintain resilience against infections and illnesses.

5. Antioxidant and Anti-Inflammatory Effects

Due to its high antioxidant content, Dong Quai helps protect cells from oxidative damage caused by free radicals. This is particularly important for reducing inflammation, which is often linked to conditions like arthritis, cardiovascular disease, and other chronic illnesses. By reducing inflammation, Dong Quai supports overall health and helps alleviate inflammatory pain, particularly in conditions associated with aging.

How to Use Dong Quai Tincture

Dong Quai tincture is typically administered orally, with the dosage and frequency adjusted based on individual needs. Here's how to incorporate Dong Quai tincture safely and effectively:

1. **Dosage**: The general dosage for Dong Quai tincture ranges from 1 to 2 ml (approximately 20-40 drops), taken up to three times daily. Always start with a lower dose to assess tolerance, and consult with a healthcare provider, particularly if combining with other medications.

2. **Timing**: Dong Quai tincture can be taken with or without food. However, to support menstrual health, some women find it helpful to take it a week or two before their menstrual cycle begins to help reduce PMS symptoms.

3. **Method of Consumption**: The tincture can be taken directly under the tongue for faster absorption or diluted in a small amount of water or tea for a milder taste.

It's essential to take breaks from Dong Quai tincture. For instance, using it for three weeks with a one-week break helps prevent potential dependency or reduced efficacy over time.

Making Dong Quai Tincture at Home

While Dong Quai tincture is available commercially, it can also be made at home with simple ingredients:

- **Ingredients**: Dried Dong Quai root (1 cup), high-proof alcohol (such as vodka) to serve as a solvent.

- **Instructions**: Place the dried root in a glass jar and cover with alcohol, leaving about an inch of space at the top. Seal the jar and store in a cool, dark place for four to six weeks, shaking it gently every few days. Once ready, strain the tincture through a cheesecloth or fine sieve, transferring the liquid into a dark glass bottle for storage.

Homemade tinctures generally have a shelf life of one to two years when stored in a cool, dark place. This method allows individuals to control the strength and purity of their tincture.

Safety and Side Effects of Dong Quai

While Dong Quai is generally considered safe for most people, there are important considerations and precautions to keep in mind:

- **Photosensitivity**: Dong Quai can make the skin more sensitive to sunlight due to its furanocoumarin content. It's advisable to wear sunscreen or avoid prolonged sun exposure when using Dong Quai.
- **Blood Thinning**: Due to its anticoagulant effects, Dong Quai may interact with blood-thinning medications and increase the risk of bleeding. Individuals on anticoagulants or those with clotting disorders should consult a healthcare provider before use.
- **Pregnancy and Lactation**: Dong Quai should not be used during pregnancy, as it can stimulate uterine contractions. It's also recommended to avoid it during breastfeeding due to limited safety data.

Integrating Dong Quai with Other Natural Remedies

For those looking to enhance the benefits of Dong Quai, combining it with other complementary herbs can provide synergistic effects:

- **For Hormonal Balance**: Combining Dong Quai with black cohosh or chasteberry can enhance its effects on hormonal regulation and provide comprehensive support for menstrual and menopausal symptoms.
- **For Stress Relief**: Adding ashwagandha or Rhodiola rosea, adaptogens known for their stress-relieving properties, can improve mood stability and reduce the emotional impact of hormonal fluctuations.
- **For Circulatory Health**: Pairing Dong Quai with ginger or ginkgo biloba, both known for their circulatory benefits, can further support cardiovascular health and boost energy levels.

When combining herbs, it's advisable to work with a healthcare provider to determine safe and effective dosages.

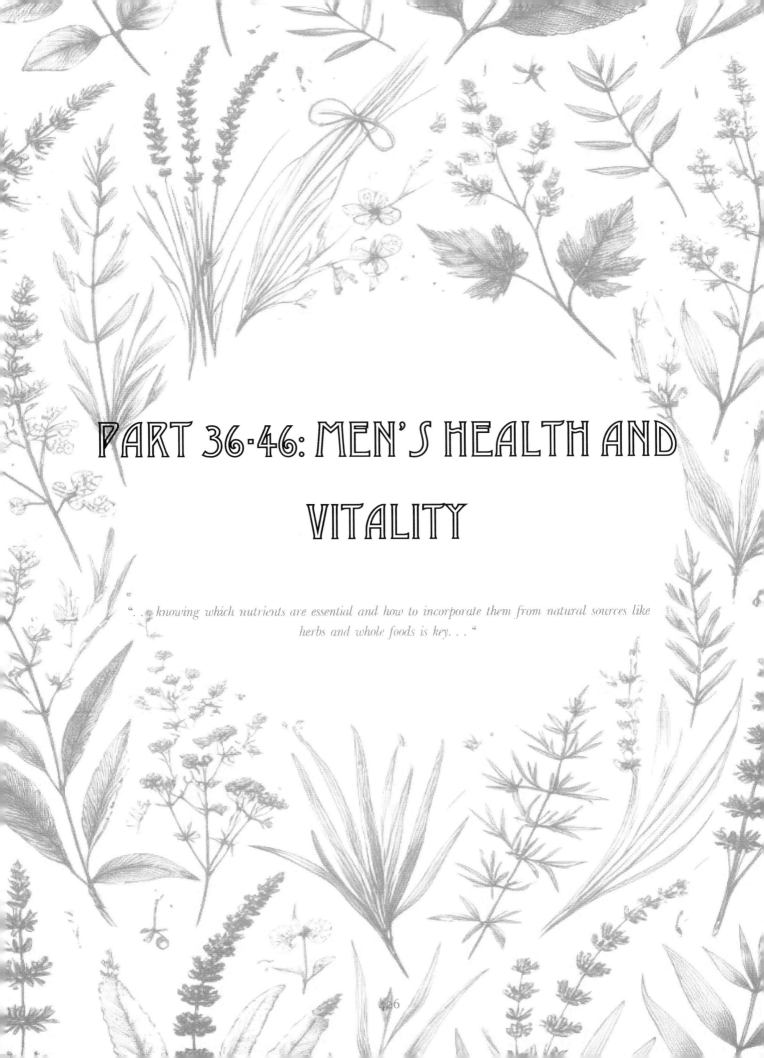

PART 36-46: MEN'S HEALTH AND VITALITY

". . . knowing which nutrients are essential and how to incorporate them from natural sources like herbs and whole foods is key. . . "

Chapter 1: Men's Health Essentials

Nutrition plays a foundational role in overall health, impacting everything from energy levels to immune function, brain health, and even mood. Understanding key nutritional needs is essential for supporting the body's daily functions, preventing disease, and promoting longevity.

Key Nutritional Needs

For individuals interested in natural health approaches, knowing which nutrients are essential and how to incorporate them from natural sources like herbs and whole foods is key.

Macronutrients: The Building Blocks

Macronutrients include carbohydrates, proteins, and fats, each serving distinct but interconnected roles in the body.

Carbohydrates

Carbohydrates are the primary energy source for the body, especially for the brain and muscles. Unlike other macronutrients, carbohydrates can be rapidly broken down to provide fuel for intense physical activities. For optimal health, focus on consuming complex carbohydrates from sources like whole grains, vegetables, and legumes. These provide not only energy but also fiber, which supports digestive health and helps stabilize blood sugar levels.

Refined carbohydrates, such as those in white bread and sugary snacks, should be minimized as they can lead to blood sugar spikes, energy crashes, and increased risk of chronic diseases like diabetes. Choosing natural carbohydrate sources like quinoa, sweet potatoes, and oats can provide sustained energy and essential nutrients.

Proteins

Proteins are critical for tissue repair, immune function, hormone production, and the development of enzymes. Protein needs vary depending on factors like age, activity level, and overall health, but they are indispensable for maintaining muscle mass and cellular health.

High-quality protein sources include lean meats, fish, eggs, dairy, and plant-based options like lentils, chickpeas, and tofu.

For individuals with plant-based diets, pairing plant proteins, such as rice and beans, ensures they receive all nine essential amino acids, which are typically more abundant in animal-based proteins.

Fats

Fats are vital for brain health, hormone production, and cellular integrity. Healthy fats include monounsaturated and polyunsaturated fats found in foods like avocados, olive oil, nuts, seeds, and fatty fish. These fats support cardiovascular health by lowering bad cholesterol and providing anti-inflammatory benefits. Omega-3 fatty acids, a type of polyunsaturated fat found in fish like salmon and plant sources like flaxseeds, are particularly beneficial for heart health and brain function.

Trans fats, commonly found in processed foods, should be avoided due to their negative impact on heart health and their potential to trigger inflammation. Instead, choose natural fats, which not only provide satiety but also help absorb fat-soluble vitamins.

Micronutrients: Essential Vitamins and Minerals

Micronutrients are vitamins and minerals that the body requires in smaller amounts but are crucial for proper functioning.

Vitamin A

Vitamin A is essential for vision, immune function, and skin health. It plays a critical role in forming and maintaining healthy skin and mucous membranes, which are the body's first line of defense against pathogens. This vitamin can be obtained from animal sources like liver and dairy or from plant sources high in beta-carotene, like carrots, sweet potatoes, and spinach, which the body converts into vitamin A.

B Vitamins

The B vitamin family, including B1 (thiamine), B2 (riboflavin), B3 (niacin), B6, B12, folate, and biotin, supports energy production, cognitive function, and cell metabolism. B vitamins are water-soluble and must be replenished regularly through the diet. Leafy greens, whole grains, legumes, eggs, and lean meats are good sources. Vitamin B12, however, is primarily found in animal products, so vegetarians and vegans may need to consider fortified foods or supplements to meet their needs.

Vitamin C

Vitamin C is an antioxidant that supports immune health, skin health, and iron absorption. It also plays a role in collagen synthesis, which helps maintain the integrity of skin, cartilage, and bones. High concentrations of vitamin C can be found in citrus fruits, bell peppers, strawberries, and broccoli. Since the body cannot produce vitamin C, regular intake through food or supplements is necessary.

Vitamin D

Vitamin D is crucial for bone health, immune support, and mood regulation. It helps the body absorb calcium, which is essential for bone strength. While the body produces vitamin D when exposed to sunlight, food sources include fatty fish, egg yolks, and fortified dairy. Vitamin D deficiency is common, especially in regions with limited sunlight, and may require supplementation to reach optimal levels.

Vitamin E

Vitamin E acts as an antioxidant, protecting cells from damage and supporting skin and eye health. This vitamin also contributes to immune function. Sources include nuts, seeds, spinach, and avocado. Adequate vitamin E intake can support skin health by combating free radicals and maintaining skin's elasticity.

Vitamin K

Vitamin K is essential for blood clotting and bone health. It works synergistically with calcium and vitamin D to promote bone density and prevent fractures. Leafy greens, like kale and spinach, are excellent sources of vitamin K. Those taking blood-thinning medications should consult with a healthcare provider before significantly increasing their vitamin K intake due to its role in clotting.

Calcium

Calcium is well-known for its role in bone health, but it's also vital for muscle function, nerve transmission, and hormonal secretion. Dairy products are rich in calcium, but it can also be obtained from leafy greens, almonds, and fortified plant milks. Consistent calcium intake is essential, particularly for women and aging populations, to prevent osteoporosis.

Iron

Iron is required for the production of hemoglobin, which transports oxygen in the blood. It is also necessary for energy metabolism and cognitive function. Iron deficiency can lead to anemia, characterized by fatigue and weakness. Animal-based iron, called heme iron, is more easily absorbed by the body and is found in red meat, poultry, and fish. Non-heme iron, found in plant sources like lentils, beans, and spinach, can be enhanced by pairing it with vitamin C-rich foods to improve absorption.

Magnesium

Magnesium is a multifunctional mineral that plays a role in over 300 enzymatic reactions in the body, including muscle and nerve function, blood sugar control, and energy production. Magnesium-rich foods include nuts, seeds, legumes, and dark leafy greens. This mineral also promotes relaxation and may improve sleep quality.

Potassium

Potassium is an electrolyte that supports heart function, muscle contraction, and fluid balance. It helps maintain normal blood pressure by balancing sodium levels in the body. Bananas, sweet potatoes, tomatoes, and legumes are good potassium sources. A diet high in potassium and low in sodium can significantly reduce the risk of hypertension and cardiovascular disease.

Hydration: An Often Overlooked Essential

Hydration is a critical component of nutrition, impacting nearly every function in the body. Proper hydration supports digestion, nutrient transport, and temperature regulation. While water is the best hydrator, herbal teas and foods with high water content, like cucumbers and watermelon, can also contribute to daily fluid needs. Maintaining hydration is especially crucial for those living in hot climates, engaging in regular physical activity, or consuming high-protein diets, as these factors increase water requirements.

Dietary Fiber

Fiber is a type of carbohydrate that the body cannot digest, yet it plays a vital role in digestive health. There are two types of fiber: soluble, which can help lower blood sugar and cholesterol levels, and insoluble, which aids in digestive regularity. Foods like oats, beans, apples, and flaxseeds are excellent sources of soluble fiber, while whole grains, nuts, and vegetables provide insoluble fiber. Fiber intake is associated with a reduced risk of heart disease, improved gut health, and better blood sugar control.

Antioxidants and Phytochemicals

Phytochemicals are compounds found in plants that provide various health benefits, including antioxidant properties. Antioxidants help protect cells from oxidative stress, which can lead to chronic diseases. Colorful fruits and vegetables, such as berries, tomatoes, and leafy greens, are high in antioxidants. Incorporating a variety of these foods ensures that the body receives a wide spectrum of antioxidants, which can help reduce inflammation and support overall health.

Creating a Balanced Nutritional Plan

Meeting these nutritional needs requires a well-balanced diet that includes diverse food sources. Prioritizing whole, unprocessed foods and incorporating a variety of colors on the plate can help ensure an adequate intake of essential vitamins, minerals, and macronutrients. Tracking food choices and making adjustments based on specific health goals or dietary restrictions can further support overall wellness.

This approach provides the foundation for a healthy body and mind, promoting resilience against disease and supporting long-term health outcomes.

Mental and Physical Health for Men

Men's health is increasingly recognized as a field requiring focused attention, particularly as societal roles and expectations evolve. Health challenges that men face often differ from those faced by women, with specific physical and mental aspects unique to men's health, including hormone fluctuations, stressors related to work and family, and predispositions to certain health conditions. Men are also statistically less likely to seek medical advice and often face stigmas around mental health care, which can result in unaddressed concerns that impact overall well-being. This section delves into the crucial aspects of mental and physical health for men, offering insights into natural strategies to enhance quality of life holistically.

Understanding Mental Health in Men

Mental health is as integral to wellness as physical health, yet it remains under-emphasized for men. Stress, anxiety, and depression affect men differently than women, with men often expressing these feelings through irritability, aggression, or withdrawal rather than open discussion. Social stigmas around mental health persist, creating barriers for men seeking help. This reluctance to address mental health openly can lead to chronic stress, which in turn has detrimental effects on physical health. A comprehensive approach to men's mental health includes a mix of self-care practices, supportive social connections, and natural remedies that align with holistic wellness goals.

1. **Herbs for Managing Stress and Anxiety**

Herbal remedies offer accessible and effective ways to manage stress. Adaptogenic herbs, known for their ability to help the body adapt to stress, are especially beneficial for men facing high-pressure environments. **Ashwagandha**, an adaptogen widely used in Ayurvedic medicine, has been shown to reduce cortisol levels and improve resistance to stress. Similarly, **Rhodiola rosea** supports mental clarity, reduces fatigue, and has mood-enhancing properties that make it ideal for combating stress-induced anxiety.

Using these herbs as tinctures, teas, or supplements allows for easy integration into daily routines. Consistent use of adaptogens can lead to an improved ability to handle daily stressors, ultimately contributing to a more balanced state of mind.

2. **Boosting Mood Naturally**

Men dealing with mild depression or mood fluctuations can benefit from natural supplements that support serotonin production and overall brain health. **St. John's Wort** is well-known for its antidepressant effects, primarily due to its ability to influence serotonin levels. **Omega-3 fatty acids**, found in fish oil, flaxseed, and walnuts, also play a critical role in brain health and mood regulation. Including Omega-3s in the diet or as supplements helps reduce symptoms of depression and enhances cognitive function.

Additionally, lifestyle adjustments, such as regular physical activity and a diet rich in nutrient-dense foods, contribute to mood stability. Exercise, particularly aerobic and resistance training, has been shown to release endorphins and other neurochemicals that improve mood and reduce feelings of anxiety.

Physical Health Considerations for Men

Physical health is a foundational element of men's wellness, affecting energy levels, endurance, and long-term health outcomes. Maintaining an active lifestyle, balancing hormone levels, and addressing nutritional needs are essential to supporting a strong and resilient body.

1. **Hormonal Health and Testosterone Balance**

Testosterone plays a key role in male health, influencing muscle mass, energy levels, mood, and sexual function. While testosterone naturally declines with age, stress, poor diet, and lack of physical activity can exacerbate this decline. Restoring and maintaining healthy testosterone levels naturally involves a combination of diet, exercise, and herbal support.

Certain herbs and supplements can enhance testosterone production. **Tribulus terrestris** and **fenugreek** are popular herbs that stimulate testosterone synthesis, enhance libido, and support muscle growth. **Zinc** is a critical mineral for testosterone production and is commonly found in shellfish, nuts, and seeds. Regularly consuming foods rich in zinc and magnesium helps maintain optimal hormone balance.

2. Building and Maintaining Muscle Mass

Physical activity, particularly strength training, is important for muscle maintenance and overall physical strength. Muscle mass naturally decreases with age, making resistance training essential for preserving lean tissue. Regular exercise also supports cardiovascular health, improves stamina, and boosts metabolism. A combination of weightlifting, bodyweight exercises, and high-intensity interval training (HIIT) offers well-rounded physical benefits.

Adequate protein intake is crucial for muscle repair and growth. Men should aim to consume protein-rich foods like lean meats, eggs, legumes, and dairy products. Supplements such as **whey protein** or **plant-based protein powders** can complement dietary intake, ensuring that the body has sufficient protein for recovery after workouts.

3. Cardiovascular Health

Cardiovascular disease is a leading health concern for men, often due to high-stress lifestyles, diets rich in processed foods, and lack of physical activity. To support cardiovascular health, a diet high in fiber, healthy fats, and antioxidants is essential. Including foods rich in **omega-3 fatty acids**—such as salmon, chia seeds, and walnuts—supports heart health by reducing inflammation and improving blood lipid levels.

Herbal remedies like **garlic** have long been used to support cardiovascular health by lowering blood pressure and improving circulation. **Hawthorn berry** is another potent herb for heart health, known to strengthen the heart muscle and improve blood flow.

4. Prostate Health

Prostate health becomes increasingly important with age, as conditions like benign prostatic hyperplasia (BPH) and prostate cancer are common among older men. Preventive measures include a diet rich in antioxidants, reducing intake of red meat, and consuming anti-inflammatory foods.

Saw palmetto is a natural remedy for supporting prostate health, particularly in reducing symptoms of BPH. It works by inhibiting the conversion of testosterone to dihydrotestosterone (DHT), which is associated with prostate enlargement. **Pumpkin seeds**, rich in zinc and phytosterols, are also beneficial for prostate health. Adding these natural remedies into daily routines provides proactive support for maintaining prostate health and reducing age-related risks.

Enhancing Cognitive Function and Memory

Cognitive health is an essential component of overall well-being, impacting work performance, relationships, and quality of life. Natural remedies and lifestyle adjustments that support brain health can help improve memory, focus, and mental agility.

1. Nootropic Herbs for Focus and Memory

Certain herbs, known as nootropics, support cognitive function by improving blood flow to the brain, protecting neurons, and enhancing neurotransmitter function. **Ginkgo biloba** is one of the most well-researched herbs for memory enhancement, as it improves circulation and protects against cognitive decline. **Bacopa monnieri**, another nootropic, has been shown to reduce anxiety while improving memory and cognitive performance.

Regularly incorporating nootropic herbs through teas, tinctures, or supplements can improve focus, enhance problem-solving abilities, and support long-term cognitive health.

2. Sleep and Rest as Cognitive Enhancers

Sleep quality profoundly affects cognitive health. Sleep is when the body and brain repair, consolidate memories, and prepare for the next day. Insufficient sleep is linked to reduced concentration, poor memory, and a higher risk of mood disorders. Natural sleep aids such as **valerian root** and **melatonin supplements** can support restful sleep, particularly for men experiencing stress-related insomnia.

3. Dietary Factors and Brain Health

Brain health is closely tied to diet. Nutrient-dense foods that support brain function include dark leafy greens, berries, and healthy fats from avocados, nuts, and seeds. Antioxidants from fruits and vegetables protect neurons from oxidative stress, while omega-3 fatty acids support brain cell function.

Additionally, consuming foods rich in **B vitamins**, especially **B6**, **B12**, and **folate**, aids in the production of neurotransmitters and supports brain cell function. These vitamins can be found in whole grains, eggs, and fortified cereals.

Strategies for Long-Term Wellness

Sustaining mental and physical health as a man involves building habits that promote resilience, strength, and vitality over time. Adopting a holistic approach that includes regular exercise, a balanced diet, stress management, and proactive health screenings can enhance overall quality of life. Integrating natural remedies, such as herbal supplements and dietary adjustments, complements these practices, offering men a comprehensive toolkit for maintaining health and well-being at every stage of life.

Each individual's health journey is unique, and the combination of strategies that works best will vary. Working with a healthcare provider to personalize a wellness plan ensures that men receive guidance tailored to their specific needs, making it easier to navigate health challenges and prioritize long-term vitality. By incorporating these natural health practices into daily life, men can achieve a more balanced, fulfilled, and resilient state of well-being.

Stress Management Techniques

Stress has become an almost inevitable part of modern life, affecting individuals across all age groups and lifestyles. Chronic stress can lead to numerous health issues, from headaches and insomnia to more serious conditions such as cardiovascular disease, diabetes, and mental health disorders. Developing effective stress management techniques is essential to mitigate these risks and improve quality of life. This section explores various methods to manage stress holistically, focusing on natural remedies, mindful practices, physical activity, and lifestyle adjustments.

Understanding Stress and Its Effects on the Body

Stress is the body's natural response to perceived threats or challenges, activating the "fight-or-flight" response. During this response, hormones like adrenaline and cortisol are released, preparing the body to respond to danger. While this response is beneficial in short-term situations, chronic stress can lead to prolonged high cortisol levels, which negatively affect physical and mental health.

Chronic stress can lead to various symptoms, including muscle tension, fatigue, digestive issues, sleep disturbances, and emotional challenges like irritability and depression.

Understanding the mechanisms of stress helps in choosing appropriate management techniques that target both mind and body.

Mindfulness Meditation and Relaxation Techniques

Mindfulness meditation is one of the most effective ways to manage stress. This practice encourages individuals to focus on the present moment, cultivating a non-judgmental awareness of thoughts, feelings, and bodily sensations. By regularly practicing mindfulness, individuals can reduce anxiety, improve focus, and gain better control over their reactions to stressors.

How to Practice Mindfulness Meditation

Begin by finding a quiet space and sitting in a comfortable position. Close your eyes and focus on your breath, taking slow, deep breaths in and out. Allow any thoughts to come and go without judgment, gently redirecting your focus back to your breathing if your mind begins to wander. Start with a few minutes a day and gradually increase the duration.

For beginners, guided meditations are available through apps like Headspace or Calm, which offer various lengths and themes, from gratitude to stress relief.

Physical Activity as a Stress Reliever

Exercise is another powerful tool for managing stress. Physical activity stimulates the production of endorphins, chemicals in the brain that act as natural mood lifters. Exercise also reduces levels of the body's stress hormones, such as adrenaline and cortisol, promoting relaxation and reducing tension.

Types of Exercise for Stress Management

- **Cardiovascular Exercise**: Activities such as running, swimming, or dancing increase heart rate and stimulate endorphin production, leading to immediate and long-lasting mood improvements.
- **Strength Training**: Lifting weights or practicing bodyweight exercises helps individuals focus their energy and clear their minds, providing a mental break from stressors.

- **Yoga**: Combining physical postures, breath control, and meditation, yoga is highly effective for reducing stress and promoting relaxation. Poses like the "child's pose" or "corpse pose" can help release tension from specific areas like the shoulders and back.

Engaging in physical activity regularly, even if it's a short walk or a few minutes of stretching, can significantly reduce stress and improve overall mental clarity.

Herbal Remedies for Stress Relief

For those interested in natural solutions, certain herbs are known for their calming properties and ability to support the body's stress response.

Adaptogens: Nature's Stress Relievers

Adaptogenic herbs help the body adapt to stress by modulating cortisol levels and improving resilience. Popular adaptogens for stress relief include:

- **Ashwagandha**: Known for its anti-anxiety properties, ashwagandha helps lower cortisol levels, reduce anxiety, and improve overall well-being.
- **Rhodiola Rosea**: This herb enhances mood, improves focus, and decreases fatigue. Rhodiola is especially helpful for individuals dealing with high-pressure environments.
- **Holy Basil**: Often referred to as "Tulsi," holy basil is effective for reducing anxiety and helping the body cope with physical and emotional stress.

These herbs are available in various forms, such as teas, tinctures, or capsules, making them easy to incorporate into a daily routine.

Deep Breathing Techniques

Deep breathing exercises can instantly calm the body and mind by slowing the heart rate and lowering blood pressure. Practicing deep breathing helps reduce muscle tension, calm the nervous system, and increase the flow of oxygen to the brain.

Box Breathing Technique

One effective technique is called "box breathing," which involves taking deep breaths in a rhythmic pattern:

1. Inhale through your nose for a count of four.
2. Hold your breath for a count of four.
3. Exhale slowly through your mouth for a count of four.

4. Hold again for a count of four.

Repeat this cycle several times, focusing on the rhythm of your breath. This practice can be done anytime stress arises and serves as an excellent way to regain composure.

Cognitive Behavioral Techniques for Stress Management

Cognitive-behavioral techniques (CBT) help individuals identify and change negative thought patterns that contribute to stress. By practicing cognitive restructuring, people can learn to view challenges as manageable and reduce self-imposed stressors.

For instance, if an individual constantly feels overwhelmed by their workload, CBT encourages them to break down tasks into smaller, achievable steps. This method helps prevent the mind from becoming overwhelmed and allows for steady progress.

Practicing Gratitude

Incorporating gratitude practices, like keeping a journal or noting down three positive experiences each day, can shift focus away from stress and cultivate a positive mindset. Studies show that gratitude can enhance mental resilience and reduce stress.

Aromatherapy for Relaxation

Aromatherapy is an ancient practice that uses essential oils to improve well-being. Inhaling essential oils stimulates the limbic system in the brain, which is responsible for emotions and memory, making it an effective method for reducing stress and anxiety.

Recommended Essential Oils for Stress Relief

- **Lavender**: Known for its calming and sedative properties, lavender oil helps alleviate anxiety and promote better sleep.
- **Chamomile**: Chamomile oil has a mild sedative effect, making it useful for calming nerves and promoting relaxation.
- **Bergamot**: This citrusy essential oil is known to uplift mood and reduce stress.

To use these oils, add a few drops to a diffuser or a warm bath, or dilute with a carrier oil for a calming massage.

Establishing a Relaxing Evening Routine

Creating a relaxing evening routine can help signal the brain and body that it's time to wind down, improving both stress levels and sleep quality. Disconnecting from electronics, taking a warm bath, or reading a book are examples of activities that can aid relaxation.

A calming routine before bed helps prevent the mind from racing at night, allowing for more restorative sleep and lower stress levels the following day.

Journaling as a Stress Outlet

Writing down thoughts and feelings can be a therapeutic way to process emotions and gain perspective. Journaling provides an outlet for self-reflection, helping individuals identify sources of stress and develop strategies for managing them.

Daily journaling doesn't have to be lengthy; even a few lines about the day's events and feelings can be beneficial. Writing down concerns helps externalize thoughts, making it easier to let go of stress.

Practicing Self-Compassion

Self-compassion involves treating oneself with kindness and understanding, especially during times of stress. Recognizing that everyone experiences stress and allowing oneself to rest without guilt is essential for mental health. Practicing self-compassion reduces self-criticism and encourages a healthier perspective on challenges.

Setting Boundaries

Many people experience stress due to over-commitment. Learning to set boundaries, both personally and professionally, allows individuals to prioritize their well-being without feeling obligated to take on more than they can handle. This can include saying "no" to extra work, setting limits on screen time, or designating certain days for self-care.

Setting boundaries reduces burnout, improves relationships, and fosters a greater sense of control over one's time and responsibilities.

Social Support and Connection

Human beings are social creatures, and maintaining strong connections with family and friends can provide a powerful buffer against stress. Talking to someone about personal challenges can provide new perspectives and emotional support. Sharing moments of laughter and joy also releases endorphins, creating natural relief from stress.

Nutrition's Role in Stress Management

Eating a balanced diet is critical for supporting the body's ability to handle stress. Nutrients like magnesium, omega-3 fatty acids, and complex carbohydrates play roles in stabilizing mood and energy. Consuming foods rich in these nutrients, such as nuts, leafy greens, and fatty fish, can support mental health and improve resilience to stress.

Reducing caffeine and sugar intake, which can cause energy crashes, also helps maintain a balanced mood throughout the day.

Endurance and Energy

Endurance and energy are foundational to an active, fulfilling lifestyle. Whether you're looking to support athletic performance, maintain vitality through daily tasks, or simply improve your overall stamina, understanding how to build and sustain energy levels is essential. In today's fast-paced world, natural methods for boosting energy and endurance have become increasingly popular, offering long-lasting benefits without the crash associated with stimulants like caffeine or sugary foods. This section explores natural strategies, including specific herbs, dietary changes, and lifestyle adjustments, to support sustained energy and resilience.

Understanding the Body's Energy Systems

The body generates energy through a complex network of systems, primarily driven by the mitochondria within cells. Known as the cell's powerhouse, mitochondria produce ATP (adenosine triphosphate), the energy currency that powers nearly all bodily functions. The quality of fuel (nutrition), oxygen levels, and overall cellular health are key factors in maintaining efficient ATP production. Natural strategies to enhance endurance and energy focus on supporting mitochondrial health, improving blood flow, and balancing hormones that play a role in energy regulation.

To enhance both endurance and energy, the approach should be multi-faceted, combining nutrition, herbal support, hydration, and physical conditioning.

Herbal Allies for Endurance and Energy

Several herbs have long been valued for their ability to boost endurance and energy naturally. Many of these plants are classified as adaptogens, which help the body adapt to physical, mental, and environmental stressors.

1. **Ginseng (Panax ginseng and Panax quinquefolius)**

Known as a traditional tonic for vitality, ginseng is one of the most researched herbs for enhancing endurance and energy. Panax ginseng (Asian ginseng) and Panax quinquefolius

(American ginseng) have slightly different profiles but both contribute to energy and stress resilience. Asian ginseng is more stimulating, providing a direct energy boost, while American ginseng is milder, supporting endurance and reducing fatigue over time.

Studies have shown that ginseng can increase oxygen uptake and support mitochondrial function, which are essential for sustained energy during physical activities. This herb is beneficial for those who engage in regular exercise or demanding physical labor, as it helps reduce muscle soreness and improves recovery time.

2. Ashwagandha (Withania somnifera)

Ashwagandha is an adaptogen celebrated for its ability to reduce stress while simultaneously increasing energy levels. By lowering cortisol, a stress hormone that can sap energy and lead to fatigue, ashwagandha promotes balance within the body's adrenal system, which plays a central role in managing energy and endurance.

Taking ashwagandha regularly helps to enhance muscle strength and improve cardiorespiratory endurance. This herb is particularly beneficial for those experiencing burnout or adrenal fatigue, as it provides long-lasting energy without overstimulation.

3. Rhodiola (Rhodiola rosea)

Rhodiola is another powerful adaptogen with a unique ability to combat fatigue, improve focus, and increase physical stamina. Often used by athletes and military personnel, Rhodiola has been shown to enhance performance by reducing perceived exertion, allowing individuals to push through strenuous activities with less mental and physical strain.

The herb also promotes efficient energy production at the cellular level, which supports sustained endurance. Rhodiola is ideal for those who need a mental and physical boost without the jitteriness associated with stimulants.

4. Cordyceps (Cordyceps sinensis)

Known as a "medicinal mushroom," cordyceps has been used in traditional Chinese medicine to enhance athletic performance, reduce fatigue, and increase stamina. This fungus supports oxygen uptake and increases blood flow, which is essential for high-intensity activities and endurance sports.

Studies suggest that cordyceps improves aerobic capacity, making it beneficial for long-distance runners, cyclists, and swimmers. It is also valuable for anyone experiencing age-related declines in energy, as it supports cardiovascular and respiratory function.

Dietary Strategies for Sustained Energy

In addition to herbal support, diet plays a crucial role in maintaining consistent energy levels. The body relies on nutrient-dense foods that provide complex carbohydrates, proteins, healthy fats, vitamins, and minerals essential for cellular energy production.

1. **Complex Carbohydrates for Steady Fuel**

Unlike simple sugars that lead to rapid energy spikes and crashes, complex carbohydrates provide a steady release of glucose, the body's primary energy source. Foods such as oats, quinoa, brown rice, and sweet potatoes are excellent choices for sustained energy. They have a low glycemic index, meaning they release glucose gradually, helping to prevent sudden drops in blood sugar.

2. **Healthy Fats for Endurance**

Fats are a dense source of energy, and including healthy fats in the diet can support endurance by providing a slow-burning fuel. Foods rich in omega-3 fatty acids, like salmon, chia seeds, and flaxseeds, not only support energy production but also reduce inflammation, allowing for quicker recovery after physical exertion.

3. **Protein for Muscle Repair and Energy**

Protein is essential for muscle repair and growth, making it a key dietary component for those focused on endurance. Protein-rich foods such as lean meats, eggs, legumes, and nuts provide amino acids necessary for repairing muscle tissue and promoting recovery. For athletes or those engaged in regular physical activity, consuming protein after workouts can reduce muscle soreness and support sustained energy levels.

4. **Hydration and Electrolytes**

Dehydration is a common cause of fatigue and low energy. Water alone is often not enough; the body also requires electrolytes like potassium, magnesium, and sodium to maintain proper hydration at a cellular level. Natural sources of electrolytes include coconut water, bananas, and leafy greens, or you can create homemade electrolyte drinks using a blend of citrus juice, sea salt, and honey.

Exercise Routines to Build Endurance

Consistent physical activity, especially aerobic and resistance training, is essential for building endurance and supporting overall energy levels. Exercise improves cardiovascular health, enhances oxygen utilization, and strengthens muscles, all of which contribute to higher energy levels.

1. **Aerobic Exercise for Cardiovascular Health**

Activities like jogging, swimming, cycling, and brisk walking improve cardiovascular endurance by strengthening the heart and lungs. Engaging in aerobic exercise several times a week increases oxygen uptake, which enhances stamina for both physical and mental tasks.

2. **Resistance Training for Muscular Endurance**

Resistance training, including weightlifting or bodyweight exercises like push-ups and squats, builds muscle strength and endurance. Increased muscle mass supports metabolic health, contributing to better energy utilization and a higher basal metabolic rate. This means that even at rest, the body burns more calories, supporting overall energy levels.

3. **High-Intensity Interval Training (HIIT)**

HIIT alternates between short bursts of intense exercise and periods of rest, effectively increasing both aerobic and anaerobic endurance. HIIT can be adapted for beginners and advanced fitness levels, making it an efficient way to boost energy and build stamina in a shorter time frame.

Managing Energy with Balanced Hormones

Hormones play a central role in regulating energy, with key players including cortisol, testosterone, and thyroid hormones. A balanced hormonal profile supports consistent energy levels, mental clarity, and overall vitality.

1. **Supporting the Adrenals**

Chronic stress can lead to adrenal fatigue, where the body struggles to produce adequate cortisol. Adaptogenic herbs like ashwagandha, rhodiola, and holy basil can support adrenal function, helping to balance cortisol levels and reduce feelings of exhaustion.

2. **Thyroid Health**

The thyroid gland regulates metabolism, and an underactive thyroid can lead to fatigue, low energy, and sluggishness. Iodine-rich foods like seaweed, and selenium from Brazil nuts, support thyroid health. Additionally, managing stress and ensuring adequate rest are vital for maintaining optimal thyroid function.

3. **Testosterone for Men's Endurance**

Testosterone, a key hormone in men, influences energy, muscle mass, and endurance. Engaging in resistance training and consuming a diet rich in protein, healthy fats, and zinc supports healthy testosterone levels. Herbs like tribulus and fenugreek also aid in maintaining testosterone balance, contributing to increased endurance and vitality.

Natural Supplements for Energy Enhancement

For individuals seeking additional support, natural supplements can provide an effective way to boost energy without the crash associated with stimulants. Certain vitamins and minerals play essential roles in energy production at the cellular level.

1. **B Vitamins**

B vitamins, particularly B12 and B6, are vital for energy metabolism. They help convert food into usable energy and are essential for healthy nerve and blood cell function. Vitamin B12 is especially important, as a deficiency can lead to fatigue, weakness, and mood changes.

2. **Magnesium**

Magnesium is involved in over 300 enzymatic reactions in the body, including those related to energy production. It helps reduce muscle cramps, improves recovery, and enhances sleep quality. Foods rich in magnesium include dark leafy greens, nuts, and seeds.

3. **Iron for Oxygen Transport**

Iron is essential for producing hemoglobin, the molecule that carries oxygen in the blood. Low iron levels can lead to anemia, resulting in fatigue and low endurance. Iron-rich foods like spinach, red meat, and legumes, or an iron supplement if needed, support energy levels by ensuring efficient oxygen transport to muscles.

Lifestyle Habits to Maintain Energy and Endurance

Endurance and energy are not solely dependent on diet and exercise; lifestyle habits also play a critical role in maintaining vitality. Regular sleep, stress management, and mindful relaxation practices can enhance energy levels and support a resilient body and mind.

- **Prioritizing Sleep**: Quality sleep is essential for recovery and sustained energy. Aim for 7-9 hours per night to support the body's natural repair processes.
- **Stress Management**: Practices such as mindfulness meditation, deep breathing exercises, and journaling can help reduce stress, supporting balanced cortisol levels and preventing burnout.
- **Mindful Breaks**: Taking breaks throughout the day prevents burnout and maintains energy. Simple practices like stretching, walking, or deep breathing help recharge mental and physical energy, making it easier to sustain endurance throughout the day.

Chapter 2: Nutrition for Prostate Health

Maintaining a heart-healthy diet is one of the most effective ways to reduce the risk of cardiovascular disease, which remains a leading cause of death in the United States. A diet focused on heart health includes balanced nutrients, mindful choices, and understanding how specific foods impact the cardiovascular system.

Heart-Healthy Diet Tips

This section explores dietary strategies to protect heart health, with practical advice on selecting, preparing, and consuming foods that support cardiovascular wellness.

The Importance of a Heart-Healthy Diet

A heart-healthy diet does more than reduce the risk of cardiovascular disease; it also helps manage cholesterol levels, blood pressure, and inflammation. Heart disease often begins with factors like high blood pressure and high cholesterol, which can lead to atherosclerosis, a condition where plaque builds up in the arteries, narrowing them and increasing the risk of heart attacks and strokes. Diet can influence these factors significantly, offering a preventive approach to managing heart health.

Prioritizing Healthy Fats

Contrary to popular belief, not all fats are harmful. In fact, some fats are essential for heart health. The key lies in choosing the right kinds of fats.

Unsaturated Fats

Unsaturated fats, especially monounsaturated and polyunsaturated fats, help reduce bad cholesterol levels (LDL) while increasing good cholesterol (HDL). Foods rich in these fats include:

- **Avocados**: Containing monounsaturated fats, avocados are great for heart health, and they also contain potassium, which helps lower blood pressure.
- **Nuts and Seeds**: Almonds, walnuts, chia seeds, and flaxseeds are packed with omega-3 fatty acids, which help reduce inflammation.

- **Olive Oil**: Extra virgin olive oil is high in antioxidants and heart-healthy fats. Using olive oil in cooking or as a dressing is an excellent way to boost heart health.

Omega-3 Fatty Acids

Omega-3 fatty acids are a type of polyunsaturated fat that has been shown to reduce triglycerides, prevent arrhythmias, and lower blood pressure slightly. Fatty fish like salmon, mackerel, and sardines are rich in omega-3s. For those who prefer plant-based sources, chia seeds, flaxseeds, and walnuts are also good options.

Reducing Saturated and Trans Fats

While some fats are beneficial, others can be detrimental to heart health. Saturated fats, found in red meat and dairy products, and trans fats, found in many processed foods, can raise LDL cholesterol levels, leading to artery clogging.

- **Limit Red Meat**: Choose lean meats like chicken and turkey or opt for plant-based proteins. When consuming red meat, choose cuts labeled "lean" and keep portions small.
- **Avoid Processed Foods**: Processed foods like baked goods, fried snacks, and margarine often contain trans fats, which are known to increase the risk of heart disease.
- **Read Labels Carefully**: Trans fats may be listed as "partially hydrogenated oils" in ingredient lists. Avoid foods with these ingredients to protect heart health.

Emphasizing Whole Grains

Whole grains are high in fiber, which is essential for heart health. Fiber helps reduce cholesterol levels and improve digestion, lowering the risk of heart disease.

Choosing Whole Grains

Whole grains retain all parts of the grain, including the bran, germ, and endosperm, which makes them more nutritious than refined grains. Excellent choices for whole grains include:

- **Oats**: Rich in beta-glucan, a type of soluble fiber, oats help lower cholesterol levels.
- **Quinoa**: A complete protein and high in fiber, quinoa supports heart health and offers sustained energy.
- **Brown Rice**: Containing more nutrients than white rice, brown rice is a better option for those looking to manage blood sugar and cholesterol levels.

Avoiding Refined Carbohydrates

Refined carbohydrates, such as white bread, pastries, and sugary snacks, cause spikes in blood sugar, which can contribute to weight gain and heart disease over time. Opt for whole-grain versions of bread, pasta, and rice to support a heart-healthy diet.

Managing Sodium Intake

Excessive sodium intake is linked to high blood pressure, a major risk factor for heart disease. Most people consume more sodium than needed, primarily from processed foods and restaurant meals.

Tips for Reducing Sodium

- **Cook at Home**: Preparing meals at home allows for better control over salt levels.
- **Use Herbs and Spices**: Flavoring food with herbs and spices, such as garlic, rosemary, or cumin, adds taste without extra sodium.
- **Read Labels**: Foods labeled "low sodium" or "no added salt" are often better choices. Aim for foods with less than 140 mg of sodium per serving.

Increasing Fiber Intake

Fiber is crucial for heart health, as it helps lower cholesterol levels, improve digestion, and regulate blood sugar. Foods high in soluble fiber, such as fruits, vegetables, and legumes, are particularly beneficial.

Fiber-Rich Foods for Heart Health

- **Fruits**: Apples, oranges, berries, and pears are high in fiber and rich in antioxidants.
- **Vegetables**: Leafy greens like spinach and kale, as well as root vegetables like carrots and sweet potatoes, provide ample fiber.
- **Legumes**: Beans, lentils, and chickpeas are not only high in fiber but also provide plant-based protein.

Increasing fiber intake can be as simple as adding more fruits and vegetables to each meal and choosing whole grains over refined options.

Focusing on Antioxidant-Rich Foods

Antioxidants protect cells from damage caused by free radicals, which contribute to heart disease. Incorporating a variety of antioxidant-rich foods in your diet can support heart health.

Best Sources of Antioxidants

- **Berries**: Blueberries, strawberries, and blackberries are loaded with antioxidants, particularly anthocyanins, which have been shown to reduce blood pressure and inflammation.
- **Dark Chocolate**: In moderation, dark chocolate with at least 70% cocoa is a good source of antioxidants and may help improve blood flow.
- **Green Tea**: Rich in catechins, green tea has been linked to reduced cholesterol levels and improved heart health.

Incorporating Plant-Based Proteins

Switching to plant-based proteins helps reduce saturated fat intake and increases fiber. Plant-based diets have been shown to improve heart health by lowering cholesterol and blood pressure.

Plant-Based Protein Sources

- **Beans and Lentils**: High in fiber and protein, beans and lentils make excellent meat substitutes.
- **Tofu and Tempeh**: Both are versatile and low in saturated fat, offering high-quality protein.
- **Nuts and Seeds**: Almonds, chia seeds, and pumpkin seeds provide heart-healthy fats and protein.

Incorporating plant-based meals into your diet, even a few times a week, can make a significant difference in heart health.

Limiting Sugar Intake

High sugar consumption is linked to obesity, diabetes, and heart disease. Excess sugar leads to weight gain, increased triglycerides, and higher blood pressure, all of which can strain the heart.

Tips for Reducing Sugar

- **Choose Whole Fruits**: Unlike fruit juices and snacks, whole fruits contain fiber, which helps slow the absorption of sugar.
- **Avoid Sugary Beverages**: Soft drinks, energy drinks, and even certain fruit juices contain high levels of sugar. Opt for water, herbal teas, or sparkling water.

- **Read Ingredient Labels**: Sugar is often added to foods under names like corn syrup, fructose, and sucrose. Aim to avoid products with added sugars, particularly as one of the first ingredients.

Drinking in Moderation

While moderate alcohol consumption has been associated with certain heart health benefits, excessive drinking can lead to high blood pressure, heart failure, and other serious conditions.

- **Moderate Consumption**: For most people, moderate drinking means up to one drink per day for women and up to two for men.
- **Heart-Healthy Choices**: Red wine contains resveratrol, an antioxidant that may support heart health, though more research is needed.

If you do consume alcohol, doing so in moderation is key to maintaining heart health.

Planning Balanced Meals

Creating balanced meals with a variety of nutrients helps support heart health and overall well-being.

- **Half Plate of Vegetables**: Start with a base of colorful vegetables to provide fiber, vitamins, and antioxidants.
- **Lean Protein**: Choose lean sources of protein, such as chicken breast, tofu, or legumes.
- **Whole Grains**: Incorporate whole grains like brown rice or quinoa for sustained energy.
- **Healthy Fats**: Add a source of healthy fat, such as avocado, olive oil, or nuts.

This balanced approach ensures that you receive essential nutrients for heart health in every meal.

Staying Hydrated for Heart Health

Hydration is often overlooked, but it plays an essential role in heart health. Proper hydration helps the heart pump blood more efficiently, supports digestion, and maintains energy levels.

- **Water First**: Make water your primary beverage choice, as it helps maintain the body's fluid balance without adding calories or sugar.

- **Limit Caffeinated Beverages**: While moderate caffeine can be part of a heart-healthy diet, excessive intake may lead to increased heart rate and blood pressure.
- **Hydrating Foods**: Foods like cucumbers, watermelon, and oranges contribute to hydration and provide vitamins and antioxidants beneficial for the heart.

Maintaining a heart-healthy diet is about making consistent, mindful choices that support the cardiovascular system. Through these dietary practices, you can support long-term heart health and well-being.

Foods to Support Vitality

Vitality, or the state of feeling energized and robust, is influenced significantly by the foods we consume. A nutrient-rich diet not only provides the essential building blocks for energy but also helps maintain mental clarity, physical strength, and emotional stability. While each person's nutritional needs vary, certain foods have universal benefits that support vitality through their high concentration of vitamins, minerals, antioxidants, and other bioactive compounds.

In this section, we will explore a variety of foods known to support vitality, delve into their unique nutritional profiles, and examine how they contribute to sustained energy and overall wellness.

The Foundations of Vitality in Nutrition

For optimal vitality, the body requires a balance of macronutrients (carbohydrates, proteins, and fats) and micronutrients (vitamins and minerals). Carbohydrates provide the primary fuel, proteins build and repair tissues, and fats offer long-lasting energy. Meanwhile, vitamins like B-complex aid in energy metabolism, and minerals such as iron and magnesium support cellular processes that drive stamina and resilience.

Maintaining this balance also requires a focus on nutrient density. Choosing foods that are packed with essential nutrients per calorie is key to supporting vitality, as these foods promote optimal health without the excess calories that could lead to sluggishness.

Vitality-Boosting Foods and Their Benefits

1. **Leafy**   **Greens**

   Leafy greens like spinach, kale, and Swiss chard are often referred to as "superfoods" because of their dense nutritional profiles. They are rich in vitamins A, C, E, and K, as well as essential minerals like calcium, magnesium, and potassium. These nutrients collectively support cellular energy production and help reduce oxidative stress, a known factor in fatigue.

Spinach, in particular, contains high levels of iron, which is essential for producing hemoglobin, a protein in red blood cells that carries oxygen throughout the body. Oxygen is crucial for energy at the cellular level, making leafy greens a cornerstone of any vitality-boosting diet.

2. **Berries**

   Blueberries, strawberries, raspberries, and blackberries are loaded with antioxidants, particularly vitamin C and flavonoids, which help neutralize free radicals that cause cellular damage. Berries are also high in fiber, which supports digestive health and ensures a steady release of glucose into the bloodstream, preventing energy crashes.

The polyphenols in berries have been shown to improve cognitive function, supporting mental vitality and focus. Studies suggest that regularly consuming berries can improve memory, making them especially valuable for those who seek not just physical vitality but mental clarity as well.

3. **Nuts**   **and**   **Seeds**

   Almonds, walnuts, flaxseeds, chia seeds, and pumpkin seeds are rich in healthy fats, protein, and fiber, making them an excellent source of sustained energy. The high levels of omega-3 fatty acids in walnuts and flaxseeds also support brain health and help reduce inflammation, which can cause fatigue over time.

Seeds like chia and flax also contain lignans, a type of antioxidant that has been shown to support hormonal balance. For individuals facing energy dips related to hormonal fluctuations, incorporating these seeds into the diet can provide a steady source of fuel while promoting hormonal stability.

4. **Avocado**

   Avocados are nutrient powerhouses, providing healthy monounsaturated fats, fiber, and potassium. The fats in avocados support cell membrane health, making it easier for nutrients to enter cells and waste products to be expelled. This process enhances cellular efficiency, which is essential for sustained energy levels.

Additionally, avocados are rich in B vitamins, which are involved in energy metabolism. Their potassium content helps regulate blood pressure and electrolyte balance, both important for preventing fatigue, especially after physical exertion.

5. **Quinoa**

Quinoa is a complete protein, meaning it contains all nine essential amino acids that the body cannot produce on its own. This makes quinoa a fantastic choice for supporting muscle repair and energy. It is also a good source of complex carbohydrates, providing a steady release of glucose.

Furthermore, quinoa contains magnesium, a mineral essential for ATP production, the molecule that provides energy to cells. Magnesium also plays a role in muscle relaxation, making quinoa a valuable food for both energy production and muscle recovery.

6. **Sweet** **Potatoes**

Sweet potatoes are rich in complex carbohydrates, which provide a slow and steady energy release. Unlike refined carbs, complex carbs stabilize blood sugar levels and help prevent energy crashes. Sweet potatoes are also high in beta-carotene (a precursor to vitamin A), which supports immune function and eye health.

These root vegetables are also packed with potassium, which helps maintain electrolyte balance and hydration, especially important for active individuals. The combination of fiber, vitamins, and minerals makes sweet potatoes an ideal food for sustained vitality.

7. **Fermented** **Foods**

Fermented foods like yogurt, kefir, sauerkraut, and kimchi contain beneficial probiotics that support gut health. A healthy gut is essential for energy because it ensures efficient nutrient absorption. Many people don't realize that gut health can directly impact energy levels, as an imbalanced gut microbiome may lead to inflammation and sluggishness.

Fermented foods also help balance the immune system, which is crucial for preventing illness-related fatigue. A balanced gut can improve overall vitality by supporting both digestive and immune health.

8. **Bananas**

Bananas are well-known for their quick energy boost, thanks to their high carbohydrate content. They also contain vitamin B6, which aids in the conversion of food into energy. Bananas are rich in potassium, which helps regulate muscle function and prevent cramps, especially during physical activity.

For those seeking a pre-workout snack that won't cause a rapid energy crash, bananas provide a blend of natural sugars, fiber, and essential nutrients, making them an effective source of quick and sustainable energy.

9. **Eggs**

Eggs are an excellent source of high-quality protein, choline, and various B vitamins, including B12, which are crucial for energy metabolism. The amino acids in eggs support muscle repair and growth, making them valuable for physically active individuals.

Choline, found in egg yolks, is essential for brain health and cognitive function. This nutrient supports mental vitality by helping maintain cell membrane integrity and supporting neurotransmitter synthesis, which influences mood and focus.

10. **Green** **Tea**

Green tea contains a modest amount of caffeine, which provides an energy boost without the jitteriness associated with coffee. Additionally, it is rich in antioxidants, particularly EGCG (epigallocatechin gallate), which supports metabolic health.

One of the unique compounds in green tea, L-theanine, promotes relaxation and focus, balancing the stimulating effects of caffeine. This makes green tea a powerful option for sustained vitality, supporting both physical energy and mental clarity.

Implementing a Vitality-Boosting Diet

Incorporating these vitality-boosting foods into your diet doesn't have to be complicated. A few practical steps can help you optimize your meals for sustained energy and overall wellness.

1. **Start the Day with a Balanced Breakfast**
A balanced breakfast can set the tone for the day by providing lasting energy. Consider a combination of complex carbohydrates, healthy fats, and protein. For example, a smoothie made with spinach, banana, chia seeds, and a handful of berries provides essential vitamins, minerals, and sustained energy.

2. **Include Protein in Every Meal**

   Protein is essential for muscle repair and maintaining energy levels. Adding protein to every meal helps prevent energy dips and supports metabolism. Nuts, seeds, quinoa, eggs, and lean meats are all excellent protein sources that can be included in various meals.

3. **Snack Wisely**

   Instead of reaching for processed snacks that can cause an energy spike and subsequent crash, opt for nutrient-dense options. Apple slices with almond butter, Greek yogurt with berries, or a handful of walnuts can provide a quick energy boost without the downsides of refined sugars.

4. **Stay Hydrated**

   Hydration is essential for maintaining energy. Sometimes, what feels like fatigue is simply dehydration. Incorporate hydrating foods like cucumbers, oranges, and watermelon alongside regular water intake to ensure optimal hydration.

5. **Use Herbs and Spices**

   Adding vitality-boosting herbs and spices to your meals can provide extra health benefits. Turmeric, for example, is a potent anti-inflammatory that pairs well with sweet potatoes. Cinnamon helps regulate blood sugar levels, making it an excellent addition to oatmeal or yogurt.

Foods to Avoid for Sustained Vitality

Just as there are foods that support vitality, certain foods can drain energy and leave you feeling sluggish. Reducing or avoiding these foods can help you maintain high energy levels throughout the day.

1. **Refined Sugars**

   Sugary foods cause a quick spike in blood sugar followed by a rapid drop, leading to energy crashes. Replacing refined sugars with natural sources of sweetness, like fruit, provides fiber and additional nutrients that promote lasting energy.

2. **Processed Foods**

   Processed foods are often low in nutrients and high in unhealthy fats, sodium, and additives. These foods may cause inflammation and negatively impact gut health, which can contribute to feelings of sluggishness. Opt for whole foods as much as possible to ensure nutrient intake that supports vitality.

3. **Excessive**   **Caffeine**

   While moderate caffeine can enhance focus and energy, excessive caffeine can lead to dependency and energy crashes. Green tea or herbal teas can be a better option for a gentle, sustained boost without the risk of over-stimulation.

4. **Alcohol**

   Alcohol disrupts sleep patterns and can dehydrate the body, both of which lead to fatigue. Limiting alcohol intake, particularly before bedtime, can improve sleep quality and help you feel more energized.

The Role of Lifestyle in Supporting Vitality

While diet plays a major role, other lifestyle factors also contribute to vitality. Combining a nutrient-dense diet with regular physical activity, adequate sleep, stress management, and mindful practices creates a foundation for optimal health.

Chapter 3: Herbs for Men's Health

Saw palmetto, a small palm tree native to the southeastern United States, has long been recognized for its medicinal properties, particularly in supporting men's prostate health.

Saw Palmetto for Prostate Health

Derived from the berries of the saw palmetto tree (*Serenoa repens*), this natural remedy has become one of the most popular supplements for men seeking to maintain prostate health and manage symptoms associated with benign prostatic hyperplasia (BPH), a common condition as men age. This section explores saw palmetto's effects on prostate health, how it works, and practical ways to incorporate it safely and effectively.

Understanding Prostate Health and Common Issues

The prostate is a small, walnut-sized gland that is part of the male reproductive system. It plays an essential role in producing seminal fluid, which nourishes and transports sperm. As men age, the prostate gland often enlarges, a condition known as benign prostatic hyperplasia (BPH). BPH is non-cancerous but can cause uncomfortable symptoms, including difficulty urinating, frequent urges to urinate (especially at night), and a weakened urine stream.

While the exact cause of BPH is unclear, hormonal changes are believed to play a role. Testosterone levels decline as men age, while levels of dihydrotestosterone (DHT), a hormone derived from testosterone, may increase within the prostate. DHT is thought to stimulate prostate cell growth, contributing to an enlarged prostate. Saw palmetto is believed to work by inhibiting the enzyme responsible for converting testosterone into DHT, thus helping to manage symptoms associated with BPH.

Saw Palmetto: Mechanism of Action

The active compounds in saw palmetto berries are primarily fatty acids and phytosterols, which are believed to inhibit the enzyme 5-alpha-reductase. This enzyme is responsible for converting testosterone into DHT, the hormone linked to prostate growth. By blocking this enzyme, saw palmetto can potentially reduce the accumulation of DHT in the prostate, helping to slow or reduce prostate enlargement.

In addition to inhibiting DHT production, saw palmetto is also thought to have anti-inflammatory properties, which may further support prostate health by reducing inflammation in the prostate tissue. Some studies suggest that saw palmetto can even help relieve symptoms of BPH, such as frequent urination and nighttime urination, which can significantly improve quality of life for men experiencing these issues.

Benefits of Saw Palmetto for Prostate Health

Saw palmetto has been widely studied for its potential benefits in supporting prostate health, especially in relation to BPH. Below are some of the key benefits of saw palmetto based on scientific research and traditional use.

Symptom Relief for BPH

One of the primary reasons men use saw palmetto is for relief from the urinary symptoms associated with BPH. These symptoms can disrupt sleep and daily activities, making effective management crucial for a better quality of life. Research has shown that saw palmetto can:

- **Reduce urinary frequency**: By decreasing the size of the prostate or reducing the obstruction caused by an enlarged prostate, saw palmetto may help reduce the need to urinate frequently, particularly at night.

- **Improve urinary flow**: Studies suggest that saw palmetto may improve urinary flow rates, making it easier for men to empty their bladders.

- **Decrease residual urine volume**: Saw palmetto may help reduce the amount of urine left in the bladder after urination, which can reduce the likelihood of urinary tract infections and discomfort.

Natural Alternative to Medications

Many men prefer saw palmetto as a natural alternative to prescription medications, which can come with side effects. Common medications for BPH include alpha-blockers and 5-alpha-reductase inhibitors. While effective, these medications can lead to side effects such as dizziness, fatigue, and sexual dysfunction. Saw palmetto is generally well-tolerated and offers a milder approach to managing BPH symptoms, making it an attractive option for those seeking a more holistic remedy.

Anti-Inflammatory Effects

Inflammation is often linked to various health issues, including prostate enlargement. Saw palmetto has been shown to possess anti-inflammatory properties, which may contribute to its effectiveness in reducing prostate symptoms. By reducing inflammation in the prostate, saw palmetto may help alleviate pain, improve urinary function, and potentially slow the progression of BPH.

How to Use Saw Palmetto for Prostate Health

Saw palmetto is available in various forms, including capsules, tablets, liquid extracts, and teas. The most common form is a standardized extract, as it provides a consistent concentration of active compounds. The recommended dosage can vary depending on the specific product, so it is important to follow manufacturer instructions and consult a healthcare provider before starting saw palmetto.

Dosage Recommendations

For BPH symptom management, the typical dosage of saw palmetto extract is around 160 mg twice daily, standardized to contain 85-95% fatty acids. Some studies have used higher dosages or once-daily dosages, but 160 mg twice daily is a widely accepted starting point. It's essential to consult a healthcare provider before beginning any herbal supplement, as individual needs and responses can vary.

Combining with Other Supplements

Saw palmetto is sometimes combined with other herbs and nutrients that support prostate health, such as:

- **Pygeum**: Extracted from the African cherry tree, pygeum has shown promise in reducing BPH symptoms and is often used alongside saw palmetto.
- **Beta-Sitosterol**: A plant sterol found in fruits, vegetables, and nuts, beta-sitosterol has been shown to support urinary function in men with BPH.
- **Zinc**: Zinc is essential for prostate health, and a deficiency has been linked to BPH. Many prostate supplements combine saw palmetto with zinc for comprehensive support.

Practical Tips for Incorporating Saw Palmetto

- **Consistency**: Herbal supplements often work best when taken consistently over time. Saw palmetto may take several weeks to show noticeable effects.
- **Time of Day**: Taking saw palmetto with food can help prevent stomach upset. Many men prefer taking it with breakfast or dinner.
- **Monitor Symptoms**: It's essential to track symptoms while using saw palmetto. If symptoms persist or worsen, consult a healthcare provider to discuss other treatment options.

Scientific Research on Saw Palmetto

Numerous studies have investigated the effects of saw palmetto on prostate health, though results have been mixed. Some studies suggest that saw palmetto is effective in reducing symptoms of BPH, while others indicate that its effects may be modest or comparable to a placebo. It is worth noting that saw palmetto's benefits may vary depending on the severity of symptoms and individual response.

Notable Studies

1. **Journal of the American Medical Association (JAMA) Study**: A 2006 study published in JAMA found that saw palmetto did not significantly improve symptoms of BPH compared to a placebo. However, the study's participants had varying levels of symptom severity, which may have influenced the results.
2. **Complementary and Alternative Medicine (CAM) Study**: Another study published in a CAM journal found that men who took saw palmetto experienced improved urinary symptoms compared to those who took a placebo. The participants also reported fewer side effects, supporting the herb's safety and tolerability.
3. **Meta-Analysis Review**: Some meta-analyses have concluded that saw palmetto may be effective in reducing BPH symptoms, particularly urinary frequency and nocturia (nighttime urination). However, the effect size is often modest, and more research is needed to clarify the herb's efficacy.

Safety and Side Effects of Saw Palmetto

Saw palmetto is generally well-tolerated, but it can cause mild side effects in some individuals. Common side effects include stomach discomfort, nausea, and headaches. Taking saw palmetto with food can help reduce these side effects. Unlike prescription medications for BPH, saw palmetto does not appear to cause significant sexual side effects, which is one reason it is popular among men seeking natural remedies.

Precautions and Considerations

- **Pregnancy and Breastfeeding**: Although primarily used for men's health, saw palmetto should not be used by women who are pregnant or breastfeeding, as its effects on hormone levels may interfere with pregnancy.
- **Interactions with Medications**: Saw palmetto may interact with medications that affect hormone levels or blood clotting. It is essential to consult a healthcare provider if you are taking any prescription medications.
- **Medical Monitoring**: While saw palmetto may alleviate symptoms of BPH, it does not address other prostate conditions such as prostate cancer. Regular medical check-ups and screenings are important for monitoring prostate health, especially in men over 50.

Lifestyle Tips for Prostate Health

In addition to using saw palmetto, adopting a healthy lifestyle can further support prostate health. Regular exercise, a balanced diet rich in fruits, vegetables, and whole grains, and maintaining a healthy weight all contribute to prostate wellness. Reducing caffeine and alcohol intake can also help manage urinary symptoms associated with BPH.

Prostate health is a critical component of overall wellness for men, particularly as they age. By incorporating saw palmetto and other prostate-friendly habits, men can support their health naturally and manage symptoms associated with prostate enlargement effectively.

Adaptogens for Energy

In today's fast-paced world, energy demands are high, and individuals often face challenges managing stress and maintaining vitality. This is where adaptogens—natural substances that help the body adapt to stress and enhance energy—become valuable allies. Originating from herbal traditions in regions like Asia, India, and Russia, adaptogens have been used for centuries to support resilience, energy, and overall well-being. Today, these remarkable plants and herbs are studied for their effects on physical and mental endurance, stress management, and the ability to balance energy levels.

This section delves into various adaptogens known for boosting energy, exploring their unique properties, practical applications, and the scientific insights that support their efficacy.

Understanding Adaptogens and Their Mechanism

Adaptogens work by influencing the body's stress response, specifically by interacting with the hypothalamic-pituitary-adrenal (HPA) axis, which governs how our bodies react to stress. They help regulate cortisol, a key stress hormone, to prevent the extreme highs and lows associated with stress-related fatigue. By maintaining cortisol levels within a healthy range, adaptogens enable the body to stay balanced, even in stressful situations.

Adaptogens do not act as stimulants in the way caffeine or sugar might. Instead, they work to optimize energy production at a cellular level, enhancing stamina without causing spikes and crashes. For people dealing with fatigue or burnout, adaptogens offer a gentle, sustainable boost in energy, resilience, and mental clarity.

Key Adaptogens for Energy and Vitality

1. **Ashwagandha**

   Ashwagandha (Withania somnifera) is one of the most researched adaptogens and has a long history in Ayurvedic medicine for enhancing stamina and energy. This adaptogen is particularly beneficial for reducing cortisol levels, which can lead to reduced anxiety, improved sleep quality, and sustained energy levels.

Studies suggest that ashwagandha can also improve muscle strength and endurance, making it beneficial for those who engage in physical activity. Additionally, ashwagandha is known to increase the body's resilience to stress by balancing cortisol and supporting thyroid function, which is critical for metabolic health.

   o *Usage*: Ashwagandha can be taken as a powder mixed with milk or warm water, or in capsule form. A common dose is between 300-600 mg per day, often standardized to a specific withanolide content, the active compounds in ashwagandha.

2. **Rhodiola   Rosea**

   Known as the "golden root," Rhodiola Rosea is native to Arctic and mountainous regions and has been used by Russian and Scandinavian cultures to combat fatigue and enhance endurance. Rhodiola is recognized for its ability to reduce physical and mental fatigue, especially under stressful conditions. Research has shown that Rhodiola can improve exercise performance, reduce mental fatigue, and increase mental clarity.

Rhodiola works by influencing neurotransmitters like dopamine and serotonin, which affect mood and energy levels. It also has a mild stimulating effect, providing an energy boost without the crash often associated with caffeine.

- o *Usage*: Rhodiola Rosea is commonly taken in capsule form, with dosages ranging from 100-400 mg. It is generally recommended to take it in the morning or early afternoon to avoid disrupting sleep.

3. **Eleuthero   (Siberian   Ginseng)**

   Eleuthero, also known as Siberian ginseng, is widely recognized for its ability to increase stamina and resilience, especially in challenging environments. Russian athletes have used Eleuthero to enhance endurance and recovery, and studies support its role in reducing fatigue and enhancing physical performance.

Eleuthero works by modulating the HPA axis, helping the body adapt to physical and mental stress. It is particularly beneficial for individuals who need sustained energy throughout the day, as it supports both mental focus and physical stamina.

- o *Usage*: Eleuthero is available as a powder, capsule, or tincture, with common dosages around 300-500 mg daily.

4. **Holy   Basil   (Tulsi)**

   Holy basil, also known as tulsi, is another Ayurvedic adaptogen renowned for its calming effects and ability to balance energy. Unlike other adaptogens that have more stimulating effects, holy basil provides a sense of calm alertness, making it suitable for those who experience both anxiety and fatigue.

Holy basil supports mental clarity, reduces inflammation, and helps manage blood sugar levels, which can contribute to sustained energy. Its balancing effects on the nervous system make it especially beneficial for people dealing with stress-induced fatigue.

- o *Usage*: Holy basil can be enjoyed as a tea or taken in capsule form. Drinking tulsi tea throughout the day can provide a gentle, steady boost in mental clarity and resilience.

5. **Maca   Root**

   Originating from the Andes mountains in Peru, maca root has been used for centuries to enhance energy, fertility, and stamina. Maca is known to help balance hormones, which can positively impact energy levels, particularly for individuals dealing with hormonal imbalances or adrenal fatigue.

Maca is rich in vitamins, minerals, and amino acids, making it a nutritional powerhouse that supports physical vitality. Its energy-boosting effects are not immediate but build over time, making maca an ideal adaptogen for long-term energy and endurance support.

- o *Usage*: Maca is typically consumed as a powder that can be added to smoothies, coffee, or oatmeal. The recommended dosage varies, but around 1-3 teaspoons per day is common.

6. **Schisandra**

Schisandra, often referred to as the "five-flavor berry," has been used in Traditional Chinese Medicine to increase endurance, reduce fatigue, and support liver health. It is unique among adaptogens for its ability to support both mental and physical endurance, making it beneficial for people with demanding lifestyles.

Schisandra is known to enhance concentration, improve coordination, and increase resistance to stress. Its liver-supporting properties also help in detoxification, which indirectly contributes to better energy by preventing toxin buildup.

- o *Usage*: Schisandra is commonly available as a tincture or in capsule form. A typical dosage is around 500 mg daily.

7. **Cordyceps**

Cordyceps, a type of medicinal mushroom, is famed for its energy-enhancing properties. This adaptogen supports ATP (adenosine triphosphate) production, the body's primary energy currency, making it especially useful for physical endurance and recovery. Cordyceps is popular among athletes and has been shown to improve oxygen utilization, which enhances stamina.

Unlike stimulants, Cordyceps provides a natural, sustainable boost in energy without causing jitters or crashes. It also supports the immune system, helping the body stay resilient in the face of physical stress.

- o *Usage*: Cordyceps is commonly taken in capsule or powder form, with typical dosages between 500-1000 mg daily.

Practical Tips for Using Adaptogens to Boost Energy

To harness the full benefits of adaptogens, it's essential to understand how and when to use them. Here are some practical strategies to consider:

- **Consistency is Key**: Adaptogens work best when taken consistently over time, as their effects are cumulative rather than immediate. Most adaptogens are safe for long-term use, although it's often recommended to take occasional breaks.
- **Choose the Right Form**: Adaptogens are available in various forms, including capsules, powders, and tinctures. The form you choose depends on personal preference and lifestyle. Powders are versatile and can be mixed into smoothies or coffee, while capsules are convenient for on-the-go use.
- **Timing Matters**: While some adaptogens like Rhodiola are stimulating and best taken in the morning, others like holy basil provide a calming effect and can be consumed in the evening. Pay attention to how each adaptogen affects your energy levels and adjust timing accordingly.
- **Combine Adaptogens for Synergy**: Some adaptogens work well together, enhancing each other's effects. For example, combining ashwagandha and Rhodiola can provide a balanced approach to energy and stress resilience, while Cordyceps and maca root together can offer robust physical endurance.

The Role of Adaptogens in Stress and Energy Management

One of the primary benefits of adaptogens is their ability to support energy levels by modulating the body's response to stress. Chronic stress drains the adrenal glands, leading to adrenal fatigue and, ultimately, low energy. By balancing cortisol and other stress hormones, adaptogens prevent the body from depleting its energy reserves in response to ongoing stress.

Adaptogens also support neurotransmitter balance, influencing mood and mental clarity. Adaptogens like Rhodiola and Schisandra, which impact dopamine and serotonin levels, can enhance motivation and concentration, crucial for sustained energy and productivity.

Incorporating Adaptogens into a Balanced Lifestyle

While adaptogens provide valuable support for energy, they work best when combined with a healthy lifestyle. Adequate sleep, balanced nutrition, hydration, and regular physical activity are all essential components of a high-energy lifestyle. Adaptogens complement these habits by enhancing resilience, reducing stress-related fatigue, and improving stamina.

Incorporating adaptogens into daily routines can also foster a more mindful approach to energy management, encouraging individuals to listen to their bodies and make adjustments as needed.

Precautions and Considerations

Adaptogens are generally safe for most people; however, certain considerations should be kept in mind:

- **Start Slowly**: When introducing a new adaptogen, it's wise to start with a low dose to observe how your body responds.
- **Consult a Healthcare Provider**: If you have any underlying health conditions or are pregnant or breastfeeding, consult a healthcare professional before using adaptogens.
- **Quality Matters**: Purchase adaptogens from reputable sources to ensure they are free from contaminants and contain active compounds.

Adaptogens offer a powerful, natural approach to enhancing energy and resilience. By supporting physical and mental stamina, they allow individuals to thrive, even in the face of life's demands.

Chapter 4: Men's Health Recipes

P umpkin seed oil, derived from the seeds of the pumpkin (*Cucurbita pepo*), has gained recognition for its health benefits, particularly in supporting prostate health, urinary function, and heart health.

Pumpkin Seed Oil Capsules

Rich in essential fatty acids, vitamins, and minerals, pumpkin seed oil provides a natural remedy with a variety of therapeutic properties. This section explores the benefits of pumpkin seed oil capsules, their applications, and practical ways to incorporate them into a daily health regimen.

Nutritional Composition of Pumpkin Seed Oil

Pumpkin seed oil is packed with nutrients that contribute to its therapeutic benefits. Key components of pumpkin seed oil include:

- **Essential Fatty Acids**: Pumpkin seed oil is a rich source of omega-6 fatty acids, particularly linoleic acid, which supports heart health, brain function, and cellular health. It also contains omega-9 fatty acids (oleic acid), which have anti-inflammatory properties.
- **Phytosterols**: These plant compounds help support prostate health and may contribute to lowering cholesterol levels, promoting cardiovascular health.
- **Vitamins**: Pumpkin seed oil contains vitamin E, a potent antioxidant that protects cells from oxidative damage, and is crucial for skin and eye health.
- **Minerals**: The oil is a natural source of zinc, magnesium, and potassium, minerals that play roles in immune function, muscle health, and heart health.

The combination of these nutrients gives pumpkin seed oil its powerful health-supporting properties, particularly in areas of prostate health, urinary health, and cardiovascular wellness.

Prostate Health and Pumpkin Seed Oil

One of the most common uses of pumpkin seed oil is for promoting prostate health, making it particularly beneficial for men. The prostate, a small gland in men's reproductive system, can become enlarged due to hormonal changes as men age, leading to a condition known as benign prostatic hyperplasia (BPH). This non-cancerous enlargement can cause uncomfortable urinary symptoms, including frequent urination, difficulty urinating, and an increased urge to urinate at night.

Mechanism of Action for Prostate Health

Pumpkin seed oil has been shown to benefit prostate health through several mechanisms:

1. **Inhibition of DHT**: Pumpkin seed oil may help reduce the production of dihydrotestosterone (DHT), a hormone derived from testosterone that contributes to prostate enlargement. By reducing DHT levels, pumpkin seed oil may help slow prostate growth, alleviating symptoms associated with BPH.

2. **Anti-Inflammatory Properties**: The fatty acids in pumpkin seed oil, particularly oleic and linoleic acids, exhibit anti-inflammatory effects. This can help reduce inflammation in the prostate gland, providing relief from urinary discomfort and other symptoms associated with prostate issues.

3. **High Zinc Content**: Zinc is essential for prostate health, and pumpkin seeds are naturally high in zinc. Zinc supports immune function, reduces inflammation, and may play a role in regulating DHT levels.

Clinical Studies on Pumpkin Seed Oil and Prostate Health

Several studies have examined the effects of pumpkin seed oil on prostate health, particularly in men with BPH. For instance, a study published in *Urology International* found that men with BPH who took pumpkin seed oil over a 12-month period experienced significant improvements in symptoms, including reduced urinary frequency and improved flow rate. Another study published in the *Journal of Medicinal Food* demonstrated that men who took pumpkin seed oil had improved quality of life due to the reduction in urinary symptoms.

These studies highlight pumpkin seed oil's potential as a natural supplement for men seeking relief from BPH symptoms without the side effects often associated with prescription medications.

Heart Health Benefits of Pumpkin Seed Oil

In addition to its prostate-supporting properties, pumpkin seed oil is beneficial for cardiovascular health. Its high content of essential fatty acids, phytosterols, and antioxidants contribute to heart health in several ways:

- **Blood Pressure Regulation**: Pumpkin seed oil contains potassium and magnesium, two minerals essential for maintaining healthy blood pressure. Potassium helps balance sodium levels in the body, while magnesium relaxes blood vessels, aiding in blood pressure control.
- **Cholesterol Management**: Phytosterols found in pumpkin seed oil are similar in structure to cholesterol and can help lower LDL cholesterol levels by blocking its absorption in the intestines. This can reduce the risk of atherosclerosis, a condition characterized by plaque buildup in the arteries.
- **Anti-Inflammatory Effects**: Chronic inflammation is a risk factor for heart disease. The anti-inflammatory properties of pumpkin seed oil can help reduce inflammation in blood vessels, promoting better circulation and cardiovascular health.

Supporting Urinary Health with Pumpkin Seed Oil

Pumpkin seed oil is known for its ability to support urinary tract health, especially in men and women experiencing frequent urination or incontinence. By promoting bladder health, pumpkin seed oil helps reduce urinary frequency and may improve bladder function.

How Pumpkin Seed Oil Supports Urinary Health

- **Strengthening the Bladder**: The fatty acids and phytosterols in pumpkin seed oil can help strengthen the bladder, reducing overactivity and improving control over urinary frequency.
- **Reducing Inflammation**: For those experiencing irritation or inflammation in the bladder, the anti-inflammatory properties of pumpkin seed oil can provide relief.
- **Promoting Healthy Hormone Balance**: Pumpkin seed oil may have mild hormone-modulating effects, which can help with conditions related to hormone imbalances that affect urinary health.

How to Use Pumpkin Seed Oil Capsules

Pumpkin seed oil is available in various forms, including capsules, liquid extracts, and culinary oils. Capsules are a convenient option for those who prefer a measured dosage without the need for measuring or tasting the oil.

Dosage Recommendations

The standard dosage for pumpkin seed oil capsules can vary, but most supplements recommend a dose of around 1,000 mg per day, typically taken in divided doses with meals. For prostate health and urinary support, consult with a healthcare provider to determine the appropriate dosage for individual needs.

Tips for Incorporating Pumpkin Seed Oil Capsules

- **Consistency is Key**: Like many herbal supplements, pumpkin seed oil often works best when taken consistently over time. It may take a few weeks to notice the full effects.
- **Take with Food**: Taking pumpkin seed oil capsules with a meal can help improve absorption and reduce any mild digestive discomfort.
- **Monitor Symptoms**: Track any improvements in prostate health, urinary symptoms, or cardiovascular health while using pumpkin seed oil. Consult with a healthcare provider if symptoms persist or worsen.

Safety and Side Effects of Pumpkin Seed Oil Capsules

Pumpkin seed oil is generally safe and well-tolerated, with minimal side effects. However, it is essential to be aware of any potential reactions and to follow dosage recommendations carefully.

Common Side Effects

Some individuals may experience mild gastrointestinal discomfort, such as bloating or nausea, especially when taking pumpkin seed oil on an empty stomach. Taking the capsules with food usually alleviates these symptoms.

Precautions and Considerations

- **Pregnancy and Breastfeeding**: While pumpkin seed oil is safe for general use, pregnant or breastfeeding women should consult a healthcare provider before incorporating it into their regimen.

- **Allergies**: Individuals with allergies to pumpkin or related plants should exercise caution when using pumpkin seed oil.
- **Interactions with Medications**: Pumpkin seed oil may interact with certain medications, particularly those that affect hormone levels or blood clotting. Consult a healthcare provider if you are taking any prescription medications.

Choosing a High-Quality Pumpkin Seed Oil Supplement

When selecting pumpkin seed oil capsules, it is essential to choose a high-quality product to ensure maximum potency and effectiveness. Here are some tips for choosing a reliable supplement:

1. **Look for Cold-Pressed Oil**: Cold-pressed pumpkin seed oil retains more nutrients and antioxidants than oils processed with heat, which can degrade essential compounds.
2. **Choose Organic**: Organic pumpkin seed oil capsules are free from pesticides and chemicals, providing a purer product.
3. **Check the Ingredient List**: A high-quality pumpkin seed oil supplement should have minimal ingredients, ideally only the oil and a capsule (usually made of gelatin or a vegetarian alternative).
4. **Consider Standardization**: Some products are standardized to contain a certain amount of phytosterols or fatty acids. Standardization ensures consistency in the potency of the active compounds.

Combining Pumpkin Seed Oil with Other Prostate-Supportive Supplements

For individuals specifically seeking prostate health support, pumpkin seed oil is sometimes combined with other herbs and nutrients to enhance its effects. These may include:

- **Saw Palmetto**: Known for its prostate-supportive properties, saw palmetto and pumpkin seed oil together can provide a comprehensive approach to prostate health.
- **Zinc**: Zinc is a critical mineral for prostate health, and combining zinc with pumpkin seed oil may enhance its benefits for men's reproductive health.
- **Lycopene**: Found in tomatoes, lycopene is an antioxidant that may help protect the prostate from oxidative damage.

These combinations offer a holistic approach to men's health, particularly for those experiencing symptoms associated with an enlarged prostate.

Summary of Benefits

Pumpkin seed oil capsules offer a natural and holistic approach to supporting various aspects of health, including prostate health, urinary function, heart health, and overall wellness. Rich in essential fatty acids, antioxidants, and minerals, pumpkin seed oil provides a nutrient-dense supplement that addresses both specific and general health concerns.

By incorporating pumpkin seed oil capsules into a daily regimen, individuals can experience a range of benefits, particularly as part of a prostate health maintenance strategy. Regular use, combined with a balanced diet and healthy lifestyle choices, can contribute to improved health outcomes, making pumpkin seed oil a valuable addition to natural health practices.

Nettle Root Tincture

Nettle root (Urtica dioica) has long been valued for its medicinal properties, particularly in supporting prostate health, reducing inflammation, and balancing hormones. Traditionally, it's been used in European and Native American herbal practices, and its popularity has only grown as scientific research validates many of its health benefits. While nettle leaves are well-known for their use in teas and soups, it's the root that provides a unique set of properties when transformed into a tincture.

A nettle root tincture captures and preserves the active compounds in the plant's root, making it a convenient and potent form of this herb. Nettle root tincture is often used as a natural remedy for men's health concerns, particularly benign prostatic hyperplasia (BPH), and is recognized for its anti-inflammatory, diuretic, and adaptogenic properties.

In this section, we'll explore the medicinal properties of nettle root, how a tincture is prepared, and the specific benefits it can offer, along with guidelines on dosage, usage, and safety.

Benefits and Medicinal Properties of Nettle Root

Nettle root contains a range of active compounds, including lignans, sterols, and lectins, each contributing to its medicinal effects. These compounds have been studied for their potential to influence hormone levels, support urinary health, and reduce inflammation.

1. **Prostate Health and Benign Prostatic Hyperplasia (BPH)**
   Nettle root is particularly known for its positive effects on prostate health. BPH, a non-cancerous enlargement of the prostate, is common in men over the age of 50 and can lead to uncomfortable symptoms, including frequent urination, weak urine flow, and a feeling of incomplete bladder emptying. Nettle root is believed to inhibit the enzyme aromatase, which converts testosterone into estrogen, helping to maintain a balanced hormone profile that supports prostate health.

Several studies have shown that nettle root can help alleviate the symptoms of BPH by reducing inflammation in the prostate and modulating hormonal effects on the gland. By reducing the effects of excessive estrogen and supporting testosterone balance, nettle root offers a natural option for men seeking relief from BPH symptoms without the side effects of pharmaceutical medications.

2. **Anti-Inflammatory** **Effects**
   Inflammation is a root cause of many chronic diseases, and nettle root has strong anti-inflammatory properties. Its active compounds work to inhibit inflammatory pathways in the body, particularly those related to the release of pro-inflammatory cytokines. Nettle root tincture can thus be beneficial not only for prostate health but also for conditions associated with inflammation, such as arthritis and muscle pain.

By reducing inflammation, nettle root may help ease joint pain and improve mobility. This property makes it an attractive option for individuals with arthritis, as well as athletes or those with physically demanding jobs.

3. **Hormonal Balance and Endocrine Support**
   The hormonal effects of nettle root extend beyond prostate health. It helps to balance sex hormones by inhibiting the enzyme that converts testosterone into dihydrotestosterone (DHT). Elevated levels of DHT are associated with conditions like BPH and hair loss in men. By reducing DHT levels, nettle root supports not only prostate health but also hair health, making it beneficial for men experiencing hair thinning or androgenic alopecia.

Additionally, nettle root's effects on the endocrine system can aid women as well. It may be beneficial for balancing estrogen levels, which is particularly useful for women experiencing symptoms of estrogen dominance, such as PMS, fibroids, or endometriosis.

4. **Urinary**   **Tract**   **Health**

    Nettle root acts as a diuretic, promoting the elimination of excess fluids and toxins through urine. This property helps prevent fluid retention and supports kidney function. Nettle root tincture may benefit individuals with mild urinary issues, as it encourages regular urination and can help flush bacteria from the urinary tract. For men, this diuretic effect further complements prostate support, as it reduces residual urine in the bladder and prevents urinary retention associated with BPH.

5. **Adaptogenic**   **Qualities**

    While nettle root is not a classic adaptogen like ashwagandha or Rhodiola, it does exhibit adaptogenic qualities, particularly in helping the body adapt to stress and promoting resilience. Nettle root supports adrenal health and helps stabilize cortisol levels, making it a valuable addition for those experiencing fatigue or chronic stress.

Preparing and Using Nettle Root Tincture

A tincture is a concentrated liquid extract made by soaking herbs in alcohol to draw out the active compounds. Tinctures are an efficient way to consume nettle root because they allow the body to absorb the active compounds quickly, bypassing the need for digestion.

1. **Ingredients**   **for**   **Nettle**   **Root**   **Tincture**

    To make a nettle root tincture, you'll need:

    - Fresh or dried nettle root (dried is more commonly available and easier to handle)
    - High-proof alcohol, such as vodka or brandy (at least 80 proof)
    - A glass jar with a tight-fitting lid
    - A dropper bottle for storage once strained

When selecting nettle root, ensure it is sourced from a reputable supplier to avoid contamination with pesticides or heavy metals.

2. **Preparation Steps**

    - *Step 1*: Chop the nettle root into small pieces to increase surface area.
    - *Step 2*: Fill a glass jar about one-third full with nettle root.
    - *Step 3*: Pour alcohol over the nettle root, covering it entirely. Leave about an inch of alcohol above the herb to allow for expansion.
    - *Step 4*: Seal the jar tightly and shake well.

- o *Step 5*: Store the jar in a cool, dark place for 4-6 weeks, shaking it daily to encourage extraction.
- o *Step 6*: After the extraction period, strain the tincture through cheesecloth or a fine sieve, and pour the liquid into a dropper bottle.

3. **Dosage** **and** **Usage**

A typical dosage of nettle root tincture is 1-2 dropperfuls (approximately 30-60 drops) taken 1-3 times per day. The tincture can be added to water, juice, or taken directly under the tongue for quicker absorption. However, individual needs and responses vary, so it is advisable to start with a lower dose and increase gradually as needed.

Safety and Precautions

Nettle root tincture is generally safe for most people when used at the recommended dosages. However, as with any herbal remedy, certain precautions should be observed:

- **Consult a Healthcare Professional**: Individuals with kidney issues, low blood pressure, or hormone-sensitive conditions should consult a healthcare provider before using nettle root tincture.
- **Allergies**: Although rare, some people may be allergic to nettle. Discontinue use if any allergic reactions occur, such as skin irritation or difficulty breathing.
- **Interactions with Medications**: Nettle root can interact with certain medications, including diuretics, blood pressure medications, and medications that affect hormone levels. If you are on any prescription drugs, it's best to consult with a healthcare professional before adding nettle root to your regimen.

Scientific Studies on Nettle Root's Benefits

Numerous studies highlight the efficacy of nettle root in promoting prostate health and managing BPH symptoms. One study published in the *Journal of Herbal Pharmacotherapy* found that nettle root significantly improved symptoms of BPH and urinary flow, with few reported side effects. Another study in *Phytotherapy Research* found that nettle root was effective in reducing inflammatory markers, supporting its role in managing conditions like arthritis.

Studies have also explored nettle root's impact on DHT and estrogen balance. By inhibiting 5-alpha-reductase, nettle root reduces the conversion of testosterone to DHT, potentially slowing hair loss in men with androgenic alopecia. Additionally, the lignans in nettle root have been shown to bind to sex hormone-binding globulin (SHBG), which helps balance hormones by preventing excess free estrogen or testosterone.

Incorporating Nettle Root Tincture into a Health Routine

Incorporating nettle root tincture into your daily routine is simple and can be tailored to individual health goals. For those focused on prostate health, taking the tincture consistently can help alleviate symptoms and improve urinary flow. Nettle root tincture can also be combined with other herbs such as saw palmetto for enhanced prostate support.

For individuals interested in balancing hormones, nettle root can be combined with other adaptogens like ashwagandha or Rhodiola. The combined effect can support overall hormone balance and resilience to stress.

In terms of daily timing, nettle root tincture can be taken with or without food, although it is often best to avoid taking it late in the day due to its mild diuretic effects. If using for adrenal support and mild energy enhancement, taking it in the morning may yield optimal benefits.

Practical Tips for Long-Term Use

For those planning to use nettle root tincture long-term, here are some strategies to maximize its benefits:

- **Rotate with Other Herbs**: To maintain its effectiveness, some herbalists recommend rotating nettle root with other adaptogens or herbs that support urinary health.

- **Stay Consistent**: While the effects of nettle root tincture can be subtle at first, consistency is key for achieving long-term benefits, especially for prostate health and hormonal balance.

- **Monitor Symptoms**: If using nettle root for specific health concerns, keep track of any changes in symptoms. This practice can help you determine the ideal dosage and timing for your needs.

Nettle root tincture offers a natural approach to managing a range of health concerns, from supporting prostate health to balancing hormones and reducing inflammation. By understanding how to use nettle root effectively, individuals can harness its benefits and improve their well-being naturally.

Maca root, often referred to as Peruvian ginseng, is a superfood with a long history of traditional use in South American cultures, particularly in the Andes. Known for its unique nutrient profile and adaptogenic qualities, maca root is celebrated for its ability to support energy levels, hormonal balance, mood enhancement, and endurance. This section delves into the benefits of maca root, specifically in the form of a smoothie, a delicious and convenient way to incorporate this powerhouse ingredient into daily routines.

Nutritional Profile of Maca Root

Maca root is nutrient-dense, containing an array of vitamins, minerals, and bioactive compounds that contribute to its energizing and health-promoting effects. Some of the primary nutrients in maca root include:

- **Vitamins**: Maca is rich in vitamins B1, B2, C, and E, which play key roles in energy production, immune health, and antioxidant protection.
- **Minerals**: It contains essential minerals such as calcium, potassium, magnesium, and zinc, all of which contribute to muscle function, bone health, and immune support.
- **Amino Acids**: Maca is a source of essential amino acids, which are the building blocks of protein and are vital for muscle recovery, mental function, and hormone production.
- **Antioxidants**: Maca is packed with natural antioxidants, which help reduce oxidative stress and protect cells from damage.
- **Adaptogens**: These compounds help the body adapt to stress, enhancing resilience, mental clarity, and physical stamina.

The synergy of these nutrients makes maca a valuable addition to smoothies, especially for those looking to improve energy, hormonal balance, and overall wellness.

Health Benefits of Maca Root

Maca root is valued for its potential to support several aspects of health, particularly due to its adaptogenic properties, which help balance the body's stress response. Below are some of the specific benefits of maca root.

Energy and Stamina

Maca root is well-known for its energizing effects, making it an ideal choice for those looking to enhance their physical performance and stamina. Unlike caffeine, which provides a short-term energy boost followed by a potential crash, maca root supports sustained energy throughout the day. This makes it a great pre-workout addition to smoothies or simply a way to combat fatigue without stimulants.

Hormonal Balance

One of maca root's most renowned benefits is its ability to support hormonal balance, especially for those dealing with hormonal fluctuations. Maca works as an adaptogen, helping the endocrine system balance hormone production. This is particularly beneficial for women experiencing symptoms of menopause, PMS, or irregular menstrual cycles. Men can also benefit, as maca has been associated with improvements in libido and testosterone levels, enhancing reproductive health.

Mood and Mental Clarity

Maca is known for its mood-enhancing properties. Its adaptogenic nature helps reduce the impact of stress and anxiety, promoting a balanced mood and improving focus and mental clarity. This effect can be especially beneficial for individuals dealing with mental fatigue, brain fog, or stress-related emotional imbalances.

Bone Health

Due to its high calcium and magnesium content, maca root is also a supportive ingredient for bone health. These minerals play a crucial role in maintaining bone density, making maca a beneficial addition for individuals looking to support skeletal health and prevent osteoporosis.

Preparing a Maca Root Smoothie

Incorporating maca root into a smoothie is a straightforward and effective way to enjoy its benefits. Maca root is typically available as a powder, which blends easily with various fruits, vegetables, and liquids.

Basic Maca Root Smoothie Recipe

Below is a basic maca root smoothie recipe that can be customized according to taste preferences and dietary needs:

Ingredients:

- 1 tablespoon maca root powder
- 1 cup almond milk (or any preferred milk alternative)
- 1 banana (for natural sweetness and creaminess)
- ½ cup spinach or kale (for additional nutrients)
- 1 tablespoon almond butter (optional, for added protein and healthy fats)
- ½ teaspoon cinnamon (for flavor and additional antioxidants)
- 1 teaspoon honey or maple syrup (optional, for added sweetness)

Instructions:

1. Add all ingredients to a blender.
2. Blend on high until smooth and creamy.
3. Adjust sweetness to taste, and add more liquid if a thinner consistency is desired.
4. Serve immediately to enjoy the fresh flavors and maximum nutrient content.

This smoothie is nutrient-dense and filling, making it an excellent choice for breakfast or as a post-workout snack.

Variations of the Maca Root Smoothie

To suit different dietary preferences and nutritional goals, the maca root smoothie can be customized in various ways. Here are a few ideas for specific health goals:

Energy Boost Smoothie

For an added energy boost, consider adding ingredients like chia seeds, which are rich in fiber and omega-3 fatty acids, or a small serving of oats, which provide sustained-release carbohydrates.

Ingredients:

- 1 tablespoon maca root powder
- 1 cup coconut water (for electrolytes)
- 1 banana
- 1 tablespoon chia seeds
- ½ cup oats

This variation supports sustained energy release, making it ideal for a busy day or before physical activities.

Hormone Balance Smoothie

For those looking to balance hormones, consider adding flaxseeds or pumpkin seeds, which are rich in lignans and zinc. Both contribute to hormone regulation and support overall reproductive health.

Ingredients:

- 1 tablespoon maca root powder
- 1 cup unsweetened almond milk
- 1 tablespoon ground flaxseeds
- ½ cup berries (such as blueberries or raspberries for antioxidants)

This smoothie variation is particularly beneficial for women experiencing hormonal imbalances.

Muscle Recovery Smoothie

After a workout, a maca root smoothie can support muscle recovery and reduce soreness. Adding a high-quality protein powder, along with anti-inflammatory ingredients, can maximize recovery benefits.

Ingredients:

- 1 tablespoon maca root powder
- 1 scoop of plant-based or whey protein powder
- 1 cup almond milk
- ½ cup pineapple (for natural enzymes and sweetness)
- ½ teaspoon turmeric (anti-inflammatory)

This smoothie is designed to provide the necessary nutrients for muscle repair and reduce inflammation.

Tips for Using Maca Root in Smoothies

While maca root is a powerful addition to smoothies, there are a few tips to ensure you're getting the most out of this superfood:

1. **Start with a Small Amount**: If you're new to maca, start with a smaller amount (like ½ teaspoon) and gradually increase to 1 tablespoon. This can help your body adjust to maca's adaptogenic effects.

2. **Avoid Using Excessive Heat**: Maca powder is best consumed raw, as cooking may reduce its nutritional properties. Blending it into smoothies or mixing it into yogurt and cold dishes preserves its active compounds.

3. **Consistency is Key**: For best results, incorporate maca root regularly into your diet, as adaptogens typically require consistent use to build up in the system.

4. **Experiment with Flavor Pairings**: Maca has an earthy, slightly nutty flavor. It pairs well with naturally sweet ingredients like bananas, dates, and honey, as well as with spices like cinnamon and ginger.

Potential Side Effects and Precautions

While maca root is generally safe and well-tolerated, it's important to be aware of potential side effects and considerations.

- **Hormonal Effects**: Due to its hormone-balancing properties, individuals with hormone-sensitive conditions, such as breast cancer or endometriosis, should consult a healthcare provider before using maca.

- **Sleep Sensitivity**: Some people experience increased energy levels from maca, which could potentially interfere with sleep if taken late in the day.

- **Pregnancy and Breastfeeding**: While maca is generally considered safe, pregnant or breastfeeding women should consult a healthcare professional before using maca root.

Choosing a Quality Maca Root Powder

When selecting maca root powder for smoothies, quality is essential to ensure maximum benefits. Here are some tips to consider:

- **Look for Organic**: Organic maca powder is free from pesticides and is generally a safer choice, especially for long-term use.

- **Check for Gelatinized Maca**: Gelatinized maca has been processed to remove starch, making it easier to digest. This option is ideal for individuals with sensitive stomachs.

- **Choose Reputable Brands**: Purchase maca root powder from reputable brands that test for quality and potency.

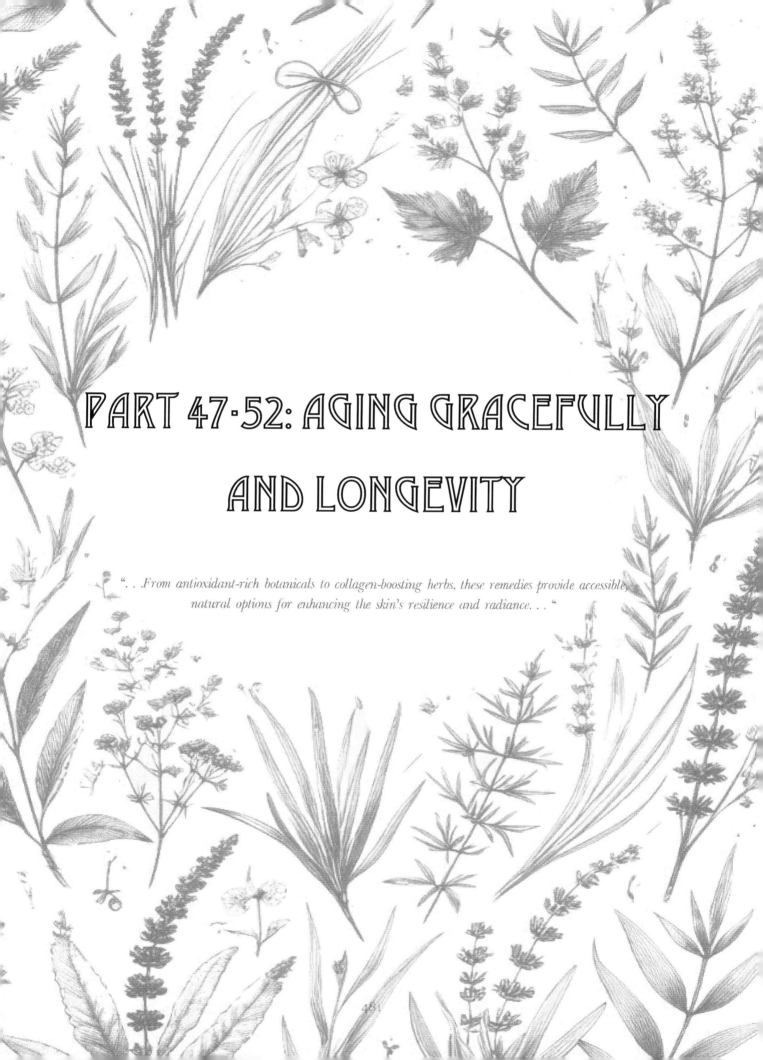

PART 47-52: AGING GRACEFULLY AND LONGEVITY

". . .From antioxidant-rich botanicals to collagen-boosting herbs, these remedies provide accessible, natural options for enhancing the skin's resilience and radiance. . ."

Chapter 1: Healthy Aging Fundamentals

Skin health and elasticity are essential components of our overall well-being and physical appearance, as the skin is our largest organ and primary barrier against the environment.

Skin Health and Elasticity

Maintaining youthful, resilient, and healthy skin requires a combination of proper nutrition, hydration, and, in many cases, the support of natural remedies. For many people, natural solutions offer a gentler approach to skin care without harsh chemicals or synthetic compounds, harnessing the power of herbal remedies to enhance elasticity, reduce signs of aging, and protect the skin from environmental damage.

In this section, we'll explore the importance of maintaining skin elasticity, the factors that influence it, and natural remedies that can help support and improve skin health. From antioxidant-rich botanicals to collagen-boosting herbs, these remedies provide accessible, natural options for enhancing the skin's resilience and radiance.

The Importance of Skin Elasticity

Skin elasticity is the skin's ability to stretch and then return to its original shape. It plays a crucial role in maintaining a youthful appearance and preventing sagging, wrinkles, and fine lines. When skin loses its elasticity, it can become looser, making wrinkles and folds more pronounced. Elasticity is largely determined by the presence of collagen and elastin, two proteins that give skin its structure and bounce.

1. **Collagen   and   Elastin**

   Collagen and elastin are fibrous proteins that form a network in the dermis, the skin's middle layer. Collagen is responsible for the skin's firmness and structure, while elastin provides flexibility and resilience. As we age, collagen production naturally decreases, leading to reduced elasticity and the formation of wrinkles. Sun exposure, pollution, and lifestyle factors can further accelerate the breakdown of collagen and elastin, making it essential to support skin health with nutrients and remedies that promote these proteins.

2. **External and Internal Factors Affecting Skin Health**
   Both external and internal factors can impact skin health and elasticity. External factors include exposure to UV rays, pollution, harsh skincare products, and smoking, which all contribute to the degradation of collagen and elastin. Internally, factors like hydration, diet, hormonal balance, and genetics play significant roles. Dehydration and poor nutrition can make skin appear dull and prone to wrinkling, while imbalances in hormones can lead to changes in skin texture and elasticity.

3. **Aging and the Natural Decline in Elasticity**
   The natural aging process causes a gradual decline in collagen production, resulting in a loss of elasticity and firmness. While aging cannot be stopped, there are ways to slow its visible effects through dietary and lifestyle choices, including the use of natural remedies to nourish the skin and support elasticity.

Natural Remedies to Support Skin Health and Elasticity

Using herbs and natural compounds can be a gentle yet effective way to support skin health. Certain botanicals are rich in antioxidants, which fight free radical damage, while others provide nutrients that stimulate collagen production, protect elastin fibers, and help the skin retain moisture. Below, we discuss some of the most beneficial herbs and natural remedies for enhancing skin elasticity.

1. **Aloe Vera**
   Aloe vera is well-known for its soothing and hydrating properties. The gel of this succulent contains vitamins C and E, which are powerful antioxidants that help combat free radical damage. Aloe also contains polysaccharides, compounds that help retain moisture and stimulate the skin's fibroblasts, cells that produce collagen and elastin. Regular application of aloe vera gel can help keep the skin hydrated, improve elasticity, and reduce fine lines.
   o *Usage*: Fresh aloe vera gel can be applied directly to the skin as a moisturizer. For a deeper treatment, apply the gel as a mask, leaving it on for 10-15 minutes before rinsing off with lukewarm water.

2. **Rosehip**   **Oil**

Rosehip oil is a highly nourishing oil derived from the seeds of the wild rose bush. It is rich in essential fatty acids, vitamin A, and vitamin C, all of which support skin elasticity and repair. Vitamin C is crucial for collagen production, while vitamin A promotes cell regeneration, helping the skin maintain its structure and resilience. Rosehip oil also helps even out skin tone, reduce the appearance of scars, and soften fine lines.

   o *Usage*: Apply a few drops of rosehip oil to the skin before bed, gently massaging it in to allow deep absorption overnight. Regular use can lead to smoother, firmer skin with a radiant glow.

3. **Gotu   Kola   (Centella   Asiatica)**

Gotu kola is an adaptogenic herb renowned for its ability to stimulate collagen synthesis. It contains compounds called triterpenoids, which boost collagen production and strengthen the skin. Gotu kola has been used in Ayurvedic and traditional Chinese medicine for centuries to improve wound healing and enhance skin elasticity. Its anti-inflammatory properties also make it suitable for sensitive skin prone to redness.

   o *Usage*: Gotu kola can be applied topically in creams or serums that contain the extract. It can also be taken as a supplement or consumed as a tea for internal support of skin health.

4. **Green   Tea   Extract**

Green tea is packed with polyphenols, particularly epigallocatechin gallate (EGCG), which is one of the most potent antioxidants known. EGCG helps neutralize free radicals that damage collagen and elastin fibers, thereby slowing down the breakdown of these proteins. Green tea extract can improve skin elasticity and reduce inflammation, making it ideal for individuals with aging or sensitive skin.

   o *Usage*: Green tea extract can be found in serums and creams, or you can use cooled green tea as a natural toner by applying it to the skin with a cotton pad.

5. **Sea   Buckthorn   Oil**

Sea buckthorn oil is rich in omega-7, a fatty acid that promotes skin hydration and elasticity. This oil also contains antioxidants like vitamin E and carotenoids, which protect the skin from environmental stressors. Sea buckthorn oil can support collagen structure and prevent the skin from losing moisture, making it especially beneficial for dry and mature skin types.

- o *Usage*: Sea buckthorn oil can be applied directly to the skin or added to creams and lotions. Due to its bright orange color, it's best to mix it with a carrier oil before applying it to avoid staining the skin.

6. **Horsetail**   **(Equisetum**   **arvense)**

Horsetail is a natural source of silica, a mineral essential for collagen synthesis and maintaining skin elasticity. Silica strengthens connective tissues, helping to keep the skin firm and resilient. Horsetail also has astringent properties that tighten the skin, reduce puffiness, and refine pores, making it a versatile remedy for enhancing skin health.

- o *Usage*: Horsetail extract can be found in creams and serums, or it can be used in the form of an herbal infusion applied as a toner. Alternatively, horsetail supplements can be taken to support skin health from within.

Supporting Skin Elasticity Through Nutrition

While topical treatments play a significant role, internal support is equally important for maintaining skin elasticity. Certain nutrients are vital for collagen production, hydration, and protecting the skin from oxidative damage.

1. **Vitamin**   **C**

Vitamin C is crucial for the production of collagen. It works as an antioxidant to protect the skin from free radical damage and stimulates collagen synthesis. Foods rich in vitamin C, like oranges, strawberries, bell peppers, and broccoli, can help support skin elasticity from within.

2. **Vitamin**   **E**

Vitamin E is another powerful antioxidant that protects the skin's lipid barrier, helping it retain moisture and stay supple. Nuts, seeds, and leafy greens are excellent sources of vitamin E. Using vitamin E-rich oils or serums can also support skin elasticity and reduce the appearance of fine lines.

3. **Omega-3**   **Fatty**   **Acids**

Omega-3 fatty acids found in fatty fish, flaxseeds, and walnuts help maintain the skin's lipid barrier, keeping it hydrated and plump. They also reduce inflammation, which can help prevent collagen breakdown. A diet rich in omega-3s supports smooth, resilient skin.

4. **Zinc**

   Zinc is essential for skin repair and the synthesis of collagen. It also has anti-inflammatory properties, which make it beneficial for individuals with acne or sensitive skin. Foods like pumpkin seeds, lentils, and quinoa provide zinc, helping to support skin health from the inside out.

5. **Hyaluronic**   **Acid**

   Though not a nutrient in the traditional sense, hyaluronic acid is essential for skin hydration and elasticity. It attracts and retains water in the skin, providing a plumping effect. Foods like bone broth contain hyaluronic acid, or it can be applied topically for direct benefits.

Creating a Natural Skin Care Routine for Elasticity

To achieve and maintain skin elasticity, incorporating natural remedies into a daily skincare routine can be highly effective. Here's a sample routine:

1. **Cleansing**: Use a gentle, hydrating cleanser to remove impurities without stripping the skin of its natural oils. Avoid harsh cleansers, as they can weaken the skin barrier.

2. **Toning**: Apply a toner made from green tea or horsetail to prepare the skin for hydration and balance its pH. This step also helps tighten the pores and provides a refreshing boost of antioxidants.

3. **Moisturizing**: Apply a few drops of rosehip or sea buckthorn oil to lock in moisture and provide the skin with essential fatty acids and antioxidants.

4. **Weekly Treatments**: Once or twice a week, use a mask made from aloe vera gel or a mixture of honey and rosehip oil. These ingredients deeply hydrate and nourish the skin, helping to maintain elasticity.

5. **Internal Support**: Include foods rich in vitamins C, E, and omega-3s in your diet, and stay hydrated. Adding herbs like gotu kola and horsetail as supplements can further support elasticity from the

Bone Density and Joint Health

Bone density and joint health are fundamental aspects of physical wellness that play a critical role in our mobility, strength, and overall quality of life. As we age, the natural process of bone density loss and joint wear can lead to conditions such as osteoporosis and arthritis. Fortunately, there are natural approaches to support bone and joint health, ranging from targeted nutrients to herbal remedies, lifestyle habits, and exercises that specifically aim to improve skeletal strength and joint flexibility. This section covers the essentials of maintaining bone density and joint health, especially through natural remedies and dietary strategies, with practical guidance on how to integrate these approaches into daily routines.

Understanding Bone Density and Joint Health

Bone density refers to the amount of mineral content, particularly calcium and phosphorus, within bones. Dense, mineral-rich bones are strong and resistant to fractures. As we age, the body's ability to absorb calcium decreases, leading to reduced bone density. This loss can result in fragile bones that are more susceptible to fractures, a condition known as osteoporosis.

Joint health is equally crucial, as joints are the connections between bones that allow movement and flexibility. Over time, joints can suffer from wear and tear, inflammation, and degradation, especially in weight-bearing joints such as the knees and hips. Osteoarthritis, for instance, is a common condition where cartilage within joints breaks down, leading to pain and stiffness.

Maintaining strong bones and healthy joints requires a combination of proper nutrition, physical activity, and herbal support. Each of these factors contributes to reducing the risk of bone and joint issues, preserving mobility, and minimizing pain or stiffness.

Essential Nutrients for Bone Density and Joint Health

The following nutrients play key roles in supporting bone and joint health. A diet rich in these nutrients helps maintain bone density, strengthens connective tissues, and promotes resilience against joint-related conditions.

Calcium

Calcium is perhaps the most well-known nutrient for bone health. Approximately 99% of the body's calcium is stored in the bones and teeth, giving them structure. Foods rich in calcium include dairy products like milk, cheese, and yogurt, as well as leafy green vegetables, almonds, and fortified foods. For those who struggle to get enough calcium through diet alone, calcium supplements can provide additional support.

Vitamin D

Vitamin D is essential for calcium absorption. Without adequate vitamin D, the body cannot effectively absorb calcium from the digestive system, leading to calcium deficiency. This deficiency can weaken bones and make them more prone to fractures. Sunlight is a natural source of vitamin D, and dietary sources include fatty fish (such as salmon and mackerel), egg yolks, and fortified foods. Supplementation is also common, especially for individuals with limited sun exposure.

Magnesium

Magnesium works in conjunction with calcium and vitamin D to support bone density. It plays a role in bone formation and helps regulate calcium transport in the body. Sources of magnesium include nuts (particularly almonds and cashews), seeds, leafy greens, and whole grains. Regular magnesium intake is crucial for bone mineralization and preventing conditions like osteoporosis.

Vitamin K

Vitamin K is vital for bone health as it helps regulate bone mineralization. Specifically, it activates proteins that help bind calcium to the bone matrix, improving bone strength. Vitamin K-rich foods include leafy greens, broccoli, and Brussels sprouts. For those with higher risk of osteoporosis, vitamin K2 supplements can be considered under medical guidance.

Omega-3 Fatty Acids

Omega-3 fatty acids, known for their anti-inflammatory properties, are essential for maintaining joint health. They help reduce inflammation in the joints, making them particularly beneficial for individuals with arthritis or other joint-related conditions. Omega-3s can be found in fatty fish, flaxseeds, walnuts, and chia seeds. For joint support, including these foods in the diet helps minimize pain and stiffness.

Herbal Solutions for Bone Density and Joint Health

Various herbs offer natural support for bones and joints, either by providing additional nutrients, enhancing calcium absorption, or reducing inflammation in joints.

Horsetail

Horsetail is an herb rich in silica, a mineral that aids in calcium absorption and promotes collagen production. Collagen is essential for joint cartilage and bone flexibility, making horsetail a valuable addition for those with joint pain or osteoporosis risk. Horsetail can be consumed as a tea or in supplement form, but individuals should consult with a healthcare professional due to its potential effect on vitamin B1 absorption.

Turmeric

Turmeric is widely recognized for its anti-inflammatory properties due to its active compound, curcumin. Studies have shown that turmeric can alleviate joint pain and improve mobility, especially for individuals with osteoarthritis. Turmeric can be added to foods, smoothies, or taken as a supplement, often combined with black pepper to improve curcumin absorption.

Nettle

Nettle is a calcium-rich herb that has been used traditionally to support bone health. It also contains magnesium, iron, and vitamin K, all of which are essential for strong bones. Nettle tea or capsules can be consumed to provide these nutrients, supporting both bone density and joint comfort.

Boswellia

Boswellia, also known as Indian frankincense, has anti-inflammatory properties that can reduce joint pain and stiffness. Boswellia supplements have been shown to help individuals with arthritis experience improved joint function and reduced discomfort.

Lifestyle and Exercise for Bone Density and Joint Health

In addition to nutrition and herbal support, lifestyle habits and specific exercises play a critical role in maintaining bone density and joint health.

Weight-Bearing Exercises

Weight-bearing exercises stimulate bone formation by encouraging bone cells to grow stronger and denser. Activities such as walking, jogging, hiking, and resistance training place stress on the bones, which signals the body to strengthen bone tissue. Engaging in weight-bearing exercise regularly helps to preserve bone density, reducing the risk of osteoporosis.

Strength Training

Strength training not only improves muscle mass but also supports bone density by putting controlled pressure on bones. Lifting weights, using resistance bands, or engaging in bodyweight exercises like squats and lunges can promote bone health. Strong muscles also support the joints, reducing wear and tear over time.

Flexibility and Balance Training

Maintaining flexibility and balance can prevent falls and related fractures. Yoga and tai chi are effective practices for improving flexibility, joint mobility, and balance. Stretching also helps prevent joint stiffness and enhances the range of motion, supporting joint health over time.

Avoiding Smoking and Excessive Alcohol

Smoking and excessive alcohol intake are risk factors for bone density loss. Nicotine and alcohol disrupt the body's calcium absorption processes and impair bone formation. Reducing or eliminating these habits contributes to better bone and joint health.

Integrating Natural Remedies into a Daily Routine

Incorporating natural approaches to support bone density and joint health can be done with a few simple adjustments to daily routines. Here are some practical ways to incorporate these methods:

1. **Morning Sunlight Exposure**: Spend 10–15 minutes in sunlight daily to boost vitamin D production, which aids calcium absorption.
2. **Herbal Teas**: Include herbal teas such as nettle or horsetail in your daily beverage routine for a natural source of minerals that support bones.
3. **Smoothie Additions**: Add a teaspoon of turmeric or ground flaxseed to smoothies for an anti-inflammatory boost.
4. **Exercise Routine**: Incorporate weight-bearing exercises, such as brisk walking or resistance training, into your weekly routine.
5. **Supplement Wisely**: If dietary sources are insufficient, consider supplements like calcium, vitamin D, or Boswellia after consulting with a healthcare provider.

Chapter 2: Nutrition for Longevity

Inflammation is a natural immune response that our bodies use to heal wounds and fight infections. However, chronic inflammation, which can result from a poor diet, stress, or exposure to environmental toxins, is associated with a range of health issues, including heart disease, arthritis, diabetes, and certain cancers.

Foods That Prevent Inflammation

Preventing and managing chronic inflammation through diet has become a primary focus for many people seeking to improve their long-term health and vitality.

Fortunately, many foods possess anti-inflammatory properties due to their rich content of antioxidants, vitamins, minerals, and healthy fats. By incorporating these foods into a balanced diet, individuals can support their body's natural processes, reduce inflammation, and promote overall health.

The Role of Antioxidants in Fighting Inflammation

Antioxidants are compounds that protect the body from oxidative stress caused by free radicals. Free radicals are unstable molecules that can damage cells, proteins, and DNA. The body produces free radicals naturally, but excessive amounts can lead to chronic inflammation. Antioxidants neutralize free radicals, helping to prevent this damage and reducing the inflammatory response.

1. **Berries**

   Berries such as strawberries, blueberries, raspberries, and blackberries are among the richest sources of antioxidants, including anthocyanins, which give berries their vibrant colors. Anthocyanins have powerful anti-inflammatory effects, protecting cells from oxidative damage and reducing markers of inflammation in the body.

   - *Usage*: Berries can be added to smoothies, yogurt, or oatmeal. Their high antioxidant levels make them an excellent choice for an anti-inflammatory breakfast or snack.

2. **Green** **Leafy** **Vegetables**

Vegetables like spinach, kale, and Swiss chard are packed with vitamins A, C, and K, along with various antioxidants that reduce inflammation. These vegetables also contain fiber, which supports a healthy gut and reduces inflammation by aiding digestion and balancing blood sugar levels.

- o *Usage*: Leafy greens can be enjoyed in salads, smoothies, or lightly sautéed with olive oil and garlic. Incorporating these vegetables into daily meals helps maintain a balanced diet rich in anti-inflammatory nutrients.

3. **Fatty** **Fish**

Fatty fish, including salmon, mackerel, sardines, and trout, are rich in omega-3 fatty acids, particularly EPA (eicosapentaenoic acid) and DHA (docosahexaenoic acid). Omega-3s are essential fats that reduce inflammation by counteracting pro-inflammatory omega-6 fatty acids, commonly found in processed foods.

- o *Usage*: For optimal anti-inflammatory benefits, aim to consume fatty fish at least twice a week. Grilling or baking fish is an excellent way to preserve its omega-3 content.

4. **Turmeric**

Turmeric, a vibrant yellow spice often used in Indian cuisine, contains curcumin, a compound with powerful anti-inflammatory and antioxidant effects. Curcumin has been widely studied for its ability to reduce inflammation and alleviate symptoms of inflammatory diseases like arthritis.

- o *Usage*: Turmeric can be added to curries, soups, or teas. To enhance curcumin's absorption, combine turmeric with black pepper, as piperine in black pepper increases its bioavailability.

5. **Ginger**

Ginger is known for its digestive benefits and anti-inflammatory properties, thanks to compounds like gingerol and shogaol. These compounds reduce inflammation by inhibiting pro-inflammatory enzymes and cytokines. Studies have shown that ginger can be effective in managing arthritis pain and improving joint function.

- o *Usage*: Fresh ginger can be grated into smoothies, teas, and stir-fries, or used as a spice in cooking. Consuming ginger regularly may help manage inflammation, especially in people with inflammatory conditions.

Nutrient-Dense Foods for Inflammation Prevention

Nutrient-dense foods provide essential vitamins and minerals that support the body's immune response, making it easier for the body to fight off inflammation. Consuming a variety of these foods daily ensures that the body has the necessary nutrients to maintain optimal function.

1. **Nuts and Seeds**

   Nuts like almonds, walnuts, and seeds such as flaxseeds and chia seeds contain fiber, omega-3 fatty acids, and various antioxidants that reduce inflammation. Walnuts are particularly beneficial due to their high levels of alpha-linolenic acid (ALA), a plant-based omega-3 that can help lower inflammatory markers.

   o   *Usage*: Nuts and seeds can be eaten as snacks, added to salads, or included in smoothies. Their high fiber and healthy fat content make them an ideal addition to an anti-inflammatory diet.

2. **Olive Oil**

   Olive oil, especially extra-virgin olive oil, contains oleocanthal, a compound with anti-inflammatory effects similar to those of ibuprofen. Olive oil also contains antioxidants and monounsaturated fats, which help reduce the risk of heart disease and lower inflammation levels in the body.

   o   *Usage*: Use olive oil as a base for salad dressings, drizzled over vegetables, or for light sautéing. Olive oil is versatile and offers numerous health benefits when used in cooking or as a finishing oil.

3. **Tomatoes**

   Tomatoes are high in lycopene, an antioxidant that reduces inflammation and protects against certain types of cancer. Lycopene is more bioavailable when tomatoes are cooked, which makes tomato-based sauces and soups excellent anti-inflammatory options.

   o   *Usage*: Tomatoes can be eaten raw in salads or sandwiches, but cooking them enhances lycopene availability. For an anti-inflammatory boost, consider using tomatoes in soups, sauces, or as a topping for baked dishes.

4. **Beets**

   Beets are a vibrant source of betalains, antioxidants that help reduce inflammation and support detoxification. The fiber and vitamin C content in beets also contribute to their anti-inflammatory properties, helping to reduce the risk of chronic diseases.

- o *Usage*: Beets can be roasted, added to salads, or blended into smoothies. Their natural sweetness and vibrant color make them a versatile ingredient for a range of dishes.

Whole Grains and Fiber-Rich Foods

Whole grains contain fiber, vitamins, and minerals that support digestive health and reduce inflammation. Refined grains, in contrast, have been stripped of their fiber and nutrients, which can lead to blood sugar spikes and increased inflammation.

1. **Oats**

    Oats are a great source of beta-glucans, a type of fiber that promotes heart health and reduces inflammation. The antioxidants in oats also provide additional anti-inflammatory benefits, making them an ideal breakfast choice.

    - o *Usage*: Oats can be cooked as oatmeal, added to smoothies, or used in baking. Steel-cut and rolled oats retain more nutrients than instant oats, offering better anti-inflammatory effects.

2. **Quinoa**

    Quinoa is a complete protein that also contains fiber, magnesium, and manganese, nutrients that support overall health and help reduce inflammation. Its high protein content makes it an excellent choice for people looking to add more plant-based options to their diets.

    - o *Usage*: Quinoa can be used as a base for salads, as a side dish, or even in soups. Its mild flavor pairs well with various vegetables and dressings, making it versatile in anti-inflammatory meal planning.

3. **Brown   Rice**

    Brown rice is a whole grain rich in fiber, selenium, and magnesium. These nutrients support heart health and help reduce inflammation. Brown rice has a lower glycemic index than white rice, making it a healthier choice for blood sugar regulation.

    - o *Usage*: Brown rice can be used in place of white rice in most dishes, from stir-fries to grain bowls. Its slightly nutty flavor and chewy texture complement a variety of ingredients.

Herbs and Spices for Inflammation Reduction

Certain herbs and spices are potent anti-inflammatory agents due to their high levels of antioxidants and unique active compounds. Including these in your diet can be an easy way to boost your intake of inflammation-fighting nutrients.

1. **Garlic**

   Garlic contains allicin, a compound that has been shown to reduce inflammation and enhance immune function. Studies suggest that garlic can inhibit pro-inflammatory cytokines, making it particularly beneficial for individuals with autoimmune conditions.

   o *Usage*: Garlic can be used in cooking to add flavor to sauces, soups, and stir-fries. Its anti-inflammatory benefits are most potent when raw or lightly cooked, so consider adding it toward the end of cooking.

2. **Cinnamon**

   Cinnamon contains cinnamaldehyde, a compound with anti-inflammatory and antioxidant properties. It has been shown to reduce markers of inflammation and improve insulin sensitivity, making it beneficial for people with inflammatory conditions and those at risk for type 2 diabetes.

   o *Usage*: Add cinnamon to oatmeal, smoothies, and teas. Its sweet flavor makes it a natural addition to both savory and sweet dishes.

3. **Rosemary**

   Rosemary is rich in carnosic acid and rosmarinic acid, antioxidants that help reduce inflammation. Rosemary also improves blood circulation, which can aid in reducing inflammatory responses in the body.

   o *Usage*: Use rosemary in cooking by adding it to meats, roasted vegetables, and stews. Fresh rosemary sprigs can add a unique flavor and enhance the anti-inflammatory benefits of a meal.

4. **Thyme**

   Thyme contains thymol, a compound with antibacterial and anti-inflammatory effects. It has been used traditionally to treat respiratory conditions, as it can help reduce inflammation in the airways.

- ○ *Usage*: Fresh or dried thyme can be used in soups, sauces, and marinades. Its earthy flavor complements a range of dishes and can easily be incorporated into an anti-inflammatory diet.

Practical Tips for Incorporating Anti-Inflammatory Foods

Incorporating anti-inflammatory foods into your daily routine doesn't have to be complicated. Here are a few practical strategies:

- **Plan meals around vegetables**: Start by filling half of your plate with vegetables, especially leafy greens and colorful veggies, to ensure a diet rich in antioxidants and anti-inflammatory compounds.
- **Replace refined grains with whole grains**: Swap white rice and bread for whole grains like brown rice, quinoa, and oats to improve fiber intake and support stable blood sugar levels.
- **Use herbs and spices regularly**: Keep a variety of herbs and spices on hand and experiment with them in cooking. Not only do they add flavor, but they also provide significant health benefits when used consistently.
- **Include omega-3-rich foods**: Make a habit of including fatty fish in your diet at least twice a week, or consider flaxseeds, chia seeds, and walnuts as plant-based sources of omega-3s if you prefer a vegetarian approach.

By making these small changes, you can harness the power of food to reduce inflammation and support long-term health. Through consistent effort, a diet rich in anti-inflammatory foods can contribute to a healthier, more vibrant life.

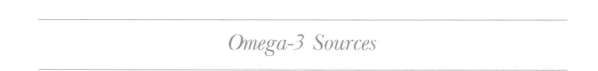

Omega-3 Sources

Omega-3 fatty acids are essential nutrients that play a vital role in maintaining overall health, particularly in supporting heart, brain, and joint function. Our bodies cannot produce omega-3s on their own, so it is crucial to obtain these fatty acids from dietary sources. Omega-3s come in three main types: ALA (alpha-linolenic acid), EPA (eicosapentaenoic acid), and DHA (docosahexaenoic acid). Each type offers unique benefits, and incorporating a variety of omega-3 sources into your diet is essential for optimal health.

The Health Benefits of Omega-3s

Research has consistently shown that omega-3 fatty acids contribute to various aspects of physical and mental health:

- **Heart Health**: Omega-3s reduce triglyceride levels, lower blood pressure, and decrease the risk of heart disease by improving endothelial function and reducing inflammation.
- **Brain Health**: DHA is a critical component of brain cell membranes, and adequate omega-3 intake is associated with improved cognitive function, reduced risk of Alzheimer's disease, and better mood regulation.
- **Joint Health**: Omega-3s have anti-inflammatory properties, which can relieve symptoms of rheumatoid arthritis and other inflammatory conditions.
- **Eye Health**: DHA is a major structural component of the retina, and adequate omega-3 levels are essential for maintaining vision and reducing the risk of age-related macular degeneration.

Understanding these benefits, let's explore some of the best dietary sources of omega-3s, both animal-based and plant-based, to help meet your nutritional needs.

Animal-Based Sources of Omega-3s

Animal-based sources are particularly rich in EPA and DHA, the two omega-3 fatty acids most readily absorbed and utilized by the body. These sources are ideal for those looking to increase their intake of these specific forms of omega-3.

1. Fatty Fish

Fatty fish are the most well-known and accessible sources of EPA and DHA. They provide a high concentration of these omega-3s and are easy to incorporate into various meals.

- **Salmon**: Salmon is one of the most nutrient-dense fish, containing high levels of EPA and DHA, as well as protein and essential vitamins such as B12 and D. Wild-caught salmon is particularly rich in omega-3s and is less likely to contain environmental toxins.
- **Mackerel**: Mackerel is another fatty fish with a high omega-3 content. It's affordable and versatile, making it easy to include in meals regularly.

- **Sardines**: Sardines are a small, oily fish that contain both EPA and DHA. They are typically consumed canned, which preserves their omega-3 content. Sardines are also rich in calcium and vitamin D, adding additional nutritional benefits.
- **Anchovies**: Although small, anchovies pack a punch in terms of omega-3 content. They can be added to salads, pizzas, or pastas for a nutrient boost.
- **Herring**: Herring is a common fish in European diets and is an excellent source of omega-3s. It can be consumed fresh, smoked, or pickled, providing flexibility in how it's incorporated into meals.

2. Fish Oil Supplements

For individuals who don't consume fish regularly, fish oil supplements are a convenient option to increase omega-3 intake. Fish oil supplements come in capsule or liquid form and are typically derived from the oils of fatty fish.

- **How to Use**: Fish oil supplements should be taken with meals to enhance absorption and reduce the risk of stomach upset. The recommended dosage varies depending on individual health needs, so it's best to follow the label or consult a healthcare professional.
- **Types of Fish Oil**: Choose high-quality fish oil supplements that are third-party tested for purity to avoid contaminants like mercury or other toxins. There are also options like krill oil, which some studies suggest may offer better absorption than traditional fish oil.

3. Cod Liver Oil

Cod liver oil, derived from the livers of codfish, is another excellent source of EPA and DHA. In addition to omega-3s, it is rich in vitamins A and D, which support immune function, bone health, and vision.

- **How to Use**: Cod liver oil can be taken in liquid form or as a capsule. Due to its high vitamin A content, it's essential not to exceed recommended dosages, as excessive vitamin A intake can be harmful.

4. Shellfish

Certain types of shellfish, such as oysters and mussels, provide omega-3 fatty acids along with additional nutrients like zinc and iron, which support immune health and energy production.

- **Oysters**: Oysters are rich in DHA and EPA and provide a unique blend of minerals, particularly zinc. They can be enjoyed raw, steamed, or grilled.
- **Mussels**: Mussels contain moderate amounts of omega-3s and are high in protein, making them a nutritious addition to a balanced diet.

Plant-Based Sources of Omega-3s

For those following a vegetarian or vegan diet, plant-based sources of omega-3s, particularly ALA, are essential. While ALA is not as readily utilized by the body as EPA and DHA, the body can convert small amounts of ALA into these active forms.

1. Flaxseeds

Flaxseeds are one of the richest plant-based sources of ALA. They also provide fiber and lignans, which have antioxidant properties and support hormonal balance.

- **Usage**: Flaxseeds should be ground before consumption, as whole flaxseeds pass through the digestive system without releasing their nutrients. Ground flaxseeds can be added to smoothies, yogurt, oatmeal, or baked goods.

2. Chia Seeds

Chia seeds are tiny, nutrient-dense seeds high in ALA, fiber, and protein. They are particularly beneficial for those looking to add plant-based omega-3s to their diet.

- **Usage**: Chia seeds can be mixed into water or plant-based milk to create a gel-like texture, perfect for puddings. They can also be added to smoothies, cereals, and baked goods for an omega-3 boost.

3. Hemp Seeds

Hemp seeds are a versatile source of ALA and contain a balanced ratio of omega-3 to omega-6 fatty acids, which can help reduce inflammation.

- **Usage**: Sprinkle hemp seeds over salads, blend them into smoothies, or mix them into yogurt. They add a nutty flavor and a dose of protein and fiber.

4. Walnuts

Walnuts are the only nut that provides a significant amount of ALA. In addition to omega-3s, they contain antioxidants and are known to support heart health.

- **Usage**: Walnuts can be eaten as a snack, added to salads, or incorporated into baking. They pair well with fruits and can enhance the texture and flavor of various dishes.

5. Algal Oil

Algal oil is a unique plant-based omega-3 source derived from algae. It provides DHA, making it one of the few non-animal sources of this essential fatty acid.

- **Usage**: Algal oil is available as a supplement, making it a great choice for vegans and vegetarians. It's especially beneficial for those looking to increase their DHA levels without consuming fish.

Comparing Animal and Plant-Based Omega-3 Sources

Both animal and plant-based omega-3 sources offer distinct benefits, and including a mix of both types in your diet can help maximize your omega-3 intake. Here's how they compare:

- **Bioavailability**: Animal-based sources of omega-3, particularly fish and shellfish, provide EPA and DHA directly, which the body can use immediately. In contrast, the ALA from plant-based sources must be converted into EPA and DHA, a process that is relatively inefficient (only about 5-10% conversion rate).
- **Environmental Considerations**: Plant-based sources of omega-3s are generally more sustainable and environmentally friendly than fish. Sustainable fishing practices can help mitigate the environmental impact of sourcing omega-3s from marine life.
- **Nutritional Variety**: Each omega-3 source offers unique nutritional benefits beyond just omega-3 content. Fatty fish provides vitamin D and selenium, while flaxseeds and chia seeds offer fiber and antioxidants.

Practical Tips for Incorporating Omega-3 Sources into Your Diet

Adding a variety of omega-3 sources to your meals can be simple and enjoyable. Here are some practical tips for integrating these foods into your diet:

- **Start Your Day with Omega-3s**: Add ground flaxseeds or chia seeds to your morning smoothie, yogurt, or oatmeal for a plant-based omega-3 boost.
- **Include Fatty Fish in Your Weekly Menu**: Aim to eat fatty fish such as salmon, mackerel, or sardines twice a week. Experiment with different recipes to keep your meals interesting.

- **Opt for Omega-3-Rich Snacks**: Nuts, particularly walnuts, make excellent snacks. You can also use a handful of hemp seeds or chia seeds as a topping for fruit or vegetables.

- **Experiment with Sea Vegetables and Algal Oil**: If you're vegan or vegetarian, consider taking algal oil supplements or adding seaweed to your diet, as these are excellent sources of DHA.

- **Read Labels on Packaged Foods**: Some foods, such as certain brands of eggs, yogurt, or juice, are fortified with omega-3s. Checking labels can help you identify products that offer additional omega-3 content.

Chapter 3: Anti-Aging Herbal Solutions

J oint health is a vital component of overall well-being, enabling mobility, flexibility, and the ability to perform daily activities without discomfort. Unfortunately, many people experience joint pain and stiffness due to aging, injury, or inflammatory conditions such as arthritis.

Herbs for Joint Health

While pharmaceutical solutions like pain relievers and anti-inflammatory drugs are commonly prescribed, they may come with undesirable side effects. Natural remedies, particularly herbal therapies, offer a gentle yet effective alternative for supporting joint health and alleviating discomfort.

Understanding Joint Pain and Its Causes

Joint pain can be caused by a variety of factors, including:

- **Inflammation**: Conditions like rheumatoid arthritis result in chronic inflammation, which damages the joint tissues over time.
- **Degeneration**: Osteoarthritis, a common age-related condition, occurs when the cartilage that cushions joints wears down, leading to pain and reduced mobility.
- **Injury or Overuse**: Strains, sprains, and repetitive motion can cause temporary or long-lasting joint pain.
- **Nutritional Deficiencies**: Lack of nutrients such as calcium, magnesium, and omega-3 fatty acids can weaken bones and joints, making them more susceptible to damage.

Herbs have been used for centuries to address these root causes. Many contain powerful anti-inflammatory, antioxidant, and pain-relieving compounds that promote joint health without the risks associated with conventional medications.

Key Herbs for Joint Health

1. Turmeric (Curcuma longa)

Turmeric is a well-known herb in the world of natural remedies, celebrated for its potent anti-inflammatory properties. The active compound in turmeric, curcumin, has been extensively studied for its ability to reduce inflammation and pain in conditions such as osteoarthritis and rheumatoid arthritis.

- **How It Works**: Curcumin inhibits inflammatory pathways by targeting specific enzymes and molecules, such as COX-2 and TNF-alpha, which play a role in joint pain.
- **Usage**: Turmeric can be consumed as a spice, added to teas, or taken as a concentrated curcumin supplement. Combining turmeric with black pepper enhances its absorption.
- **Example**: Golden milk, a warm beverage made with turmeric, milk (or plant-based alternatives), and a pinch of black pepper, is a soothing way to support joint health.

2. Ginger (Zingiber officinale)

Ginger is another herb renowned for its anti-inflammatory and analgesic properties. It has been shown to reduce pain and stiffness in individuals with arthritis and other joint conditions.

- **How It Works**: Ginger contains gingerols and shogaols, compounds that inhibit inflammatory processes and reduce oxidative stress.
- **Usage**: Fresh ginger can be grated into meals, brewed as tea, or taken as a supplement. Topical ginger compresses are also used to alleviate localized joint pain.
- **Example**: A soothing ginger tea can be made by steeping fresh ginger slices in hot water and adding honey or lemon for flavor.

3. Boswellia (Boswellia serrata)

Also known as Indian frankincense, boswellia has been used in Ayurvedic medicine for centuries to treat inflammatory conditions, including joint pain.

- **How It Works**: Boswellic acids, the active compounds in boswellia, inhibit 5-LOX, an enzyme that contributes to inflammation.
- **Usage**: Boswellia is typically consumed in capsule form or as an extract. It is often combined with other anti-inflammatory herbs for synergistic effects.
- **Example**: A boswellia supplement taken daily can significantly reduce symptoms of osteoarthritis and improve joint function.

4. Devil's Claw (Harpagophytum procumbens)

Native to Southern Africa, devil's claw is a powerful herb for reducing joint pain and inflammation. It is particularly effective for managing osteoarthritis and lower back pain.

- **How It Works**: Devil's claw contains harpagoside, a compound that has anti-inflammatory and analgesic properties.
- **Usage**: It is available as a capsule, powder, or tea. Devil's claw is often used in combination with other herbal remedies for joint health.
- **Example**: Adding devil's claw powder to smoothies or juices provides a convenient way to support joint health.

5. Willow Bark (Salix alba)

Willow bark has been used for centuries as a natural pain reliever. Its active ingredient, salicin, is a precursor to aspirin and provides similar anti-inflammatory benefits.

- **How It Works**: Salicin reduces inflammation and pain by inhibiting the COX enzymes involved in the inflammatory process.
- **Usage**: Willow bark can be consumed as a tea or taken as a supplement. It is particularly helpful for managing acute joint pain.
- **Example**: A willow bark tea can provide quick relief for joint discomfort after physical activity.

6. Nettle (Urtica dioica)

Nettle is a nutrient-rich herb with anti-inflammatory properties that make it ideal for joint health. It is particularly effective in managing the symptoms of rheumatoid arthritis.

- **How It Works**: Nettle contains compounds that reduce the production of inflammatory cytokines, easing pain and swelling.
- **Usage**: Nettle can be consumed as tea, added to soups, or taken as a tincture. Topical nettle applications can also relieve localized joint pain.
- **Example**: A warm nettle tea, consumed daily, can help reduce joint inflammation and support overall health.

7. Cayenne Pepper (Capsicum annuum)

Cayenne pepper contains capsaicin, a compound known for its pain-relieving properties. It is often used topically in creams and ointments to alleviate joint and muscle pain.

- **How It Works**: Capsaicin reduces the levels of substance P, a neurotransmitter that sends pain signals to the brain.

- **Usage**: Cayenne pepper can be added to meals for an internal boost or applied as a topical cream for direct pain relief.
- **Example**: A homemade capsaicin cream, made with cayenne pepper and coconut oil, can be applied to achy joints for natural relief.

How to Incorporate Herbs into Your Routine

Incorporating these herbs into your daily life can be simple and enjoyable. Here are some practical suggestions:

- **Herbal Teas**: Teas made from turmeric, ginger, or nettle can be sipped throughout the day to support joint health.
- **Topical Applications**: Creams and oils infused with herbs like cayenne and willow bark can be applied to joints for targeted relief.
- **Dietary Additions**: Spices such as turmeric and cayenne can be incorporated into cooking, while supplements like boswellia or devil's claw can provide concentrated doses of beneficial compounds.
- **Tinctures and Extracts**: Herbal tinctures offer a convenient way to consume concentrated doses of active ingredients. These can be added to water, juice, or tea.

Lifestyle Tips for Joint Health

While herbs provide significant benefits, combining them with lifestyle changes can further enhance joint health:

- **Stay Active**: Gentle exercises such as yoga, swimming, or walking help maintain joint flexibility and reduce stiffness.
- **Eat a Balanced Diet**: Focus on anti-inflammatory foods rich in omega-3 fatty acids, antioxidants, and essential vitamins and minerals.
- **Maintain a Healthy Weight**: Excess weight puts additional stress on joints, particularly the knees, hips, and lower back.
- **Prioritize Rest**: Adequate sleep and relaxation give the body time to repair and reduce inflammation.

Cognitive Enhancing Herbs

Cognitive function, encompassing memory, focus, and mental clarity, is central to daily life and long-term brain health. With the increasing prevalence of neurodegenerative diseases and age-related cognitive decline, many individuals are turning to natural solutions to support brain function. Cognitive-enhancing herbs have emerged as a promising area of study and practical application for improving mental performance and preventing cognitive impairment.

Herbs with cognitive benefits often work by enhancing blood flow to the brain, supporting neurotransmitter production, and reducing inflammation or oxidative stress. This section explores key cognitive-enhancing herbs, their mechanisms of action, practical uses, and scientific evidence supporting their benefits.

Ginkgo Biloba: A Brain-Boosting Classic

Ginkgo biloba, one of the oldest living tree species, has been used for centuries in traditional medicine to support memory and mental clarity. The herb contains potent antioxidants, including flavonoids and terpenoids, which protect brain cells from oxidative damage and improve circulation.

How It Works: Ginkgo biloba improves blood flow to the brain by dilating blood vessels and reducing platelet aggregation. This increased circulation delivers oxygen and nutrients, enhancing cognitive performance and potentially slowing the progression of age-related cognitive decline.

Scientific Evidence: Numerous studies support ginkgo's role in improving memory, particularly in individuals with mild cognitive impairment or early-stage Alzheimer's disease. A study published in *Pharmacopsychiatry* found that ginkgo extract significantly improved attention and memory in older adults with cognitive decline.

Practical Applications: Ginkgo biloba is commonly available as a tea, capsule, or tincture. It can be taken daily to support cognitive health, but individuals on blood-thinning medications should consult a healthcare provider due to its anticoagulant properties.

Bacopa Monnieri: The Memory Herb

Bacopa monnieri, also known as Brahmi, has a long history in Ayurvedic medicine as a brain tonic. It is particularly renowned for its ability to enhance memory, learning, and focus.

How It Works: Bacopa contains compounds called bacosides, which enhance the growth and repair of neurons. These compounds also improve communication between brain cells by supporting synaptic activity. Additionally, Bacopa reduces oxidative stress and inflammation, key contributors to cognitive decline.

Scientific Evidence: Research published in the *Journal of Alternative and Complementary Medicine* demonstrated that Bacopa significantly improved memory acquisition and retention in healthy adults. Another study in *Psychopharmacology* highlighted its effectiveness in reducing anxiety and enhancing cognitive performance.

Practical Applications: Bacopa can be consumed as a tea, powder, or capsule. For best results, it should be taken consistently over several weeks, as its effects on memory and cognition are cumulative.

Rhodiola Rosea: The Adaptogenic Ally

Rhodiola rosea, an adaptogenic herb, is prized for its ability to enhance mental clarity, focus, and resilience to stress. It is particularly effective in combating mental fatigue and improving cognitive function under stressful conditions.

How It Works: Rhodiola influences the central nervous system by modulating the production of neurotransmitters like dopamine and serotonin. It also reduces cortisol levels, helping the body adapt to stress while preserving mental performance.

Scientific Evidence: Studies have shown that Rhodiola improves cognitive performance in individuals experiencing fatigue or stress. Research in *Phytomedicine* highlighted its ability to enhance concentration, reduce mental fatigue, and improve overall cognitive function.

Practical Applications: Rhodiola is often taken as a supplement in capsule or tincture form. It can be particularly beneficial for students, professionals, or anyone seeking to maintain mental clarity during high-stress periods.

Gotu Kola: The Herb of Longevity

Gotu kola, another staple of Ayurvedic medicine, is often called the "herb of longevity" due to its role in supporting cognitive function and overall brain health. It is known for its calming properties and ability to enhance memory and concentration.

How It Works: Gotu kola enhances circulation and protects brain cells from damage caused by oxidative stress. It also supports the regeneration of neurons, making it a valuable herb for cognitive preservation.

Scientific Evidence: A study published in *Evidence-Based Complementary and Alternative Medicine* found that Gotu kola improved cognitive function and memory in older adults. It has also shown promise in reducing symptoms of anxiety, which can interfere with focus and clarity.

Practical Applications: Gotu kola can be consumed as a tea, added to soups, or taken in supplement form. Its mild taste makes it easy to incorporate into daily routines.

Lion's Mane Mushroom: A Neuroprotective Powerhouse

Lion's Mane mushroom, a unique fungi with brain-boosting properties, has gained significant attention for its ability to support neurogenesis—the growth of new neurons.

How It Works: Lion's Mane contains compounds called hericenones and erinacines, which stimulate the production of nerve growth factor (NGF). NGF plays a critical role in maintaining the health and regeneration of neurons, making Lion's Mane a valuable tool for cognitive enhancement and neuroprotection.

Scientific Evidence: Research in *Biomedical Research* demonstrated that Lion's Mane supplementation improved cognitive function in individuals with mild cognitive impairment. It also supports mood regulation, reducing symptoms of depression and anxiety.

Practical Applications: Lion's Mane can be consumed as a tea, added to soups, or taken as a supplement. It is often included in nootropic blends aimed at enhancing cognitive performance.

Ashwagandha: Stress Relief for Sharper Focus

Ashwagandha, another adaptogen, is renowned for its ability to reduce stress and enhance cognitive function. Chronic stress can impair memory and focus, making Ashwagandha a valuable ally for mental clarity.

How It Works: Ashwagandha lowers cortisol levels and enhances resilience to stress. It also supports the production of acetylcholine, a neurotransmitter involved in learning and memory.

Scientific Evidence: A study in *The Journal of Dietary Supplements* found that Ashwagandha significantly improved memory, executive function, and information-processing speed in adults.

Practical Applications: Ashwagandha is available in powder, capsule, or tincture form. It pairs well with warm beverages like milk or herbal teas for a soothing, cognitive-enhancing effect.

Rosemary: A Fragrant Memory Booster

Rosemary, often used as a culinary herb, has surprising cognitive-enhancing properties. Its essential oil is particularly effective in improving focus and memory.

How It Works: Rosemary contains compounds like 1,8-cineole, which increase the production of acetylcholine. Inhaling rosemary essential oil or consuming it in small amounts can enhance memory retention and mental alertness.

Scientific Evidence: Research in *Therapeutic Advances in Psychopharmacology* demonstrated that rosemary essential oil improved cognitive performance and mood in participants.

Practical Applications: Rosemary can be used fresh or dried in cooking. Its essential oil can be diffused or diluted with a carrier oil for topical use.

Sage: Enhancing Mental Clarity

Sage, another common culinary herb, has been shown to improve memory and cognitive performance. It contains compounds that inhibit the breakdown of acetylcholine, a neurotransmitter crucial for learning and memory.

How It Works: By preserving acetylcholine levels, sage enhances communication between neurons, supporting cognitive function and memory retention.

Scientific Evidence: Studies have shown that both fresh sage and sage oil improve memory and mood in young adults, as published in *Physiology & Behavior*.

Practical Applications: Use sage in cooking, as a tea, or in essential oil form for aromatherapy benefits.

Adaptogens for Stress Reduction

Stress is an inevitable part of modern life, affecting individuals on emotional, mental, and physical levels. Whether caused by demanding jobs, personal responsibilities, or global uncertainties, chronic stress can lead to burnout, decreased immune function, and a host of other health issues. In recent years, adaptogens have emerged as a powerful natural solution for managing stress. These unique herbs help the body adapt to stressors, promoting balance and resilience without the side effects often associated with pharmaceutical options.

What Are Adaptogens?

Adaptogens are natural substances, primarily derived from plants and mushrooms, that help the body resist stressors. These stressors can be physical, chemical, or biological. Adaptogens work by supporting the hypothalamic-pituitary-adrenal (HPA) axis and balancing cortisol levels, the primary hormone responsible for the body's stress response.

The benefits of adaptogens extend beyond stress reduction. They also enhance energy, boost immunity, and improve overall well-being. What sets adaptogens apart is their ability to provide individualized support, meaning they help bring the body back to balance, whether it is underactive or overactive.

How Adaptogens Combat Stress

Adaptogens exert their effects through several mechanisms:

- **Regulating the HPA Axis**: Adaptogens modulate the body's response to stress by balancing cortisol levels. Excessive cortisol can lead to anxiety, weight gain, and fatigue, while too little can cause exhaustion and low motivation.
- **Improving Cellular Energy**: Stress depletes cellular energy stores. Adaptogens enhance mitochondrial function, supporting energy production at a cellular level.
- **Reducing Inflammation**: Chronic stress triggers systemic inflammation. Many adaptogens have anti-inflammatory properties that protect against stress-induced damage.
- **Enhancing Neurotransmitter Balance**: Stress affects brain chemistry, leading to anxiety and mood swings. Adaptogens can help restore balance to neurotransmitters like serotonin and dopamine, promoting calmness and emotional stability.

Top Adaptogens for Stress Reduction

1. Ashwagandha (Withania somnifera)

Ashwagandha is one of the most studied adaptogens for stress relief. Known as the "king of adaptogens," it has been used in Ayurvedic medicine for centuries to calm the mind, reduce anxiety, and enhance resilience.

- **How It Works**: Ashwagandha reduces cortisol levels, helping to normalize the body's stress response. It also supports adrenal function, preventing burnout.
- **Usage**: Ashwagandha can be consumed as a powder mixed into smoothies or taken as capsules. It pairs well with warm milk or water for a calming evening drink.
- **Example**: A daily dose of ashwagandha tea or a supplement can alleviate symptoms of chronic stress, such as insomnia and fatigue.

2. Rhodiola Rosea

Native to cold climates, rhodiola rosea is a powerful adaptogen that enhances mental clarity and physical endurance while combating stress. It is particularly effective for individuals experiencing fatigue and difficulty concentrating due to prolonged stress.

- **How It Works**: Rhodiola increases the body's resistance to stress by modulating cortisol and boosting serotonin production. It also enhances oxygen utilization, improving energy levels.
- **Usage**: Rhodiola is commonly available as a capsule, tincture, or tea.
- **Example**: Taking rhodiola in the morning can help combat fatigue and enhance focus throughout the day.

3. Holy Basil (Ocimum sanctum)

Holy basil, also known as tulsi, is revered in Ayurvedic medicine for its ability to promote mental clarity and emotional balance. It is particularly effective for individuals experiencing anxiety or mild depression due to stress.

- **How It Works**: Holy basil reduces cortisol levels and protects against oxidative stress. It also supports the immune system, which can be compromised by chronic stress.
- **Usage**: Holy basil can be consumed as a tea or taken as a capsule.
- **Example**: A cup of holy basil tea in the evening can provide a sense of calm and relaxation after a stressful day.

4. Eleuthero (Eleutherococcus senticosus)

Eleuthero, also known as Siberian ginseng, is a potent adaptogen for improving resilience to stress and physical endurance. It is particularly beneficial for individuals who feel physically and mentally drained by stress.

- **How It Works**: Eleuthero enhances the body's ability to adapt to stress by modulating the HPA axis and supporting adrenal health. It also boosts stamina and immunity.
- **Usage**: Eleuthero is commonly consumed as a tea, tincture, or supplement.
- **Example**: Taking eleuthero before a challenging day can help maintain energy and focus.

5. Schisandra (Schisandra chinensis)

Schisandra is a unique adaptogen that supports mental clarity, emotional balance, and physical resilience. It is particularly effective for individuals who feel scattered or overwhelmed by stress.

- **How It Works**: Schisandra enhances mitochondrial function, improving energy production and reducing fatigue. It also supports liver detoxification, which can be compromised by chronic stress.
- **Usage**: Schisandra is often consumed as a tea or tincture. Its tart flavor makes it a popular addition to smoothies and juices.
- **Example**: A schisandra berry infusion provides a refreshing way to combat stress and enhance focus.

Practical Ways to Incorporate Adaptogens

Adaptogens are versatile and easy to incorporate into daily routines. Here are some practical suggestions:

- **Morning Boost**: Start your day with an adaptogen-rich smoothie featuring ashwagandha or rhodiola.
- **Afternoon Focus**: Combat the mid-day slump with a cup of holy basil or eleuthero tea.
- **Evening Relaxation**: Wind down with a warm drink infused with ashwagandha or schisandra.

Combining Adaptogens for Enhanced Benefits

Many adaptogens work synergistically, meaning their combined effects are greater than the sum of their individual benefits. For example:

- **Ashwagandha and Rhodiola**: This combination balances energy and reduces anxiety, making it ideal for individuals experiencing mental and physical fatigue.
- **Holy Basil and Schisandra**: These herbs enhance emotional stability and detoxification, helping individuals feel grounded and refreshed.
- **Eleuthero and Rhodiola**: Together, these adaptogens boost physical endurance and resilience to stress, making them perfect for active individuals.

Lifestyle Tips to Maximize the Benefits of Adaptogens

While adaptogens are highly effective, their benefits are amplified when combined with healthy lifestyle practices:

- **Prioritize Sleep**: Adaptogens work best when the body is well-rested. Aim for 7-9 hours of quality sleep each night.
- **Stay Active**: Regular exercise enhances the body's stress resilience. Gentle activities like yoga and walking pair well with adaptogen use.
- **Eat a Balanced Diet**: Nutrient-dense foods provide the vitamins and minerals necessary for adaptogens to work effectively.
- **Practice Mindfulness**: Techniques such as meditation and deep breathing complement the calming effects of adaptogens.

Chapter 4: Recipes for Aging Well

Ginkgo biloba, one of the most ancient tree species on Earth, has been a cornerstone of traditional medicine for centuries. Known for its numerous health benefits, Ginkgo biloba is particularly prized for its ability to support cognitive function, improve circulation, and combat oxidative stress. One of the most popular and accessible ways to consume this powerful herb is in the form of tea.

Ginkgo Biloba Tea

Ginkgo biloba tea is celebrated for its subtle flavor and therapeutic properties, making it a staple in many wellness routines.

This section delves into the rich history, preparation methods, health benefits, and practical applications of Ginkgo biloba tea, offering a comprehensive guide for those looking to incorporate this ancient remedy into their daily lives.

The History and Legacy of Ginkgo Biloba

Ginkgo biloba, often referred to as a "living fossil," has existed for over 200 million years, predating even the dinosaurs. Native to China, the Ginkgo tree has been revered in traditional Chinese medicine for its healing properties. Historically, Ginkgo leaves were used to treat a variety of ailments, including memory loss, respiratory issues, and poor circulation. The tree itself is a symbol of resilience and longevity. Ginkgo trees famously survived the atomic bomb in Hiroshima, continuing to thrive amidst devastation. This enduring strength is mirrored in its role as a medicinal powerhouse.

The Nutritional Profile of Ginkgo Biloba Tea

Ginkgo biloba leaves are rich in bioactive compounds, including flavonoids and terpenoids, which are responsible for its health benefits. These compounds act as potent antioxidants, combating free radicals that can damage cells and contribute to aging and disease. The tea also contains ginkgolides, unique compounds that improve blood circulation and support brain health.

Drinking Ginkgo biloba tea allows these beneficial compounds to be absorbed into the body in a gentle and effective manner, making it an excellent option for daily use.

Health Benefits of Ginkgo Biloba Tea

1. Cognitive Enhancement

Ginkgo biloba is renowned for its ability to improve memory, focus, and overall cognitive function. By increasing blood flow to the brain, Ginkgo enhances the delivery of oxygen and nutrients, supporting mental clarity and reducing the risk of cognitive decline.

Scientific studies have highlighted Ginkgo's effectiveness in managing conditions such as mild cognitive impairment and early-stage Alzheimer's disease. Regular consumption of Ginkgo biloba tea may help enhance mental sharpness, particularly in older adults.

2. Improved Circulation

Ginkgo biloba tea is a natural vasodilator, meaning it helps widen blood vessels and improve circulation. This is particularly beneficial for individuals suffering from cold extremities, varicose veins, or other circulation-related issues. Enhanced blood flow also supports cardiovascular health, reducing the risk of heart disease and stroke.

3. Antioxidant Protection

The high concentration of antioxidants in Ginkgo biloba tea protects cells from oxidative stress, a major contributor to aging and chronic diseases. These antioxidants neutralize harmful free radicals, promoting cellular health and reducing inflammation.

4. Mood and Stress Management

Ginkgo biloba has adaptogenic properties, meaning it helps the body adapt to stress. Drinking Ginkgo biloba tea can promote relaxation, reduce anxiety, and improve overall mood. It is particularly effective when consumed as part of a mindful tea-drinking ritual.

5. Eye Health

The improved circulation associated with Ginkgo biloba tea benefits eye health by enhancing blood flow to the retina. This can be particularly helpful for individuals with glaucoma or macular degeneration.

How to Prepare Ginkgo Biloba Tea

Selecting the Right Ingredients

Ginkgo biloba tea can be made using dried leaves, which are widely available at health food stores or online. It is essential to source high-quality leaves from reputable suppliers to ensure safety and potency.

Step-by-Step Preparation

1. **Ingredients**:

- o 1 teaspoon of dried Ginkgo biloba leaves
- o 1 cup of boiling water
- o Optional: honey or lemon for flavor
2. **Method**:
   - o Boil water and allow it to cool slightly (to about 180°F or 80°C) to preserve the delicate compounds in the leaves.
   - o Place the Ginkgo biloba leaves in a teapot or infuser.
   - o Pour the hot water over the leaves and let steep for 5-7 minutes.
   - o Strain the tea and add honey or lemon if desired.
3. **Serving Suggestions**:
   - o Ginkgo biloba tea can be enjoyed hot or iced, making it suitable for all seasons. Pair it with a moment of relaxation or meditation for maximum benefit.

Practical Tips for Incorporating Ginkgo Biloba Tea

- **Daily Routine**: Drink Ginkgo biloba tea in the morning to kickstart your day with enhanced focus or in the afternoon as a calming, stress-relieving ritual.
- **Blending Options**: Combine Ginkgo biloba leaves with other herbs like chamomile, green tea, or peppermint for added flavor and health benefits.
- **Mindful Drinking**: Use the preparation and consumption of Ginkgo biloba tea as an opportunity to practice mindfulness, savoring the aroma and taste while focusing on the present moment.

Safety and Precautions

While Ginkgo biloba tea offers numerous health benefits, it is important to consume it responsibly. Some individuals may experience side effects such as headaches, dizziness, or stomach upset. Additionally, Ginkgo biloba has anticoagulant properties and may interact with blood-thinning medications. Always consult a healthcare provider before incorporating Ginkgo biloba tea into your routine, especially if you are pregnant, nursing, or taking medication.

Ginkgo Biloba Tea and Sustainable Wellness

Incorporating Ginkgo biloba tea into your wellness routine not only supports personal health but also aligns with sustainable practices. Many suppliers now offer ethically sourced Ginkgo leaves, ensuring the preservation of this ancient tree species and its habitats. Choosing sustainable options allows you to enjoy the benefits of Ginkgo biloba tea while contributing to environmental conservation.

Schisandra Berry Smoothie

Schisandra berries, often called the "five-flavor fruit," are a cornerstone of traditional Chinese medicine. Revered for their adaptogenic properties, these berries are not only nutrient-rich but also play a significant role in boosting energy, supporting mental clarity, and enhancing the body's resilience to stress. Incorporating these berries into your diet can be as simple and enjoyable as creating a Schisandra berry smoothie. This section explores the benefits of Schisandra berries, details the step-by-step process of preparing a smoothie, and highlights how this adaptogenic treat can support holistic health.

The Power of Schisandra Berries

Schisandra berries are a unique fruit known for their five distinct flavors: sweet, sour, salty, bitter, and pungent. This complexity makes them a fascinating addition to herbal remedies. In traditional medicine, these berries are prized for their ability to:

1. **Enhance Energy Levels**: Schisandra berries are adaptogens, meaning they help the body adapt to stress and restore balance. By modulating the release of cortisol, these berries combat fatigue and promote sustained energy.

2. **Support Liver Health**: Rich in lignans, compounds that support liver detoxification, Schisandra berries help cleanse the body of toxins. This makes them an essential ally for maintaining optimal metabolic function.

3. **Boost Cognitive Function**: Schisandra is celebrated for enhancing mental clarity, memory, and focus. It is often used as a natural nootropic to improve concentration and reduce brain fog.

4. **Promote Skin Health**: The antioxidants in Schisandra combat oxidative stress, helping to maintain youthful, radiant skin by reducing the effects of environmental damage.

5. **Strengthen Immunity**: With its high concentration of vitamins C and E, along with other phytonutrients, Schisandra boosts the immune system and supports overall wellness.

Crafting the Perfect Schisandra Berry Smoothie

A Schisandra berry smoothie is a delicious and easy way to integrate these powerful berries into your daily routine. Unlike capsules or teas, a smoothie allows for creative customization and the inclusion of complementary ingredients that amplify the benefits of Schisandra.

Ingredients for the Smoothie

- **Schisandra Berry Powder or Extract**: One tablespoon of powdered Schisandra or a teaspoon of its concentrated extract serves as the base for this smoothie.
- **Frozen Berries**: Add a cup of mixed berries (blueberries, raspberries, and strawberries) to complement the tangy notes of Schisandra and provide additional antioxidants.
- **Leafy Greens**: A handful of spinach or kale enhances the smoothie's nutrient profile without overpowering the flavor.
- **Plant-Based Milk**: Almond, coconut, or oat milk acts as a creamy base while keeping the smoothie dairy-free.
- **Banana**: A ripe banana adds natural sweetness and a smooth texture, balancing the tang of the Schisandra.
- **Adaptogenic Boosters**: Adding a teaspoon of maca powder or ashwagandha enhances the adaptogenic effects.
- **Optional Sweetener**: A touch of honey or maple syrup can be used for added sweetness, though it's not always necessary.

Step-by-Step Preparation

1. **Prepare the Ingredients**: Wash the greens thoroughly, measure out your ingredients, and ensure the frozen berries are ready to use.
2. **Blend the Base**: Start by adding the plant-based milk to the blender, followed by the Schisandra powder or extract. Blend until the powder is fully dissolved.
3. **Incorporate the Fruits and Greens**: Add the frozen berries, banana, and greens. Blend on high speed until the mixture is smooth and creamy.
4. **Add Optional Boosters**: If using maca powder, ashwagandha, or sweeteners, add them now and blend briefly to incorporate.
5. **Serve and Enjoy**: Pour the smoothie into a glass and garnish with fresh mint leaves or a sprinkle of chia seeds for an added touch of elegance.

Nutritional Benefits of the Smoothie

This Schisandra berry smoothie is more than just a refreshing drink—it's a powerhouse of nutrition. Every ingredient works synergistically to support your body's needs:

- **Antioxidants**: The combination of Schisandra and mixed berries provides a rich source of antioxidants that fight free radicals, reduce inflammation, and support cellular health.

- **Vitamins and Minerals**: Leafy greens add essential nutrients like vitamin K, folate, and magnesium, which are crucial for bone health, blood clotting, and energy production.

- **Adaptogenic Support**: The smoothie's adaptogens—Schisandra, maca, and ashwagandha—help regulate the body's stress response, improve energy, and promote emotional balance.

- **Digestive Health**: The banana contributes natural fiber, which aids in digestion and supports gut health.

- **Hydration**: The liquid base ensures hydration, an essential aspect of maintaining energy levels and cognitive function.

The Role of Schisandra in Modern Wellness

While Schisandra has been a staple in traditional medicine for centuries, its popularity has surged in the wellness industry. Adaptogenic herbs like Schisandra are now celebrated for their ability to counteract the effects of modern stressors. For individuals juggling busy schedules or dealing with chronic stress, incorporating Schisandra can make a noticeable difference in both mental and physical resilience.

The beauty of Schisandra is its versatility—it can be integrated into various recipes, including teas, tonics, and smoothies. Its tangy flavor pairs well with both sweet and savory ingredients, making it a flexible addition to your diet.

Tips for Incorporating Schisandra Smoothies into Your Routine

1. **Morning Boost**: Start your day with a Schisandra smoothie to energize your body and mind. Its adaptogenic properties help set a balanced tone for the day.

2. **Pre-Workout Fuel**: The smoothie's combination of natural sugars, vitamins, and adaptogens makes it an excellent pre-workout drink to enhance endurance and performance.

3. **Stress Relief Snack**: Enjoy a Schisandra smoothie as an afternoon pick-me-up to combat fatigue and improve focus.

4. **Bedtime Ritual**: For those who struggle with sleep, adjusting the smoothie to include calming ingredients like chamomile or valerian root can make it a soothing nighttime beverage.

Customization Options

The versatility of the Schisandra berry smoothie allows for endless customization. Here are some ideas:

- **Protein Boost**: Add a scoop of plant-based protein powder for a more filling option, perfect for post-workout recovery.
- **Nut Butter**: A tablespoon of almond or peanut butter provides healthy fats and a creamy texture.
- **Citrus Zest**: A touch of orange or lemon zest can enhance the tangy notes of Schisandra while adding vitamin C.
- **Superfood Additions**: Sprinkle in a teaspoon of chia seeds, flaxseeds, or hemp hearts for extra omega-3s and fiber.

Schisandra and Long-Term Wellness

Regular consumption of Schisandra berries, whether in smoothie form or other preparations, offers long-term benefits. From reducing stress and enhancing energy to supporting skin health and immunity, Schisandra is a holistic powerhouse. It's a testament to the effectiveness of natural remedies and their ability to complement modern lifestyles.

Chapter 5: Conclusions

Embracing Natural Wellness: A Holistic Path to Healing
The journey through **Natural Herbal Remedies** has been a deep dive into the transformative power of nature's bounty. This book was designed for you—the proactive, health-conscious individual eager to embrace a lifestyle that prioritizes natural wellness, sustainable choices, and time-tested remedies. Whether you're new to the world of herbal medicine or seeking to deepen your understanding, this book has provided an expansive guide to living in harmony with nature while addressing the challenges of modern life.

The Foundation of Holistic Health

At the heart of this book is the belief that true wellness is multidimensional, encompassing physical, mental, and emotional well-being. The remedies and practices discussed throughout are not merely treatments for isolated symptoms; they represent a comprehensive approach to healing that considers the interconnectedness of the body, mind, and environment.

By addressing foundational principles such as nutrition, hydration, exercise, and stress management, this book encourages a shift from reactive health care to a preventive, proactive approach. These foundational strategies are complemented by targeted remedies for specific concerns, ensuring that your wellness toolkit is both broad and practical.

Empowering Readers with Knowledge

A central goal of this book was to empower you with the knowledge needed to take control of your health. Each section was crafted to provide detailed, actionable insights, rooted in both traditional wisdom and modern research. From understanding the adaptogenic properties of herbs like Schisandra and Ashwagandha to exploring practical applications such as **Nettle Root Tincture** or **Schisandra Berry Smoothies**, every chapter aimed to demystify herbal remedies and make them accessible for everyday life.

The recipes and remedies provided throughout are adaptable, practical, and designed for integration into a busy lifestyle. You now have the tools to prepare tinctures, teas, and balms, as well as the knowledge to use these remedies effectively for a wide range of health concerns.

Tailored for Every Stage of Life

Health is not static—it evolves as we age, as our lifestyles change, and as new challenges arise. This book acknowledges these shifts, providing guidance for every stage of life. Whether you're seeking natural solutions for hormonal balance during menopause, boosting vitality and endurance, or improving joint health as you age, this book equips you with age-appropriate strategies.

This adaptability ensures that the knowledge you've gained here will continue to serve you and your family, no matter where you are on your wellness journey.

Aligning with Modern Needs

The modern world presents unique challenges: chronic stress, inflammation, and a growing reliance on synthetic solutions that often treat symptoms but not root causes. The remedies in this book are a counterbalance to these trends, offering natural, sustainable solutions that work with the body's inherent healing abilities.

For example:

- **Adaptogens** are highlighted for their ability to help the body manage stress and restore balance.
- **Anti-inflammatory foods** provide a natural defense against the chronic conditions linked to inflammation.
- **Omega-3 sources** and **joint-supporting herbs** address the physical wear and tear of modern living.

By integrating these strategies into your daily life, you're building resilience—not just against illness but against the physical and emotional stressors of a fast-paced world.

Reconnecting with Nature

At its core, this book is a celebration of the healing power of nature. From the vibrant nutrients in anti-inflammatory foods to the gentle strength of herbal tinctures, nature provides us with everything we need to thrive. Embracing this philosophy goes beyond personal health—it's also a commitment to living more sustainably, respecting the planet, and preserving its resources for future generations.

Through remedies like **Valerian Root Tea**, **Schisandra Berry Smoothies**, and **Arnica Muscle Rub**, you've been invited to cultivate a deeper connection with nature and its rhythms. These practices are not just about healing; they're about honoring the symbiotic relationship between humans and the natural world.

A Holistic Lifestyle for the Future

This book also emphasizes the importance of a lifestyle that supports long-term health. Incorporating hydration strategies, balanced nutrition, regular movement, and mindfulness practices creates a foundation for wellness that is sustainable and effective. These practices not only enhance physical health but also nurture mental clarity and emotional stability.

The inclusion of recipes and routines, such as **Schisandra Berry Smoothies** and tips for crafting herbal tinctures, bridges the gap between knowledge and action. By making these practices a part of your daily life, you're fostering habits that will serve you for years to come.

Building Resilience and Community

Finally, this book is a reminder that health is not a solitary pursuit. The knowledge you've gained can be shared, inspiring others to embrace natural remedies and holistic practices. Whether it's preparing a soothing tea for a loved one, recommending a nutrient-rich smoothie, or introducing friends to the benefits of adaptogens, you're contributing to a community that values wellness and sustainability.

By choosing natural remedies, you're also voting with your dollars—supporting ethical sourcing, sustainable agriculture, and the preservation of traditional practices. Together, these choices ripple outward, creating a healthier world for all.

Your Journey Continues

The path to wellness is ongoing, and **Natural Herbal Remedies** is a companion for every step of the way. Use this book as a resource, a guide, and an inspiration as you continue to explore the incredible potential of herbal medicine. The tools, recipes, and strategies within these pages are meant to empower you to make informed, confident choices for your health and well-being.

You've already taken the first step by seeking out this knowledge. Now, it's time to integrate these practices into your life, adapt them to your unique needs, and share them with those you care about. The possibilities are endless, and the rewards—greater vitality, resilience, and connection—are within your reach.

Made in the USA
Las Vegas, NV
16 December 2024

14386274R00289